DEC 09

MAR 2009

Nature's Prozac

Natural therapies and techniques to
rid yourself of anxiety, depression,
panic attacks, & stress.

Judith Sachs

An Authors Guild Backinprint.com Edition

Nature's Prozac

Natural Ways to Achieve Peak Mental and Emotional Health

Copyright © 1997, 2008 by Judith Sachs

iUniverse books may be ordered through booksellers or by contacting:

iUniverse
1663 Liberty Drive
Bloomington, IN 47403
www.iuniverse.com
1-800-Authors (1-800-288-4677)

ISBN: 978-0-595-53554-5 (pbk)

Printed in the United States of America

iUniverse rev. date: 10/15/2008

MAR   2009

Nature's Prozac

Natural therapies and techniques to
rid yourself of anxiety, depression,
panic attacks, & stress.

Judith Sachs

DEDICATION

For my dearest Bruno, who gives me space to bounce off the medians every once in a while.

ACKNOWLEDGMENTS

I gratefully acknowledge the enormous support and help given me by the following specialists in alternative therapies:

Michal Ben-Reuven, Feldenkrais Institute, Princeton, NJ
Nancy Hokenson, L.Ac.
Dr. Phillip Bonnet
Brian Logan, D.C.
Dori Sieder, Ph.D.
Phyllis Cooper, Ph.D.
Dr. Sandra Leiblum
Susanna and Guy DeRosa
Kenneth I. Frey, Institute of Physical Therapy, New York, NY
Joan Klynn

and would like to express my gratitude to those who opened their hearts and shared personal healing stories:

Karen C.	Steve A.
Jo W.	Teubel B.
Ray L.	Lois G.
Cathy C.	Lois H.
Carla C.	Yetta A.
Dick D.	Rose P.
Judy B.	Fran L.
Cecelia O.	Carole C.

CONTENTS

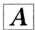

B

C

D

E

F

G

I

J

$\boxed{S}$

$\boxed{T}$

$$Y$$

Appendix

Resource Guide

FOREWORD

I took care of children for most of my professional life. It was exciting and fun because the children often grew out of their "phases" and there was not much we had to do except to alert the parents that when this "terrible twos" age disappeared, there would be a few other difficult times to go through. It was as if Mother Nature was getting the parents ready for adolescence, the last bit of craziness before the kid left home for work or college. Thank God.

I made an effort to find something wrong with a child if a mother had too many complaints about his behavior. It often turned out that the miscreant was sensitive to milk, or he had pinworms, or she was anemic, or there had been some "subtle" hurt to the nervous system, or—one of the best dodges—it was genetic and the child was going to be like Uncle Ed, the uncle from the other side of the family.

In my effort to relieve guilt, because the mother did not want to believe that she was the cause of this screw-up, I made an effort to find a physical cause for the out-of-control mischief. These parents wanted this child, they fed and cuddled him, they applied discipline that was not too punitive, but was appropriate and consistent. What went wrong? I even had the child get a brainwave test to see if odd electrical waves could explain the unruliness. If the neurologist found some odd waves between lead 16 and 22 on the test, I would point this out to the parents and say, "See. This is because he fell when he was two and hit his head on the coffee table." (Every kid has hit the coffee table at some time during his growing up.) I would have them try Dilantin or phenobarbital to see if it would calm down the non-compliance. Sometimes it even worked. Or was it that the parents got off the child's back while they waited for the drug to do its magic? I have since found out that the brain wave test can be different depending on whether the person has eaten breakfast or not. (Hypoglycemia.)

So I was almost obsessed with the idea that there was a drug for every condition. Needless to say, the pharmaceutical companies cultivated that attitude, and my medical school training was based on that paradigm: make a diagnosis and prescribe a drug. Penicillin for infections. Antihistamines for allergies. Anti-spasmodics for cramps. Anti-whatevers for whatevers. I was also fortunate to have been a student at the feet of Dr. Charles Bradley who discovered the paradoxical calming effect of stimulants for the hyperactive kid back in the 1930s.

I did have a little trouble trying to make a diagnosis based on the parents' evaluation of the child's behavior, especially if the aberrant behavior was not manifest right there in my office. I asked an internist how he was to figure out if an adult was sick enough for a mood elevator or the psychiatrist's couch. He said, "I ask if the patient is comfortable most of the time. We all have headaches, sleepless nights, anxieties, worries, and bad days, but if they are coping and feel good most of the time, I figure nothing needs to be done."

I translated that into pediatric terms. I began to ask the parents, "Does he/she laugh and smile more than he/she cries and frowns?" I figured the ratio should be about three parts fun to two parts grumpiness. That was a help, but I did not know what to do with the information if I had corrected all the correctables. Right about then I was handed an Adelle Davis book, *Let's Have Healthy Children*. Although her ideas are antithetical to standard allopathic medicine, I did read it and most of it made sense. I began to try the methods, and was delighted with the results.

In the last twenty-five years I have used nutrition and diet manipulation on my patients but still used the basic method of diagnose and treat with—not a drug this time—but with a nutrient. I studied with chiropractors, and naturopathic doctors, and became aware that my medical training was not complete. I did not understand the body/mind/spirit forces that determine our health. I did not know there are so many ways to move people into a healthy state. I have been too long locked into the idea of finding a cause and then providing the remedy. If you go to a medical doctor, you are most likely to get a prescription. It is standard allopathic training.

I attended a seminar a few years ago. The wise doctor who conducted the conference pointed out that we have the potential of self-healing, but we cannot use our cortex, the thinking and left-brain, logical approach, or we would have done it the first time we suspected we were on tilt. He pointed out that we must get down to the unconscious part of nervous system to find the answers. That is not a conscious exercise. We have to use the methods clearly and simply described in this book by Judith Sachs. Call it meditation, self-hypnosis, behavior modification, or introspection, it is at this subconscious level that the body uses to get well. Chinese and Ayurvedic methods have mastered this approach. Freud was close and Christian Science touches on it. My mother's chicken soup along with love got me through the measles and a mastoid infection when I was six years old. I believed Mom even though she was just a placebo. She was practicing psychoneuroimmunology.

In the 1960s and 1970s I was busy treating kids with Ritalin and Dexedrine because the teachers said the children were hyperactive. The teachers knew it worked, and the parents were tired of fighting with the kids to "Sit still and learn." I began to notice that those patients so touched were usually boys, and they were ticklish and most were sensitive to dairy products. With a little experimenting, I found that more than 60 percent responded to magnesium, vitamin B_6, and a diet change. (Don't let the child eat anything he likes: sugar, dairy, corn, chocolate.) More recently I have discovered that most chronically sick children and adults are somewhat alkaline and some safe nutrients and acidifiers will usually get them back to homeostatic balance.

With these changes they no longer needed medicine. This book is just what I need at this time in my search for the truth. Ms. Sachs feels it is cheating to take drugs. I agree. Drugs are band aid and only cover up the symptoms. But if you take drugs to modify your thoughts and behavior, and they work, it means that you are capable of being a reasonably normal human being, laughing and smiling more than fifty percent of the time. Then you must make up your mind—if you want to get and stay healthy—to correct the chemical screw-up from your lifestyle and diet, and do some self-affirmations to lift your self-esteem. Then you should be able to handle the downers in your life.

Remember the famous words of one of the pioneers of the pharmaceutical industry, Ely Lilly, "A drug is not a drug if it does not have side-effects." The list of adverse effects noted in the brochures from the drug companies is often longer than the symptoms the drug was designed to control.

This book should be used as a textbook for medical students, whether allopathic, naturopathic, or chiropractic. It has clear descriptions of how homeopathy works, what herbs can be used, what aromatherapy is, when to get with AA, and how to find support groups. She is not afraid to tackle sexual function and how to enhance it. She gives a few case histories to show the benefits of natural therapies. She is practical: use checks; don't carry credit cards. She suggests that many of us may benefit from short-term therapy or counselling.

As I read through this book, I have the feeling that she wants us—and encourages us— to try to find the joy we should have had when we were children. Recall those fun times when you abandoned yourself to the enjoyment of splashing in the mud, catching snowflakes with your tongue, making a gravy crater with the mashed potatoes, putting peanuts up your nose, picking the scabs off your knee, and drawing a dirty picture of teacher.

Don't lose your childhood with drugs.

Lendon Smith, M.D.

INTRODUCTION

A merry heart doeth good like a medicine.
But a broken spirit drieth the bones.

Proverbs 17:22

Can you remember one day in your life—or perhaps just an hour or two—when you were perfectly, magically, wonderfully happy and content with your lot in life? Capture one of these moments in your memory and roll it around your brain. Doesn't it fill you with warmth and energy? We all have a terrible nostalgia for those extraordinary times, probably because we have so many days when we feel neutral, blah, not-so-hot, rotten, or just plain bored. But who wants to be happy *all* the time? If life had no flaws, we would have no real bead on what "happy" means. If the sun always shone and the birds always sang, we'd want to throw something, make some trouble, go on a bender, swear a lot.

What most of us cherish and can't always manage is the ability to feel whole—cheerful but contemplative, silly but sad, enthusiastic but realistic. We would like to feel better than we do now. And we can. This book will point the way toward a new way of seeing and being; it will provide you with an exciting perspective on the self you thought you couldn't change. But it's doable and possible—without drugs. A merry heart doesn't come in a prescription bottle; rather, it comes from the desire to make a difference in the way we take on the world and make it our own.

A merry heart does take some work, however. It would be nice if we could ensure happiness genetically or tap into a brain function that would make us feel great whenever we wanted. But none of us is completely content with our lot in life, and many of us who are walking around may have moments when we don't technically qualify as "sane." That "merry heart" is an elusive prize: it's a lot more common in our society to feel lousy, anxious, depressed, furious, or just plain "blue." We live in an overcrowded, stress-filled, difficult world that sometimes seems to take away our basic sense of well-being. Our personal lives are never neat and orderly, but rather, seem to grow more confused and confusing as we get older. Still, there are very few of us who are willing to scrap it all and run away to a desert island (of which there are increasingly few) to escape the madding crowd.

Most of us cannot tolerate depression and anxiety, even for a few miserable hours. So what do we do? In our longing for peace and calm, we try to shut out what's angry and unpleasant. We opt for the easy solution, the quick fix. Most harried individuals manage to deaden the sensations they dislike with a variety of distractions, including sleep, food, alcohol, tobacco, and a blatant lack of awareness of others as well as themselves. But these are only temporary—and usually self-destructive—band-aids for real problems.

The medical establishment believes that there is a biochemical link to almost every mental ailment known to man or woman, that personality traits, inborn and developed, often lend themselves to moodiness or hyperactivity or any number of behaviors.

It may be true that we cannot escape our inborn traits. But the good news about mental and emotional problems is that they do not necessarily doom one to a life of despair. There are a variety of excellent solutions for nearly every syndrome, compulsion, or dread, and you will find them right here in *Nature's Prozac*.

Should we actually attempt to eradicate mental and emotional problems? Studies have shown that some of the most creative and brilliant individuals have also been some of the most tortured people; their very unhappiness may have spurred them to reach higher than they might have had they been content with their lives. But it's no longer fashionable to be neurotic, so doctors offer cures: They want to make us believe that our inner turmoil can be alleviated rather than blocked; it can be molded so that it's ultimately helpful rather than harmful. The medical establishment is hot on drugs for the blues.

More and more these days, doctors are prescribing medications that purport to bring out the "real person." Prozac, Wellbutrin, Xanax, Paxil, Zoloft, Luvox, Effexor and a host of other chemical fine-tuners are given out like candy to the hungry masses.

And the masses have responded with incredible enthusiasm. Why bother spending thousands of hours and dollars on a psychiatrist's couch when you can pop a pill and be . . . *happy*. Why agonize over whether you are screwed up because of what your parents did or didn't do to you when you can bypass Go and collect the two hundred dollars? The promise of Prozac and other drugs like it is that you can be more than you ever were before, find and keep a mate, be a magnanimous tiger on the job but a squishy teddy-bear at home, and discover inner peace without having to make much effort at all. Millions of Americans are medicating themselves—sometimes for the rest of their lives—in order to feel good, better, best, regardless of the fact that it may be the medication and not their innate self that they show to the rest of the world.

There *is* no quick fix for emotional turmoil. Sometimes it's a stage you have to go through, sometimes it's simply your darker side coming up to the light that begs to be acknowledged. You can do so much more for yourself than mindlessly taking a pill to cheer up. If you rely on a "magic bullet," you will be shortchanging yourself from learning how to take charge of your feelings and just, well . . . *feel* them.

You can do it yourself, and enjoy every minute of it. Regardless of how you feel today, you can change the way you look at life, and that will alter the way you look at yourself and others, and even at the lousy things that befall you. Every human being deserves the wonderful experience of creating his or her own version of happiness, and that is what you will learn from this book.

■ *How Do You Know If You Need Help?*

Are you coping with life? If you are, congratulations. If you're not, you can learn. Many people interviewed for this book said that they realized they were in trouble when their psychological turmoil began to erode their ability to cope with daily life. They were too exhausted (read, "depressed") to get out of bed in the morning; they were too nervous to drive a car at night; they were so preoccupied with a love relationship gone wrong that they couldn't concentrate on work and lost a promotion.

Other signs and symptoms for which you may need help are

- overeating or undereating
- sleeping too much or too little
- feelings of paranoia (that everyone is out to get you)
- persistent thoughts of death or suicide

- lowered sex drive or compulsive sexual behavior
- pervasive sense of fatigue or hyperactivity
- hopelessness
- inability to control emotions, that is, hair-trigger temper or bursting into tears at the slightest provocation

Evidently, mental and emotional disturbances don't exist in a vacuum. There may be physical reasons for all of the above symptoms—a chronic disease state, medication (either over-the-counter or prescription) from which you are having severe side effects, or some particular life event or trauma that suddenly throws you into a tailspin.

But there is a way out of the maze of turbulent, unsettling feelings: You can actively work to change your situation. The first step is to ascertain the state of your general health. If you don't feel balanced, if you are feeling unlike yourself, you should have a medical checkup to make sure you are in good physical condition. If you are, it may be time to see a professional counselor or therapist to talk about your problems and how you'd like to deal with them.

The good news is that you're probably not as badly off as you might imagine. The ups and downs you view as a dizzy roller-coaster ride are perfectly normal, *unless you find that they are interfering with your life.* One way to discover whether your problem is serious or benign is to monitor yourself with a diary for three days. Record the events that occur and your reactions to them, so that you can make an assessment at the end of the time as to whether you are coping or falling apart. If every little thing is such a burden that you can't deal with it at all and avoid it, or overreact so that others question your ability to "get a grip," then you need help. If, on the other hand, you feel lousy but still proceed with your chores in a routine manner, you are simply a healthy person having a bad day.

The goal of this book is to show you that you don't need drugs to feel good—*nor do you need to feel perfect all the time.* The natural therapies that are offered for your consideration will help you to get on track and shine a new light on your worries and concerns. None of them are panaceas; none of them will actually shift your appreciation of a glass as half full if you have always seen it as half empty.

But that's okay. If you think of life as a 12-lane highway, you have a lot of room for error. Unless you're bouncing off the medians, you are probably in good enough shape to treat yourself, with some guidance from professionals in the natural-therapy fields. If, however, you cannot stir yourself to make the effort to use these therapies, you should seriously consider placing yourself in the hands of a professional therapist or psychologist. Together, you may be able to find a way out of the darkness so that you can take over and take charge of your well-being.

▨ *Where Do Emotional Problems Come From?*

The current medical theory on disorders such as depression, anxiety, compulsiveness, and so forth, is that we are all borne with the propensity to develop emotional problems. That doesn't mean we have to live with a cloud hanging over us, worrying that at any moment mental illness may strike. Just as we may inherit a predisposition to heart disease, pattern baldness, or poor vision, we still have a lot of say in what we do with our inheritance. Since our brain and emotions are enormously complex, we have the chance to strengthen and improve them from day to day and year to year.

A thick concoction of genetics, biochemistry, temperament, personality, and social and environmental factors are at the root of what we term, "mental and emotional illness." They are also at the root of what we designate as mental and emotional health.

Some people feel they have to fight from the day they're born about anything and everything, and they thrive on their combativeness. Others have little to worry about, yet they worry incessantly. The development of unsettling symptoms resulting from psychological syndromes comes about, we think, because certain individuals are born without an ability to cope with stressful situations. Let's take the case of a woman who comes from a poverty-stricken single-parent household and is forced to care for her younger siblings while her mother flits from one boyfriend to another. She manages to grow up self-sufficient, responsible, and organized. She does brilliantly as a manager of an insurance office and gets one promotion after another. But when it comes to developing a romantic relationship, she falls apart. She selects abusive, uncaring men who always disappoint her, and she blames it on herself. It is possible, then, that something in her basic emotional makeup allowed her to do well with managing others but left her unable to manage herself and her deeper needs. In order for her to change, she will have to implement some of the therapies in this book that will allow her to develop emotionally. She might try meditation or bodywork, or a type of exercise that challenges her to climb higher, run faster, take care of herself better.

We all have our own triggers, the threshhold over which we can't hold on anymore. This is nothing to be ashamed of. Far from implying that we are all doomed to follow the proddings of our unruly genes, the biological theory means that once we have self-knowledge we can make substantial changes in our behavior. And armed with that knowledge, we can accomplish great emotional feats. Even if you're so painfully shy you can't leave the house, there are ways to approach the outside world. Using behavioral and cognitive techniques to improve self-esteem, working with homeopathic remedies or light therapy, you can change your internal energy so that it reaches outward. Even if you feel angry at everyone and everything, you can learn to turn that passion around and use it constructively. You might practice yoga and learn to breathe; you might get a pet and see how being around animals naturally lowers your blood pressure. For every problem you may have, there are multiple avenues of dealing with them—naturally, easily, without medication.

Peter D. Kramer, in his book *Listening to Prozac,* says that "when we call a person 'sensitive,' we will come to mean that the person we are discussing has a slight biological derangement, one that must be taken into account in assessing his behavior or opinions." If you are aware that you are touchy and that you always take every little comment or implication personally, you may learn by using meditation or biofeedback or by improving your nutritional or exercise status how it's possible for you to bypass your initial reactions and move onto better ways of coping. You may find, after a while, that what used to bug the hell out of you no longer even presses a button. This doesn't mean that you won't have severe reactions to more stressful problems in your life, but you will be an infinitely stronger individual by then and ready for some real slings and arrows that previously would have laid you low.

All of us go through bad times: we may experience the death of a loved one, divorce, loss of a job or financial security, our children or parents getting into some trouble, or just plain old "I can't get out of bed today" blues. But unless these feelings are chronic and disabling and intensify over time, we all come out on the other side of them.

While we're going through bad times, we may experience a range of emotions that feel alien to us. Actually, even when we don't feel like "us," these depths and heights of rage, sadness, terror, or a little of all three may simply be a deeper version of our everyday personality. It's possible that what seems like "craziness" or "depression" is actually a loosening up of feelings that we've repressed up to now. They are like the fever that announces the presence of flu in your body—you have to sweat it out and let the immune system do its work to heal, regardless of how lousy it makes you feel.

▓ *How to Use This Book*

Nature's Prozac will give readers the tools they need, not just to feel better, but to *be* sounder in mind, body, and spirit, and to do it without drugs. The natural methods outlined in this book have no side effects or contraindications, will save you a great deal of money, and will perhaps teach you more about yourself than you could ever have learned had you not felt the need to make a change in the way you handle your inner *angst*.

The A-to-Z listing offers an alphabetical guide to the various mental and emotional problems you may be experiencing as well as the treatments and therapies that may help you to cope with them. Although each listing will have several therapies or treatments, you don't need to practice all of them in order to get relief. Start simple and see if the easiest suggestion works for you. Give it a chance—that is, try it more than twice. Make sure you understand the methods and select those that seem most comfortable for you. If you aren't getting the complete effect you hoped for, move onto some of the more esoteric therapies. Where there is one particular method that is tried and tested for one condition, it will be listed first.

The listings include 100 common problems, including 11 major syndromes. The problems usually overlap, so you will find treatments for one that apply to several others as well. First read the general heading under the major problem such as depression, anxiety, or stress. This will give you an overview of the condition you may have and will list all the various symptoms and treatments that apply, with page numbers directing you to the treatments for the symptom or symptoms you're experiencing. All the therapies and treatments are explained under the individual symptoms.

Under the listing for your particular symptoms, we'll offer a variety of techniques and therapies you might try to alleviate them. If you can't find your particular symptom, read the entry for one or several that most closely match your own.

There are 45 therapies discussed within the A-to-Z listing, ranging from nutrition and exercise to homeopathy, light therapy, acupuncture, and various types of bodywork such as dancing and Feldenkrais therapy. You will also find certain types of psychotherapy listed, which you may wish to investigate first on your own by reading a book suggested in the resource section, or perhaps in short-term therapy with a professional.

The Appendix offers you ways to get off medication if you are currently taking it and feel either that you'd like to take a more natural route to your wellness or fear that you have become too dependent on chemical maintenance for your daily survival and sense of well-being. If you are truly concerned not just about your mental and emotional health but also how you achieve it, you will need to study this section for easy suggestions on weaning yourself slowly onto drug-free therapies. Each type of antidepressant and serotonine reuptake inhibitor will be discussed briefly here, so you'll understand what your brain is doing when it responds—well or badly—to medication.

Finally, the Resource Guide is your personal directory to natural mental health, with dozens of places to go and organizations to contact nationally and in your area. A listing of books on various therapies and emotional problems will give you access to specific information on your condition and ideas on how to handle it.

Because we are human, we have within us the potential for enormous pain and also for enormous healing. It's not always pleasant to deal with the demons that possess us occasionally and make us act and react in ways that seem beyond our control. But when we have a handle on our feelings and understand a little of where they come from, they aren't as scary. The challenge of working through them supplants the terror of facing the unknown inside us.

So let us bravely lead the way to a brighter emotional future. Without drugs, without constraints, we can learn to be bigger and stronger individuals who feel love, hate, hope, and fear and enjoy each day to its fullest.

A BUSE OF SUBSTANCES

see also Agitation, page 21; Alienation, page 28; Anxiety, page 43; Mental Confusion, page 100; Victim Mentality, page 433

Ever since the cave people discovered that certain plants had hallucinogenic properties that could alter their feelings and physical reactions, our civilization has relished the brief escape that mind-altering substances can provide. The list ranges from the more commonly used alcohol, tobacco, and marijuana to the higher-priced spreads—cocaine, heroin, methamphetamines, PCP, LSD, and even common household inhalants such as glue and paint.

■ What Happens When You Abuse Substances

You may experience an inability to get through the day or part of a day without the substance, be it nicotine, caffeine, alcohol, or drugs. You may be preoccupied with getting and consuming this substance. You may be irrational about using money appropriately, for example, going without meals in order to afford a pint of whisky or carton of cigarettes.

An addiction to a substance is possibly more dangerous and more difficult to cure than was previously thought. A new study on smoking at the Brookhaven National Laboratory shows that any addictive substance causes an increase of dopamine in the brain. This brain chemical produces a feeling of euphoria just like that caused by cocaine and amphetamines. There is also a strong relationship between smoking and alcohol consumption, which means that multiple addictions could increase your risk of depression and other mood disturbances.

A couple of glasses of wine or two beers a night after a long day is not addiction, unless you cannot get through the night without them. If you *have* to ingest or inhale something in order to restore your sense of well-being and harmony, then you have a problem.

Most people react to stress or depression by trying to make it go away, and if they can't do it alone, they take on a companion—a cigarette to hold onto when times are bad, a bottle to stare into when no one seems to care. If we get into the habit of using a substance in place of finding a solution or—more commonly—living with the unresolved dilemma, we may suddenly be hooked by a lure we didn't even know was there.

Addiction is a pernicious enemy because it tricks the addict into believing that everyone is out of step but him or her. The classic symptom of substance abuse is *denial,* and this inability to see dependence can pervade your entire life and all your relationships. It is only when you have decided to acknowledge your need for the substance that gives you relief that you have a chance at recovery.

The best programs for substance abuse work on a combination of healing factors: Both mind and body must change radically.

Change the Way You Act Around Drugs

The behavioral approach has been found to be helpful, as long as you are really motivated and have the support and steely disapproval of friends and family when you fall behind in the therapy. You must first know you have a problem in order to get rid of a problem, whether the addiction is to drugs, alcohol, cigarettes, sex, or any number of other abusive pastimes. Recognition comes usually when you are at rock bottom, physically, financially, and emotionally. And only then can you start to help yourself.

You will give yourself six weeks to change your behavior; it will take much longer to rid yourself of the substance, but all you need at first is a small change.

The first step is to chart the times of day and situations around which you abuse a substance. At first you'll find that you do it all the time, but as you begin to write down instances of use, you'll discover that there are patterns. If you smoke most frequently when you're drinking coffee, sitting in a bar, talking on the phone, or when you're around certain people who also do this behavior, you must avoid those situations entirely.

For the first week monitor the behavior and don't try to do anything about it except to point it out to yourself and others around you. Write down the instance in your logbook. During the second week, you will be allowed to do the activity only when you are not alone. During those solo times when you feel a craving, you will set up a reward system so that you can do something positive when you're impelled to do something negative. Instead of smoking a cigarette, you will occupy your hands by lathering yourself in a bubble bath, doing a crossword puzzle, or knitting.

During the next two weeks, you will modify your public behavior and keep up with your private behavior. Remember, it's not unusual to fall off the wagon, but by making changes in the setting and environment that you are accustomed to, you'll discover that the activity isn't as satisfying as it was.

On your last week of the program, you will attempt to eliminate the behavior entirely and will now write down the settings and situations that still give you trouble.

After six weeks the program hasn't ended, but rather, has just begun. At this point, you are primed to alter the behavior because you've had experience doing without it.

Your Best Friend Will *Tell You*

A support group can be the best way to bolster your own resolve to stop doing the destructive activity you've been doing. When you have people around who really care what you do, you owe something to them. As you help others in the group with their problem, you find that you are helping yourself.

The enormous success of Alcoholics Anonymous and other 12-step groups argues for joining. The meetings are available everywhere—in churches and synagogues, community groups, on college campuses, even on the job in many corporations. If you have trouble with the philosophy of AA, which is that you are in the hands of something or someone bigger than yourself who can help you, you can start your own informal group based on your own ideas. It's essential, however, that you all be accessible to one another and agree to maintain some of AA's rules. The buddy system, for example, where you can call a designated friend at any hour for continued support, has kept many individuals on track.

Put Something Else in Your Mouth

If you crave a cigarette or a drink, chew sugarless gum, a carrot stick, or have a glass of sparkling water with a slice of lemon.

Jog When You Want a Drink

Exercise can be a cure for addiction. It has been found that the discipline of getting out and moving around foils the mind's ritualistic patterns of needing abusive stimulation. Exercise also works on the cardiovascular system, the musculoskeletal system, the endocrine system, and strengthens the immune system, which puts you in better general health. Aerobic movement (that which gets the heartbeat up near its maximum for 20 minutes) triggers the release of beta endorphins in the brain—the neurotransmitters that act as natural opiates and flood us with a sense of well-being. When the brain can manufacture its own health-giving drug, it's redundant and dangerous to overmedicate with a synthetic.

Use Pressure Points

To stop cravings, use the point at the opening to the ear in the hollow formed when the mouth is open (SI 19), and the point on the back of the hand at the place where the thumb and index finger meet (LI 4). To detoxify the body, press on the point halfway between the knee and top of thigh bones on both legs.

Acupuncture combined with intensive psychotherapy has been found very helpful in the treatment of addiction. Only qualified professionals in organized substance-abuse programs will be able to provide this treatment.

Take a Yoga Posture

The following yoga postures are beneficial for clearing toxins from the liver:

LOCUST POSE: Lie on your stomach on a mat and bring your hands under your body, linking them in fists and trying to hide your elbows under you. Inhale and hold your breath, then lift your legs without bending your knees. Let the weight of your body rest on your chest and arms. Slowly lower your legs as you exhale. Relax and repeat.

SHOULDER STAND: Lie on your back with your hands alongside your body. Pressing your palms into the floor, lift your legs to a vertical position. Gently lower your legs over your head and press your chin into your chest so that your spine is completely straight. (If you cannot do this, you can rock back and forth on your sacrum until you can roll up onto your shoulders.) Breathe while in this position. Roll down slowly, one vertebra at a time.

PLOUGH POSE: This is the logical continuation of the shoulder stand. When you are completely vertical, lower your legs slowly until your toes touch the floor behind you. Breathe while in this position. Roll down slowly, one vertebra at a time.

FISH POSE: To reverse the torque of the spine after the last two poses, you should finish with this pose. Lie on your back with your palms on top of your thighs. Bend your head back, arching your spine, until you can rest the top of your head on the floor. Open your chest and breathe. Slowly let your head slide back onto the floor.

The Healing Touch

It's been found that "laying on of hands" or the simple power of another's touch can alleviate some of the stress and anxiety that impels people to abuse substances. The human bond we feel with others is part of what keeps us getting up each morning, no matter what the day might hold in store.

So ask a friend or partner to spend some time gently working on all the tension-filled areas of your body. If they don't have time for a full-body massage, an excellent remedy for those who have addictive tendencies is a head massage. The head, an incredibly sensitive area, is the source of much of the nervous-system activity that is currently out of balance.

Your partner should begin by getting you to lie flat on your back. He or she will sit behind you, taking the weight of your head in his or her hands. Your partner will work around the base of your skull and up into your hair; then around to the pressure points at your temples, then very lightly around your sinuses, and down to the sides of your nose and your mouth. The flat of the fingers can be used as well as the knuckles—smooth strokes and light pats are also effective on the head and face.

Let Go and Let God

The great success of the 12-step programs lies in the fact that we can rely on something larger than us or our own feeble attempts to cure ourselves. Many addicted individuals claim that prayer works brilliantly. By giving yourself up to a higher power, you are not abdicating responsibility for yourself but rather are enlisting the aid of a force that can dispel the strongest resistance.

You don't have to believe in God to pray for the strength to hold back when you really think you *need* a drink but actually only *want* one desperately.

Sit in a quiet place and try to clear your mind of peripheral thoughts. Concentrate on the warmth and nourishment that you imagine coming to you from the universe. Make a conscious effort to ally yourself with this power and give up the desires and cravings just for the period of time that you are praying.

You will find that the more often you pray, the easier it will be to adjust your priorities and learn to care for yourself. Praying can be a way to get in touch with a deeper side of you that has better awareness and better control over your emotions. After awhile, you will find that when an unpleasant situation arises at work or home, your first thought won't be to reach for a drink, a smoke, or a drug, but rather, to meet the problem head-on and work with it as best you can at the time.

Glance into Trance

Self-hypnosis may be the only way that people ever stop smoking (or drinking or taking drugs) for good. But in order for this technique to work (see Self-hypnosis, page 383), you must first be extremely motivated and practice going into a trance state daily.

When you are ready to work on your substance-abuse problem, write yourself a list of powerful forces that would anchor your commitment to stop. (It is much more helpful to use positive rather than negative reasons to get rid of your problem.)

First, write down that you respect your mind and body and must protect it from smoking (drinking, drugs, and so forth), which is a poison to your body. Second, tell yourself that you cannot live without your body—it is the vehicle through which you experience life. And as your body's guardian, you have obligations to keep it safe from harm. Third, you must teach others the benefit of having a body that is not polluted. Fourth, tell yourself that if you can accomplish this feat, you can do anything in life you choose.

Study your list as you prepare to put yourself into trance. Let your eyes roll up, close your eyes, let your right arm feel so light it begins to float up. Then, as you concentrate deeply in trance, recall the four items on your list. Practice this brief self-hypnosis ten times daily—every couple of hours—at the beginning. As you have increasing success, you can reduce your practice to eight and then five times daily. Soon you will see that you cannot tolerate the substance the way you used to. Hypnosis will help with the other measures you've put into place to end your addiction.

Acupuncture/Acupressure

Acupuncture, an ancient Chinese art with a few modern updates, has been known for centuries to be invaluable in the treatment of pain. In addition, it has been found that this treatment, which uses flexible, stainless-steel needles placed along certain energy pathways of the body, can alter neurochemical reactions. It is therefore often used in the treatment of addiction, depression, cardiovascular disease, pulmonary disease, and many other physical and mental disorders.

The many acupuncture points (at least 360 are commonly used, and there are many more) can be found at small dips in the skin known as gates. As the needles enter these gates, they gain access to the circulation of two vital elements: blood and *chi,* or life energy. The chi moves through the body's 14 pathways or meridians that run from the skin to the internal organs. We can access energy by needling acupoints along these meridians that transmit healing power throughout body and mind.

Chinese medicine follows the Taoist philosophy of *yin* and *yang*—the concept that the universe and everything in it is designated either as receptive and yielding (yin) or strong and untiring (yang). At the same time, there is yang within yin and yin within yang. For example, a rushing river is yang because of its powerful movement; however, when it freezes over in winter, it becomes yin when it is fixed and unchanging. Similarly, the body and mind both contain within them elements of yin and yang.

The Chinese perception of acupuncture is that it either activates or inhibits the flow of chi and blood along meridian pathways. When treating a patient, the practitioner will place needles of different thicknesses and lengths along various points on certain meridians and will manipulate them down to specific depths in the skin and tissue. If there's something wrong with one organ, for example, the brain, the problem will show up along the entire meridian. The action of the needles affects the chi as well as the blood in the meridians and therefore eventually affects all the organs in the body. Acupuncture balances our yin and yang by taking away excess, increasing a deficiency, warming a cold problem or cooling a hot problem, or increasing circulation by getting a stagnant area back in motion.

From the standpoint of Western medicine, acupuncture has several different benefits: It apparently triggers the release of neuropeptides known as beta endorphins, the natural opiates in the brain that alleviate pain and give us a sense of well-being. A second explanation for acupuncture's success lies in the close proximity of sensory thresholds for pain and pleasure in the brain. This is known as the gate theory and works on the principle that when the pain gate is closed, only pleasure can be experienced, and vice versa. Needle stimulation shuts down the gate and prevents the transmission of pain from the brain to an affected organ. But research indicates that the immune system is also involved.

A study in Shanghai showed that the use of acupuncture caused an increase in the production of immunoglobulin and specific antibodies to fight disease and keep the body healthy. Other studies show that acupuncture affects many aspects of circulation, rhythm and stroke volume of the heart, and production of red and white blood cells. It also assists in gastrointestinal peristalsis and secretion of stomach acids.

Acupuncture does not work like a drug, targeting a symptom and curing it. Rather, it interferes with or challenges the existing patterns of dysfunction and rearranges the flow of energy throughout the body.

Acupressure follows the same healing pathway, except that finger or knuckle pressure replaces needle stimulation. (*Shiatsu* is the Japanese method of finger pressure, using a thrusting and pressing type of manipulation.) Acupressure allows you to treat yourself, up to a certain point. Whereas acupuncture needles are placed very specifically, right on the points to various depths in the skin and tissue below, fingers can press only superficially. Acupressure does relieve muscle tension and allows more blood and oxygen to flow through your tissues to your brain. However, the effects are brief, and in order to get any relief, you must press the points for at least five minutes each time.

If you wish to use acupressure to alleviate emotional or mental problems, use the acupuncture charts to locate the correct point you are going to stimulate with your finger. And if you decide that you want more dramatic results, you may wish to consult an acupuncturist or Chinese medical practitioner for a consultation and treatment.

Standard Meridian Abbreviations

Lu	Lung	CV	Conception Vessel
LI	Large Intestine	Ki	Kidney
Sp	Spleen	Pe	Pericardium
TB	Triple Burner	UB	Urinary Bladder
St	Stomach	GB	Gallbladder
SI	Small Intestine	Li	Liver
Ht	Heart	GV	Governing Vessel

The 14 meridians are named for eight of the body's internal organs (although Chinese medicine never targets one organ for treatment) and four other locations:

Abbreviation Key

Lu. = Lung
L.I. = Large Intestine
St. = Stomach
Sp. = Spleen
Ht. = Heart
S.I. = Small Intestine
U.B. = Urinary Bladder
Ki. = Kidney
Pe. = Pericardium
T.B. = Triple-Burner
G.B. = Gallbladder
Li. = Liver
G.V. = Governing Vessel
C.V. = Conception Vessel
E.P. = Extra Points

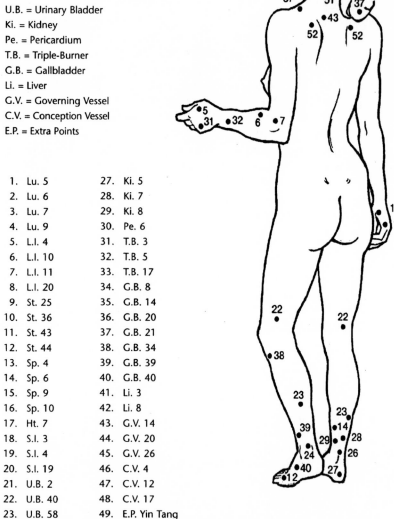

1. Lu. 5	27. Ki. 5
2. Lu. 6	28. Ki. 7
3. Lu. 7	29. Ki. 8
4. Lu. 9	30. Pe. 6
5. L.I. 4	31. T.B. 3
6. L.I. 10	32. T.B. 5
7. L.I. 11	33. T.B. 17
8. L.I. 20	34. G.B. 8
9. St. 25	35. G.B. 14
10. St. 36	36. G.B. 20
11. St. 43	37. G.B. 21
12. St. 44	38. G.B. 34
13. Sp. 4	39. G.B. 39
14. Sp. 6	40. G.B. 40
15. Sp. 9	41. Li. 3
16. Sp. 10	42. Li. 8
17. Ht. 7	43. G.V. 14
18. S.I. 3	44. G.V. 20
19. S.I. 4	45. G.V. 26
20. S.I. 19	46. C.V. 4
21. U.B. 2	47. C.V. 12
22. U.B. 40	48. C.V. 17
23. U.B. 58	49. E.P. Yin Tang
24. U.B. 60	50. E.P. Tai Yang
25. Ki. 1	51. U.B. 10
26. Ki. 3	52. U.B. 36

Abbreviation Key

Lu. = Lung
L.I. = Large Intestine
St. = Stomach
Sp. = Spleen
Ht. = Heart
S.I. = Small Intestine
U.B. = Urinary Bladder
Ki. = Kidney
Pe. = Pericardium
T.B. = Triple-Burner
G.B. = Gallbladder
Li. = Liver
G.V. = Governing Vessel
C.V. = Conception Vessel
E.P. = Extra Points

1.	Lu. 5	26.	Ki. 3
2.	Lu. 6	27.	Ki. 5
3.	Lu. 7	28.	Ki. 7
4.	Lu. 9	29.	Ki. 8
5.	L.I. 4	30.	Pe. 6
6.	L.I. 10	31.	T.B. 3
7.	L.I. 11	32.	T.B. 5
8.	L.I. 20	33.	T.B. 17
9.	St. 25	34.	G.B. 8
10.	St. 36	35.	G.B. 14
11.	St. 43	36.	G.B. 20
12.	St. 44	37.	G.B. 21
13.	Sp. 4	38.	G.B. 34
14.	Sp. 6	39.	G.B. 39
15.	Sp. 9	40.	G.B. 40
16.	Sp. 10	41.	Li. 3
17.	Ht. 7	42.	Li. 8
18.	S.I. 3	43.	G.V. 14
19.	S.I. 4	44.	G.V. 20
20.	S.I. 19	45.	G.V. 26
21.	U.B. 2	46.	C.V. 4
22.	U.B. 40	47.	C.V. 12
23.	U.B. 58	48.	C.V. 17
24.	U.B. 60	49.	E.P. Yin Tang
25.	Ki. 1	50.	E.P. Tai Yang

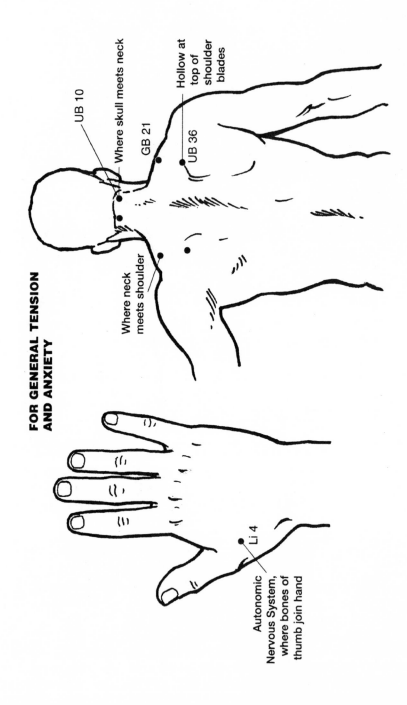

FOR GENERAL TENSION AND ANXIETY

UB 10

Where skull meets neck

GB 21

Hollow at top of shoulder blades

UB 36

Where neck meets shoulder

Li 4

Autonomic Nervous System, where bones of thumb join hand

- The Triple Burner is the pathway linking lungs, spleen, kidneys, small intestine, and bladder.
- The Pericardium is the outer, protective membrane of the heart.
- The Governing Vessel runs up the spine from the coccyx, passes through the brain, and comes over the top of the head, ending at the upper lip.
- The Conception Vessel runs from the perineum between the legs up the midline of the body to the lower lip.

ADD *(Attention Deficit Disorder)* AND ADHD *(Attention Deficit Hyperactive Disorder)*

see also Impulse Control, page 246

This common condition is usually first noted in childhood, when a teacher will be aware that a child can't listen to instructions and finds it nearly impossible to concentrate on the activity at hand. It is more prevalent in boys than in girls.

■ *What Happens When You Have ADD or ADHD*

Kids with this condition have trouble finishing anything— schoolwork or a play project—and are easily distracted. They are impulsive and may speak without raising their hand, which brands them as troublemakers in the classroom. You can spot an ADD child tapping a pencil or his foot on the floor, unable to retain what's been said for even a few minutes. ADD children can be enormously smart, but it can be difficult for them to get through school, where compliance and good organizational skills are valued.

ADHD children have the added disadvantage of being hyperactive as well as distracted. They are all over the place, running constantly, unable to keep still, frequently getting out of their seats. Hyperactive children are exhausting for parents and teachers because they can go for hours without running out of steam, finally collapsing in a tantrum or bout of whining. They generally don't sleep well and refuse to nap.

ADHD children are also difficult for their peers to take, since they can't play as equals but tend to bully or dominate others.

This syndrome usually manifests itself before the age of seven—some kids grow out of it as they mature, but others retain ADHD into adulthood, where they may become impulsive, reckless individuals. Problems such as substance abuse and criminal behavior are sometimes seen in ADHD adults.

The grownup who has ADD also has problems, since the condition is often connected to minor neurological imbalances that are generally overlooked.

It's been the rule for the last ten years to treat such disturbances with stimulant drugs—Ritalin (methylphenidate) being the most commonly used. Although it might appear counterproductive to stimulate a hyperactive child, the reason that it's effective is that the drug works on two neurotransmitters—dopamine and norepinephrine—which help to organize brain activity. But the past few years, Ritalin has been used as a cure-all for children who may not have ADD but other types of behavior problems that don't need to be medicated. Too many parents are told that this is the only solution for their children, and approximately 10 to 12 percent of all boys in the United States between the ages of 6 and 14 are now on this drug. This is an astoundingly large percentage, given the fact that long-term use of Ritalin may potentially lead to adolescent addiction.

A child who does suffer from ADD or ADHD may need to take this drug in order to function; however, there are complementary natural remedies that can work hand in hand with the medication. It is also possible that after a program of holistic change is in place, the drug can be tapered off or the dosage reduced.

Focus on Food

Nutritional change is almost mandatory—the chemical additives in most foods can be incredibly destructive to a sensitive child. The debate about whether sugar makes children hyperactive continues to rage; suffice it to say that sugar should be doled out in moderation and not in great doses. Most ADD children are very sensitive to foods, which means that you should eliminate anything made with artificial flavor and color, chocolate, MSG, preservatives, and caffeine (in most sodas).

Get the Lead Out

It's a good idea to get your physician to do blood and hair tests to rule out lead and aluminum toxicity in your child. In certain studies, higher hair and blood lead levels were found in children with hyperactivity and neurological problems.

Create an Energy Outlet

Children with excess energy need a positive outlet. Create jobs you know your child can accomplish well (feeding the pets, setting the table, sorting laundry) and praise and reward the child when he or she finishes the task that's been set. If the job doesn't get done, don't nag about it, but instead challenge him or her to do it right the following day.

Move Your Body

Exercise is the next best mode of alternative treatment. It has been found that martial arts, where self-discipline and focus on a physical structure (the forms of *kung fu* or the katas of *aikido, karate* or *tae kwon do*) offer incredible benefits for children and adults with this condition.

The Odor of Calm

Aromatherapy can help a child or adult with ADD or ADHD. Try essential oils of chamomile, hyssop, rose, or verbena mixed with a carrier oil for massage or in a defuser placed by the bed at night.

Helpful Herbs

Herbal relaxants for hyperactive children, which can be added to bathwater, include red clover (a liver tonic), lime blossom (slightly stronger but still mild as a relaxant), and chamomile.

Supplementing Vitamins and Minerals

Children with this problem should take a multivitamin daily. It should include Vitamin A (with beta carotene), C, E (with selenium), and a full range of Bs (B_1, B_2, B_6, and B_{12}). In addition, you should supplement folate. A deficiency of folate has been strongly linked to neural-tube disorders in fetuses—folic acid is equally important for a strong nervous system in children. An ADD or ADHD child also needs to supplement the minerals calcium, magnesium, iron, and zinc. It's also important to test for elevated levels of copper and phosphorus.

If you have trouble getting your child to bed, give an L-tryptophan cocktail of milk and a banana an hour before bedtime. Many ADD children have a deficit of essential fatty acids, so you may wish to try 500 mg. of evening primrose oil per 5 kg. of body weight daily.

Children's dosages of supplements should be half the adult dosage until puberty. (See *Supplementation,* page 409, for adult dosages.)

Alexander Adds Poise

Posture shores up the spine; it also is a physical symbol of the way we maintain ourselves in gravity. Alexander technique (see page 27) teaches the practitioner to support the body in space and have better physical balance, which will dovetail with the sense of emotional balance. Exercises include standing, sitting, breathing, and moving while speaking in order to identify body tensions.

AFFIRMATIONS

see also Positive Self-Talk, page 350

There's a song lyric from Rogers and Hammerstein's "South Pacific" that goes, "Make believe you're brave, and the trick will take you far. You may be as brave as you make believe you are."

The theory behind this neat saying is, "Act as if." Even if you don't believe you feel well, if you tell yourself you are, it can be reassuring and helpful. By making up phrases that you repeat over and over—or using those that have been successful for others in the past—you can affirm your own positive reasons for living. For this reason, the treatment is also called "Positive self-talk," or talking to yourself in an upbeat, inspiring manner. (No, you are *not* crazy if you talk to yourself.)

The repetitive nature of these sayings also has a drone-like quality to it. It's a kind of mind training, as if you were hypnotizing yourself into a new belief. As a matter of fact, one of the most common affirmations came from a French hypnotherapist, Émil Coué, who coined the catchy saying, "Every day, in every way, I'm getting better and better."

Affirmations are useful in emergency situations. When you're walking down a dark street at night and feel panicky, or you are anxious about a job interview and can't imagine how you can think clearly, you can quickly prime your mind with a helpful phrase that may get you through this brief rough patch.

Some common affirmations you might try are:

My pure essence is good.

Love surrounds me and fills me.

I breathe universal love.

All is forgiven.

God be my guide.

I release the past and embrace the now.

I am happy, relaxed, at peace.

An interesting way to use affirmations is to apply them to your life. You might think of a series of helpful, positive words and attach people and ideas to them. For example:

"I forgive _____. I love _____. I can do _____. I will accomplish _____. I'm a good person because _____."

Fill in the blanks and repeat your resulting sentences aloud. Keep in mind that the more you fill yourself with these thoughts, the more easily you can come to believe them and make use of them to alleviate stress, anxiety, and depression.

AGING *(and Mental Health)*

see also Agitation, page 21; Alienation, page 28; Anger, Suppressed, page 31; Confusion, mental, page 100; Depression, page 112; Loneliness, page 277; Victim Mentality, page 433

The truth is that old age does not necessarily bring with it decline, depression, and mental oblivion. Yet our image of aging often colors the old people we know. Most young people think of the elderly as irritable, cantankerous, feeble, and in the way as opposed to mature, mellow, revered, respected, and at peace with themselves and the world.

Very often an image can become a self-fulfilling prophecy. Of course, there are scores of people in their eighties, nineties and hundreds who are in great mental shape, but many start to lose interest in growing and changing after the age of 65 or 70 (generally around the time they are told they are no longer wanted in the work force). A larger number are challenged by trying to feel good despite illnesses and dysfunctions, friends and partners who are ill or have died, and having nothing important to do in life. It is all too often the case that an older person who has heart disease, cancer, osteoporosis, chronic pain, or loss of eyesight, hearing, or mobility becomes a mental and emotional cripple.

Growing old is not a disease unless you become sick of yourself. It's not how old you are but *how* you grow old that is the key here—there's as much plasticity and variability in the way people age as there is in their fingerprints.

Alzheimer's disease has the most visibility when it comes to mental diseases of the aging, and occurs in nearly a third of the population over the age of 80. More prominent in women, it is actually a type of dementia due to rapid degeneration of parts of the central nervous system and neurofibrillary tangles that impede brain function. It involves the impairment of at least two cognitive abilities (either attention, learning, memory, or orientation) and also the impairment of at least one symbolic skill (calculation, abstraction, or comprehension) as well as problems in at least one essential life role (ability to relate to work, family, or peers or to function socially).

Other types of dementia may have similar symptoms—Jacob-Creutzfeldt's disease is caused by a virus and also involves dementia and difficulty walking. Korsakoff's disease is often seen in chronic alcoholics who don't eat properly and develop a thiamine deficiency. Pick's disease involves atrophy of the frontal cortex of the brain and results in behavioral and personality changes. There are certain dementias that accompany stroke and also some resulting from metabolic disorders or drug toxicity.

But it's depression that is the most common mental disease of old age. Depression in the elderly often brings with it a type of pseudo-dementia, characterized by apathy, confusion, cognitive and memory lapses, and a loss of interest in personal care. The general symptoms of depression are no different from those in any other segment of the population (see Depression page 112); however, the external triggers are more prevalent after the age of 65. Older people keep losing—they lose jobs, status, self-esteem, physical prowess, eyesight, hearing, money—and these losses weigh heavily if you can't do anything to change your situation.

The idea is to convince older people that they *can* improve their lot in life. Mastery implies that the more you do something, the better you get at it. Certainly doing something for 80 years, whether it's cooking or carpentry, is worthy of note. It is important to keep going, keep doing, and feel wanted. The most successful elderly have a drive and a will to get up each day and be useful to others as well as themselves. Physical activity seems to be a big indicator of good mental functioning, since exercise raises levels of a nerve growth factor that keeps neurons healthy. Resilience is vital to good longevity. When you have the ability and desire to bounce back from trauma and illness, it fills you with a sense of competence and self-esteem to surpass your own expectations.

Social interaction—particularly doing things for others—is another marker of good aging. If you have nothing more to do and no one to do it for, there's no reason to stick around. However, if others value your work, you can't feel useless and neglected. If you are a master—living comfortably, getting up each morning to do something significant—you can continue indefinitely.

Although the brain shrinks with age and we lose neurons that can never be replaced, unaffected parts of a healthy brain take over functions that other areas can no longer perform. There is no reason, in the absence of disease, why we shouldn't be as vibrant and active at 90 as we are at 30. Studies have shown that in the absence of central nervous system disease, the brain does not deteriorate. It has the same

blood flow, oxygen use, and metabolism that it did in its earlier years. So if you can use your brain, you won't lose it.

Mental problems in the elderly are due in great part to
the lack of use. Older people who sit and watch TV or listen
to the radio all day tend to degenerate (and tend to get out
less to shop for healthful food, to drink more alcohol to dull
pain, and to overmedicate themselves, with the assistance of
doctors who provide all those prescriptions). But elderly people who learn new skills, doing volunteer work or starting a
business in their home, for example, seem to remain on top
of their emotional health. There is a clue we can take from
those who live successfully to over age 100—all of them say
they realize their time is limited and therefore they have to
get more accomplished in a day than their younger friends
do.

Elderly people often experience a great deal of anxiety
(especially agoraphobia), paranoia, loneliness, grief, and
bereavement. And these conditions are reinforced by society's myths that you're over the hill at 60 and virtually
worthless by the time you're 80.

The three interlocking strands of mental decay—illness,
depression, and fatigue—have to be carefully picked apart.
This is sometimes the job of social workers and psychologists,
but it more commonly falls in the laps of the next genera-
tion: the middle-aged kids who can't stand seeing Mom and
Dad fall apart and don't want to put them in a nursing home.

Independent living, or separate units attached to a central facility offering assisted living, is the way to go.
Unfortunately, right now most of the senior communities are
way beyond the means of most of the elderly (who tend to be
poorer than the rest of the population as well).

More years on this planet do not guarantee senility any
more than they confer great wisdom and honor. If we can
consider the elderly just as they were at 30, but with a few
more wrinkles, we might set up the expectation for old age as
being no more than a continuation of our natural mental
health.

Treatments to try: Aromatherapy, page 46; Exercise, page
145; Herbs, page 273; Light Therapy, page 292; Meditation,
page 294; Melatonin, page 316; Nutrition, page358; Prayer,
page 417; Tai chi chuan, page 417; Visualization, page 442.

*A*GITATION

see also Abuse of Substances, page 1; Anxiety, page 43; Aging, page 17; Impatience, page 235; Irritability, page 253; Nervousness, page 304

When we are stirred up and in a state of overwhelming emotional anxiety, we are agitated. The same word is used for the action of clothes in a washing machine, and the image we get from this is apt. When we're agitated, we feel like a hunted animal who must check around, scanning the environment for dangers. Only, of course, the vigilance we keep when we're agitated really distracts us from dealing with the problem.

What Happens When You're Agitated

You're constantly on edge and impatient with yourself and others; you don't feel grounded or centered. Many agitated people also suffer from physical symptoms: They may have gastrointestinal problems, headaches, rapid pulse, high blood pressure, heart palpitations, dizziness, frequent urination, and other distressing manifestations of their highly aroused state.

Very often, elderly people become terribly agitated over what seem to be minor issues, although they are not minor to those who are suffering with them. Because so many older people feel impotent and out of touch with the rest of the world, they sometimes have to scramble to make sense of problems that range from deciding what to eat for dinner to figuring out which bus to take. If you are close to an older person who has these concerns, be sure you act patient even when he or she is not.

Breathe!

No special technique is required, just breathe! Inflate your diaphragm and lungs and let the air go with a deep sigh. Make some noise to let out some of the pent-up energy that has gotten you all riled up. Calming the agitation in your body can take care of the turmoil in your mind.

Try a Homeopathic

The following remedies can be helpful for agitation:

For emotional excitement: Ignatia, Pulsatilla, Phosphoric acid, Tuberculinum, Staphisagria

For fearful anticipation: Phosphorus, Pulsatilla, Silica, Argentum nitrate, Arsenicum, Calcarea carbonicum, Ignatia, Lycopodium, Medorrhinum

For chaotic, confused behavior: China, Nux vomica, Arsenicum album, Belladonna, Mercury

For postoperative pain agitation, especially useful in children: Aconite.

Mind Massage

The soothing touch of hands can relax you and work wonders on your blood pressure and pulse rate as well. Your partner or a professional masseur should start with the top of your head and neck, working down your body very slowly. The technique used should maintain contact at all times, as if the masseur's hands were stuck to you (as opposed to a rubdown where the hands often come off the body). It's important to establish a sense of connectedness as the hands move from one part of you to the next.

Calming Herbs

A tonic nourishes the entire body and mind and will encourage the nervous system to heal itself. You can take any of the following herbs singly or in combination: dandelion, burdock, yellow dock, or nettle. Take $1/2$ to 1 teaspoon of extract daily or $1/2$ cup of infusion.

Chamomile or lemon tea (a cup whenever the mood strikes you) is also relaxing.

If you are feeling anxious and agitated, take avena (oat), scullcap, or valerian, $1/2$ teaspoon extract two to three times daily or 1 cup of infusion twice daily.

Use Chinese Wisdom

By pressing on acupoints on the face, you can calm yourself. Use the following points for a clockwise massage:

E.P. (extra point) Yin Tang—between the brows

E.P. (extra point) Tai Yang—the fleshy hollow between the end of the eyebrow and the temple on both sides

L.I. 20—on either side of the nostrils, in the groove beneath the bone

G.B. 14—in the hollow right above the pupil when looking forward, an inch above the eyebrow

Pe. 6—on the midline of the inside of the arm, between two tendons, two inches up from the wrist

Supplement Your Nutrition

The B vitamins are known as the stress vitamins for good reason. You should be taking a multivitamin daily, but in addition, you should supplement B_1, B_2, B_3 (niacin), and especially B_6 and B_{12}, up to 100 mg. each a day.

Move Slowly in Tai Chi Form

The various forms or choreographed patterns of the Chinese meditative art, *tai chi chuan,* are designed to make you slow down and be less impatient. As you move energy from your feet up your spine to your torso and out through your arms and hands, you have a feeling that you are a hose filled with water that cannot arrive at the nozzle until it has completed its course from the faucet.

Stand with your feet shoulder-width apart, right foot facing front, left foot 45 degrees left, head suspended on top of your neck and spine. Allow your arms to lift and shoulders to drop as you hold a big imaginary beach ball in front of you. Begin to walk forward, allowing your arms to float in the air. Put all the weight on your right foot as you allow the left to peel off the ground. As your left now becomes the front foot, get all the weight on it before lifting your back foot. As you move side to side, sink your hip and release all tension in your body. Your head should remain level—do not bounce. See how patient you can be as you wait to step—the right moment to move will arise by itself.

Mind Your Manners

Use mindfulness meditation to stop scanning the horizon for nasty surprises. Take a very simple activity that might cause you anxiety, such as tying a knot and untying it. You are going to pay exceptionally close attention—feel the piece of rope and get a sense of its shape and texture. Smell the rope; put it against your face and feel the roughness of it. Then test it in your hands, pulling it taut and then allowing it to relax. Make your hands move in synch to turn the rope into a knot shape, but do not finish the knot. Examine the spaces in between the pieces of rope. Then tug the ends shut. Reverse the process, again giving every ounce of focus and attention to what you are doing.

When you can accomplish a very simple activity mindfully with this much patience, you can move on to more anxiety-filled activities, such as cleaning the litter box or making a difficult phone call.

Magnets Can Move You

While lying on a massage table for half an hour, with a 2,000-gauss strip magnet under your head, your central nervous system will be able to "tune down" and relax. North-pole energy appears to be the major influence on emotional conditions and may trigger parasympathetic reactions that can calm body and mind. The temporal lobe of the brain and metabolic function are also influenced by magnets. There are types of equipment you can use every day; there are magnets that will fit inside your shoes, hand-held devices, and mats and chair coverings as well (see Resource Guide, page 475).

AGORAPHOBIA

see also Panic Disorder; page 344; Phobias, page 346

The "fear of the marketplace" is a common anxiety-related phobia. The terror of panicking when outside can become so severe that in order to avoid the feeling, agoraphobics often turn themselves into shut-ins who never see the light of day.

▓ What Happens When You Have Agoraphobia

The actual fear is of being unable to escape, whether you're locked in a mass of people at a football game or stuck in an elevator, tunnel, a church, a theater, or even a hairdresser's or dentist's chair. Many individuals cannot travel alone, particularly to new places, and many find it impossible to take public transportation. Agoraphobia is often related to claustrophobia—feeling surrounded often makes sufferers panic.

This phobia may start after a prolonged illness where you had to be home or in the hospital, or it may come upon you with no warning at all. Two thirds of all agoraphobics are women, generally first experiencing the problem in their mid-twenties to early-thirties. They discover that anxiety keeps them from engaging in most social activities, and eventually restricts them to the only safe territory they know, which is home.

Agoraphobia is not only a socially limiting problem, it also brings with it a raft of physical symptoms, such as dry mouth, sweating, dizziness, and shortness of breath. Because it can be so disabling, it is a particularly difficult phobia to treat and you should expect, when working with natural therapies, that it will take you some time.

Don't be discouraged! You may make a little progress and slip back, but that's to be expected.

One Step Out at a Time

Desensitization, used with visualization, is the most common treatment for agoraphobia. When you begin your program, make a schedule of where you'll have to be during the day and stick to it, spending allotted time in the car, on the street, at your job, and in a friend's house. Imagine yourself in a bubble, protected from the world. You can press on the sides of it, but it won't break. (If you are currently unable to leave your house, the schedule should take you from room to room and finally, to the porch.) You will initially do better if you have a friend or relative to accompany you. Each day, extend the time spent and add a new location. When you are ready, try a brief experience that would have caused great anxiety: Walk into a church or theater, and have your friend hold the door open so that you can see the way out. At last, you can attempt the difficult places with the door shut.

The Oil of Life

It has been found that this problem can sometimes be caused by a deficiency of an essential fatty acid known as alpha-linolenic acid, commonly sold as flaxseed oil. One study, reported in the *Journal of Biological Psychiatry,* showed that agoraphobics who had suffered for ten years or more improved within two to three months after taking 2 to 6 tablespoons of this oil daily in divided doses.

The Anti-Panic Flower

The Bach flower remedy Rock Rose is used for feelings of terror or panic. Take 5 or 6 drops in half a glass of water or squeeze directly under the tongue for immediate relief.

Homeopathic Help

The following homeopathic remedies may offer help:

> For fear of crowds and public places: Argentum nitrate, Arnica, Aconite, Nux vomica, Pulsatilla
>
> For fear of busy streets: Aconite, Carcinosin, Causticum

Carry Spirits to Buoy Your Spirit

You can get a vial of spirits of ammonia at your local drugstore. If you feel very dizzy or faint, pop it open and inhale briefly. The strong odor will snap you out of your haze.

Take Ma Bell with You

A cellular phone has proven to be a real boon for people who need immediate contact. It's worth the expense to know that help is just a phone call away.

Carry a Big Stick and Wear Shades

Strangely enough, having something in your hands, like an umbrella or cane, can make you feel safer. It's also useful to hold a newspaper or briefcase, since it has a similar effect as a security blanket does for an insecure child. It also helps to have things darkened around you—you can wear sunglasses anywhere and everywhere if you like. It may also be easier for you to venture forth on rainy days or in the evening.

Affirmations

One of the best things you can do for yourself is cheer yourself on. Make a list of positive statements and play them to yourself on the tape recorder when you are home in the evening. Try,

> *I'm looking forward to going out tomorrow.*
> *I'm part of a big happy family.*
> *I enjoy feeling like an integral part of the world.*
> *The play I'm going to see will revitalize my spirits.*

A Man and Woman's Best Friend

If you don't own a dog, this is a good time to consider getting one. Walking a dog three times a day is a real commitment to seeing the outside world. And a big dog can be your buffer against whatever scares you.

*A*LEXANDER *TECHNIQUE*

This form of bodywork was developed by a nineteenth-century actor named Alexander who lost his powers of speech and found himself unable to perform. Although at first he related this physiological problem to a sudden-onset phobia about getting up in front of an audience, he later realized that he could train himself to use his voice differently, cutting through anxiety and phobic reactions.

The Alexander system puts the emphasis on correcting bad posture and alignment in order to restore function and coordination. The way we hold ourselves relates directly to the way we feel about ourselves when we are under stress or are upset. We say we are "unbalanced" when we feel we're losing our mind. The proper use of the body can restore equilibrium to the whole being. The very act of standing up straight, yet not rigid, can influence the way we handle pain and the way we are able to respond to problems. The theory is similar to that of chiropractic or osteopathic practice, where the spine is considered the focal point for all potential illness or wellness.

Alexander believed that the order in which we use our muscles is crucial. In order to establish a way to move, we must first learn to be at rest with no body part dominant over another. We also need to break old patterns of use to give the body a chance to heal.

To experiment with an Alexander exercise, lie on your back on the floor with your knees bent and feet planted shoulder-width apart. Put your hands on your hip bones. Feel whether or not your spine is straight in this position—if not, place a book or folded towel under your head so that it is lying straight (not thrown back, not hunched forward).

Now begin to concentrate on your breath, letting the air out through your nose and mouth. Feel your back move as you breathe and see how it changes over the next ten minutes.

Now put your hand under your waist and see how much closer it is to the floor than when you started. Enjoy the sensation of your shoulders flush to the floor. Slowly get up and move around, keeping the relaxed feeling you've just discovered.

When we can perform the simplest movements well, for example, lying down and getting up off the floor, or sitting in a chair and standing up again, we are better prepared to work with our body, inside and out.

A course of Alexander will take you back to the basics: how to lie down, sit down, hold your chin up, look straight, turn, and so forth. As you become comfortable with new ways of standing and moving, your autonomic nervous system will respond in kind, realigning the nerves and muscles so that stress reactions cannot take hold.

A LIENATION

see also, Aging, page 17; Depression, page 112

When we don't care about anything, we are alienated. The word *alien* means someone who's not one of us, a stranger in every sense of the word. If we are in the midst of a trauma or a spell of chronic misery, it may be impossible to acknowledge that things are as bad as they are, so we suppress them. The outward exterior of an alienated person may be dull, expressionless, affectless. Under the surface, however, usually lurks a sea of boiling emotion.

▦ *What Happens When You're Alienated*

You experience a lack of interest in life, in other people, and in yourself. You have a sense of distance, as though you are looking at yourself from far away without any expectation of closing the gap. Alienated people can hear about horrendous events (murders, earthquakes, death, and destruction) and barely bat an eye. What has really happened is that the emotive part of the person has separated from the one who is in charge of daily life. In order to protect the vulnerable self, an alienated individual hides in a shell of unconcern that is rarely pierced by a laugh or cry.

Many teenagers are alienated, and often with good reason. If they've been subjected to terrible home lives with parents who don't care what happens to them, a school system where no one cares if they pass, fail, or never show up, and a world that denigrates them for their rotten language, music, and fashion, it's understandable that they would stop feeling. If no one cares about them, why should they care about themselves?

And many elderly individuals are terribly alienated. Society has cast them out, and they are often too tired and sick to be emotional about their condition. So they pass their days in an anesthetized haze, hardly tasting their food, hardly hearing the messages coming from the television, which may be their only companion.

In order to be less alienated, we have to persuade ourselves that it's okay to join in. So the therapies that are most useful are those that will shake you up and make you care again.

Play Like a Child

Play therapy is a type of treatment that once was used exclusively with children, but is now found beneficial for adults as well. The idea is to remove yourself from the restrictions and limitations of self-analysis and delve into the problem concretely. You can use props (such as Legos, paints, balls, or dolls), and you must really abandon all self-consciousness and throw yourself into the event.

Let's imagine that you are going to use dolls to represent different aspects of yourself. You might have one that is shy and uncomfortable, one that is cold and unfeeling, one that plays the arbitrator, and one that is hopeless, almost dead to life. You might set up a tea party and find words to describe what each doll is feeling. Let them talk it out among themselves.

Finger paints are particularly useful for getting out what's buried inside. You are going to get really messy, covering your hands, arms, even your nose or knees in paint. Give yourself a huge canvas and move around on it, letting your body describe the emotions you can't voice.

You may find that play brings you back to experiences or problems you've had since childhood and have been unable to express. Because this type of work can bring up a lot of darkness and fear, it's important to have a good friend or therapist to call should you be unable to handle some of the feelings.

Take Time to Smell the Flowers

The Bach flower for alienation and apathy is Wild Rose. People who need this flower seem wilted, "lacking in sap." Take 5 or 6 drops in a glass of water or directly under the tongue.

A Fire in the Belly

Try spicy and unusual foods you may not be familiar with— a hot curry from India, a spicy bowl of chili from Mexico, or an Indonesian or African dish with herbs that will delight your palate. Try to take your foods very hot or very cold (within comfort range, of course) and see if the change in diet will enliven your mood.

Work on Your Self-esteem

When you think there's nothing going on, it's usually because you've removed yourself from the picture. By thinking differently about your actions and your effect on others, you may be able to put yourself back in focus.

Pretend that you are at your own "roast," similar to that given at a banquet or graduation. Make a list of all the significant people in your life and write a brief statement that each one would say about you. The words aren't yours, remember, they are the beliefs and opinions of others. You cannot be critical or uncaring—you must put yourself in the shoes of your friends and relatives and come up with accolades that fit.

When you are finished, consider the truth of what others might say and see if that doesn't raise your self-esteem. Even if you take what they say with a pound of salt, there is some merit in you that others can appreciate and that you can, too.

Use Your Body and Mind to Feel Intact

The bioenergetic method of working on alienation is to try and move the spirit that is sluggish or imprisoned. The wall that you set up inside is undoubtedly mirrored outside as well. Look at yourself carefully in a mirror or allow a therapist to work with you on this. Examine yourself for a clenched jaw, a stiff neck, hunched shoulders, a rigid pelvis. You will need to use some of the most physical techniques to work your way out of the tension that keeps your spirit—just like your body—locked up inside.

Get a small stool and placed a rolled-up towel on top of it. Kneel in front of it and slowly stretch your arms up and back. Let the stool support the small of your back. Now breathe deeply as you stretch your neck and head backwards. The position is uncomfortable and will become more so as you tap into the suppressed feelings you are holding. Now when you breathe, let out some sound—it may be a moan or a shout. The more you can let go, the more you will sense the dullness and alienation passing from you.

Tape the Trouble

Don't write yourself a script, but rather, sit or stand in a room and describe the events of one day, from the most minuscule (brushing your teeth) to the most important (having a job interview). Don't attempt to censor your words; just let them flow. Speak as quickly as you can, trying not to think things out. The tape recorder not only plays back words, but also the intonation of your voice, the hesitation, the malapropisms, and a great deal more that you may not intend. The final product may be a useful key to what you're hiding and why you feel so out of touch.

ANGER

see also Depression, page 112; Stress, page 407; and manifestations of stress such as Gastrointestinal Disorders, page 189; Headaches/Migraines, page 209; Rage, page 363; Shortness of Breath, page 397; Trembling, page 428; Violence/Aggressive Behavior, page 437

We are all angry people—some of us just show it more than others. When we expect one thing and don't get it, it disorients us, often making us mistrustful of those who promised what they didn't deliver. Anger is often a part of depression: When we cannot manage the unfairness of life, we lash out and let everyone else feel a little of the rage we have been carrying inside. There's nothing wrong with being angry—however, when it pervades most aspects of your daily life and turns other people off, you have to do something to control it or manage it.

■ What Happens When You're Angry

You are in a state of readiness to defend yourself against all comers. You may explode, rant, and rave, or if you suppress the anger, you may seethe inside, planning revenge.

If you cover your anger, you may become passive-aggressive in your attitude toward others. You may forget important dates, always show up late, be careless, or procrastinate. Passive-aggressive behavior can drive other people away just as easily as overt rage can.

Anger is usually triggered by something—a word, a person's behavior, an event, or our interpretation of an event. It sets off our stress hormones—adrenaline, noradrenaline, and cortisol—and rouses uncomfortable tension in the body.

Holding onto anger is even worse than vomiting it out. Suppressed or internalized anger can lead to high blood pressure, headaches, gastrointestinal disorders, depression, and a lowered tolerance for pain. Enough years of living with this type of poison inside us can help bring on a heart attack or make us susceptible to certain cancers.

So since you have to live with your anger, you might as well make it a partner in your journey to get to know yourself better.

Decide to Be Cool

In many ways, letting the anger take over is a conscious choice. You can blow your stack, or you can contain it. Using anger to confront another person or a problem you're having is positive; misusing it as aggression or hostility is negative.

There are several ways of being angry. You can go insane for a little while as you vent at the world or another individual. You can mask the rage by suppressing your anger with passive-aggressive behavior, where you get back at someone by not showing up at an important meeting or by not paying a bill. The best way to deal with anger, however, is to meet it head-on. Confront your anger, own it, and get it out in the open. This way, you can start to direct it toward a solution.

Count to ten, taking deep breaths all the way. Give yourself some affirmations, such as, *I am doing fine and will not explode* or *I know my mind, and I am stronger than I used to be.*

Calm your face—if necessary by looking in a mirror—and consciously talk in a low voice.

Take the fury to another level. Say you are angry, but you want to find a solution to whatever it was that ticked you off. Brainstorm about what you and others can do with this anger. Treat it as though it were a potentially dangerous animal that must be both respected and handled.

Find Your Bombs and Defuse Them

When you know you always get angry if someone is late, or you get into a rage every time your partner spends money without asking you, you can do something about your behavior. First make a list of the triggers, then explore different ways of reacting to them. Instead of an explosion or a hurtful comment, or throwing a dish against a wall, decide that you will take a run around the block, ask your partner for a massage to alleviate the tension, or spend a quiet half hour in meditation before attempting to deal with the source of your anger.

Use a Prop

Take a towel and start to wring it between your hands. Say aloud that you are wringing someone's neck. Use it to thrash a wall or a piece of furniture. Say (or yell) aloud that you are getting back at _____ for all the misery he or she has caused. You may find that the screaming turns to tears—that the anger is really masking pain that you have been feeling for some time.

The Flower of Choice

The Bach Flower remedies are Cherry Plum for a fear of loss of control; Impatiens for excessive reactions and irritability. Take 5 or 6 drops in a half glass of water or directly under the tongue. You can also use the aromatherapy oil, Rose, in your bath or for massage.

Cool Foods

If you are a heavy meat eater, you are also in a high-risk category for a heart attack. Meat (especially red meat) is larded with animal fats, which raise your LDL (bad) cholesterol and lower your HDL (good) cholesterol. The effect of too much of the wrong kinds of fats is that plaque deposits are able to adhere to the insides of artery walls, thus blocking the passage of blood. Change your diet to include many more fruits and vegetables. Avoid caffeine and nicotine completely.

Run Around Sue

Or John or Mary. . . The best way to deal with anger is to channel that energy toward something constructive. As you run, row, or bike, you can get out those feelings that have been bottled up inside. Hitting something—a bat or a heavy bag in a gym—can also be a positive expression of a negative feeling.

Have an Herbal Cocktail

A recommendation for acute stress is to mix 2 parts tincture of scutellaria laterifolia with two parts tincture of valeriana officinalis and one part avena sativa. Combined, the three should equal 5 ml. of tincture. Drink this nervine tonic and relaxant as needed, mixed in a glass of water.

Another herb to calm a rage is motherwort, which is particularly good to soothe heart palpitations when anger takes over. Use 8 to 10 drops of the fresh plant tincture three times daily.

Pray Over It

If we feel we're the only ones who can handle a problem, we are taking on a lot of responsibility. But by asking a higher power to assume at least part of the cost, we can lower our own risk. You don't have to invoke God; simply acknowledge that you are in need of outside assistance every time you feel the monster welling up inside you. Close your eyes for a moment and allow the burden to be taken off your shoulders. Understand that you are not alone and that you can have all the help you ask for.

Anorexia Nervosa

see also Eating Disorders, page 139

A mental problem that results in a physical decline of the body and often leads to death, cases of anorexia were recorded as far back as the Middle Ages, and the condition probably existed even before that. Although it is the least common of all the eating disorders, prevalent in only about 1 percent of the population, it is arguably the most dangerous.

▦ *What Happens When You Are Anorectic*

This extremely serious eating disorder involves a refusal to take in nourishment, even for survival. The anorectic sees herself (and it is usually a female) as imperfect, fat, or misshapen, and repulsive to herself and others. She will mete out food (a lettuce leaf, a piece of celery) carefully, or when asked to eat with the family or in a public place, she will push food around the plate, appearing to eat but actually putting nothing in her mouth. Anorectics are difficult to help because they deny their problem—they are fixated on their "monstrous" body and will cover up with baggy clothes so that it is difficult to tell that they've lost a great deal of weight until, often, it's too late. Anorexia can lead to death.

Anorexia is a developmental crisis involving the whole family and centers around the parents' reluctance to allow their daughter to grow up. This disease is a manifestation of a severe lack of self-esteem and an obsessive need to be perfect. Anorectic girls are often smothered by their parents, who want to take over their lives. Only by controlling food intake does the sufferer control her own world and, of course, her parents. She may be plagued by depression and may also have lost the desire to live.

Anorexia is far more common in adolescent and preadolescent girls than in any other groups; however, it is becoming more prevalent in adolescent boys and reproductive-age women. The most typical characteristics of someone with anorectic behavior are a refusal to maintain weight appropriate for age and height and a distortion of perceived body size and shape. Most teenaged anorectic girls have stopped menstruating—if they ever started—and appear socially and physically much younger than their peers.

This disease can be devastating to the rest of the body. Most girls with anorexia are malnourished and therefore have slow metabolic rates. Their body temperature may fall to 96 or 97 degrees, and they may have cognitive problems: inability to remember things or concentrate, which can lead to difficulties in school or at work. They may suffer from fatigue, chills, dehydration, skin conditions, hair loss, heart palpitations, abdominal pain, and constipation. They may have abnormally low blood pressure and heart rates of only 30 or 40 beats per minute.

Some indications that you may be anorectic are

- restricting your calories to under 500 a day
- skipping two or more meals a day
- feeling disgusted with yourself, unable to look in a mirror, covering up your body with loose-fitting clothes
- staying home or avoiding situations where you have to eat in public
- feeling cold all the time
- chronic hair loss

Learn How to Eat Again

You have to assume that you know nothing about food or eating and must start from scratch. A directive program with a nutritionist is essential, in combination with a behavioral or cognitive/behavioral program directed by a therapist to make you take in certain nourishment at certain times of the day. You should be eating foods that are supportive of the body's systems, such as fresh fruits and vegetables, whole grains, legumes, pasta and cereals, with plenty of pure spring water, and they should be prepared in a way that's most palatable for you. If you have been barely surviving on tiny salads or a carrot a day, you will need time to accustom yourself to six very small balanced meals.

Keep an Eating Record

Everything should be recorded—the time, the amount of food, your level of hunger, the anxieties before and after eating, the feeling of "bloat," and whether you were able to finish the entire amount on your plate.

Get the Support You Need

Denial and subterfuge are common in households where anorexia holds sway, so the best thing you can do is surround yourself with people who won't let you get away with your same old routine. A group of other young women who have been or are currently going through your personal hell can serve two purposes: They can help to keep you on the right track with your eating, and they can substitute for the family that doesn't know enough to give you support.

It is particularly useful to have a buddy or mentor to call when you can't keep up with your program or feel you are slipping back to your old patterns.

Try a Remedy

There are several Bach flower remedies you can try:

> Cerato, for lack of confidence in your own decisions
>
> Cherry Plum, for fear of loss of control
>
> Larch, for inferiority complex, expecting to fail
>
> Rock Water, for those with suppressed inner needs who are very hard on themselves

Take 5 or 6 drops in half a glass of water or directly under the tongue. If the remedy you've selected offers no relief, you've diagnosed yourself incorrectly and should try another remedy.

Behavior Can Change If You Want It To

Behavioral training is often effective with anorectics who crave direction and rules. If you make up goals and rewards for yourself along the way, you can change your eating habits.

Start by making a list with your therapist or nutritionist of the foods you're supposed to have each day. The list will undoubtedly look daunting—how could anyone ever consume that amount? Set yourself six meals, at six times of day when you can find a quiet place that feels comfortable. Make sure the temperature of the room is right, put on some pleasant music, set the table, and even put a flower in a vase on the table. Never eat standing up or in front of the TV. The idea is to make eating as wonderful an experience as possible and to really pay attention to it—the smells, the tastes, the colors.

Set yourself a second goal of three weeks to be able to eat all your required food during the day.

When you begin the program, start with half a meal, or a quarter if that's too much. Eat some of your designated food, then have a drink of water, then walk around the room or the block. Put a checkmark on the meal or cross it off when you have been able to eat the whole thing.

Affirm That You're Good

Self-esteem is the core problem of many anorectics, and it can be helped with some positive reassurance. Writing affirmations that mean something to you may help you over the worst hump, when you are trying to change your behavior.
Write or say to yourself or into a tape recorder:

I am a worthwhile human being.

I am in charge of my life.

I have many things to look forward to each day.

I enjoy learning to use my senses to appreciate the world and everything in it.

Supplements Can Spur Appetite

It's been found that many anorectics are zinc-deficient, which dulls their senses of smell and taste. Supplementing 50 mg. zinc daily can improve sensory interest and appetite. Other important supplements are niacin (40 mg. three times daily), Vitamins B_1 and B_6 (thiamine and pyridoxine, 200 mg. each daily), and omega-6 essential fatty acids (EFA), which can be taken as evening primrose oil (500 mg. three times daily).

ANORGASMIA

see also Sexual Dysfunction, page 387

The inability to have an orgasm (also known as inhibited female orgasm, or IFO) is considered a dysfunction by most sexologists, although it does not necessarily interfere with a good sex life. Orgasm is, however, the gold standard of sexuality, and most individuals crave the experience. An orgasm is not just a release of muscle tension in the body, it is also an expression of freedom and exuberance.

Anorgasmia is very common—one estimate says that up to 30 percent of women experience orgasmic problems. This difficulty is most prevalent in women (although there are men who cannot have an orgasm) and is usually psychogenic in origin. Anything can stop an orgasm—fear of discovery, guilt, distractions, inappropriate touch, not getting the touch you want, a sense of being awkward, fear of letting go completely, or anger at your partner. Very often, it stems from a lack of trust in oneself and in others.

What Happens When You Can't Have an Orgasm

The major problem is enormous frustration, which can lead to anger, irritability, retreat from physical contact, and can actually bring on physiological symptoms such as congested feeling in the pelvis, or painful and sore nipples. Probably the worst consequence is feeling like a failure. The media have taken up the banner of orgasm and run with it, and many women's magazines imply that if you aren't having five orgasms a night, there's something wrong with you. This simply isn't true.

Before learning what it is you're not having, it's important to know what an orgasm is so that you can recognize one when you do have it. An orgasm is a release of physical tension that builds up due to sexual stimulation and the excitement of this particular event. Some people feel as if they are swept out of their bodies; others feel as if they're in the middle of an earthquake; still others feel as though they've been carried over a gentle wave.

Prior to orgasm, we experience desire, which makes us seek sexual release. When we are aroused, we first enter the excitement phase, in which the body prepares for this mammoth event. Blood vessels dilate (including, of course, those in the penis, vagina, and clitoris), heart rate and blood pressure rise, respiration and perspiration increase. The next stage is known as the plateau stage, in which we are trembling on the brink. A woman's nipples become erect, she lubricates profusely, the man's testes and penis swell to their fully tumescent state. Then comes the rush of orgasm, which for women may be felt in the clitoral or vaginal area or in a blend of the two areas. (Some women are able to have an orgasm from visualization and fantasy alone, without any physical stimulation.) Men experience first emission and then propulsion as they ejaculate. The final stage is resolution, in which the body returns to status and body and mind feel relaxed and satiated.

Sounds good, doesn't it? Happily, there are many effective treatments for anorgasmia. Even if you've never had an orgasm, you probably will be able to teach yourself to have one if you use some or all of the following suggestions:

Don't Take Drugs

Many over-the-counter and prescription pharmaceuticals, including antihistamines for colds and blood pressure medication, will put a damper on your erotic potential. The worst medication for good sex is Prozac, which inhibits the uptake of serotonin—that feel-good neurotransmitter that washes over us when we orgasm.

Many women who cannot come to orgasm have been sexually abused or raped, and the healing process for them is much slower. A trusting partner who does not demand anything of you but is simply there to hold and caress you is essential if you are to enjoy being touched again.

Men who have trouble ejaculating may be angry at their partner or may actually find the act of intercourse disgusting or repellent. There are also neurological factors that may inhibit male ejaculation. But generally, if a man has an erection, this indicates that he is aroused enough to have an orgasm, so usually a lot of direct stimulation by his partner—manual or oral or both—will bring him to climax.

Communicate Your Fantasies

You can't be rushed or cajoled into anything, nor persuaded to "just relax—it'll happen." Rather, you must make the rules. If you are the type of person who responds to being "taken," you must tell your lover that you want to lie back and not have to do anything actively. If you are a take-charge individual, you must explain to your lover that you will design the scenario and would like him to go along with it. Eventually, you'll be able to plan this event together, but for now, you are the leader and your partner is the follower. Be as explicit as you can be about your wants and needs—the ideas and images that excite you mentally will eventually excite you physically.

Pleasure Yourself

In order to learn how to have an orgasm, you have to find out what gives you pleasure. It's best to do this alone, when you don't have performance anxiety and when you aren't worried about holding your partner up or taking too much time. Take an hour to just lie back and explore your body and mind. Begin with your clothes on or off and start to touch yourself. You might like to read some erotica (Nancy Friday and Lonnie Barbach have excellent books full of these) or turn on some quiet music or take a bath.

Make sure you discover more about yourself than the fact that you have genitals. Many women are astounded to realize that they are very sensitive in many different areas, from their toes to the backs of their knees to their earlobes.

Massage your breasts and tweak the nipples to get them to stand up. Touch and stroke your whole genital area—from the pubic hair back to your anus. Start to pay attention to your clitoris, rubbing along the side of the shaft and on the tip—wherever you like it the best. You might like to slip a finger inside your vagina and gently move it around. If rubbing and pressure don't seem to be bringing you to an intensity that feels close to release, cup your whole hand over the vulval area and vibrate it rapidly.

Invest in a Vibrator

A vibrator is usually the key that opens the door. Many women who have never had an orgasm before are surprised and delighted to learn that help is just nine volts away. The intense stimulation generally triggers waves of pleasure that peak and subside. Vibrators come in all shapes and sizes, and some can be inserted in the vagina or anus or have attachments to stimulate both orifices at the same time.

Try a Chinese Remedy

The patent medicine *gou ji dze jiou,* Chinese wolfberry wine, is a kidney and liver tonic that boosts both male and female sexuality. It is sometimes called "the secret wine of harmonious marital relations." This formula tonifies yin energy and stimulates the production of hormones, blood, enzymes, and vital bodily fluids.

It should be prepared and taken as follows: Take 100 gm. Chinese wolfberry and place in a clean glass container with two liters of vodka, rum, or brandy. Let steep for 36 days, shaking once a week. Then strain off the liquid and discard the berries. Add a little honey if you find it bitter. Take one or two doses of 1.5 ounces daily on an empty stomach.

Practice Your Kegels

Kegel exercises tone the vaginal area and restore elasticity. For women who are anxious about sexual penetration and tend to clench their muscles, Kegels offer a great deal of benefit. A Kegel is a contraction and release of the pubococcygeal muscles between the vagina and the anus. First imagine that you are sitting on the toilet, letting go of the stream of urine. Then think about stopping the flow by tightening your muscles. That is one Kegel. You should practice these in sets of ten three times daily. You can do them slowly or quickly, and when you get really good, you'll find you can isolate your vaginal and anal muscles.

Use this exercise with your partner and begin to squeeze when he is inside you. Not only will this give him a great deal of pleasure, it will also intensify pressure on your vaginal walls, which may help to bring you to orgasm.

Watch a Dirty Movie

Most of them are terribly silly, but they can be great as an additional boost to your sexuality. There's nothing like watching a lot of churning and pounding with the person you adore—if it does nothing else for you, it will get you to laugh, which is a big part of letting go and enjoying sex. Pornographic films also sometimes get you talking about fantasies you've had and might like to act out. They can offer the kernel of an idea that can blossom into a real night of passion between you and your lover.

Get All Slippery

When you're aroused, you secrete a lot of natural lubrication in and around the vagina. The feeling of being wet heightens your arousal and gets you ready for orgasm. If you're tense and upset, you don't lubricate. But you can supply whatever lubrication you need and keep it on hand. Astroglide, Replens, GyneMoistrin, and Today Personal Lubricant are some of the best water-based lubricants around, available in most drug stores or sex shops.

Use All Your Orifices

It's been shown that very few women have an orgasm from penile penetration alone. Most have to be stimulated around or on the clitoris first even to approach orgasm. The "bridge" technique, designed by sex therapist Helen Kaplan, offers a way to get both your motors going at once. You or your partner can fondle and manipulate your clitoris while his penis is inside. You may also wish to experiment with anal stimulation—you might play with your clitoris while he touches your anus and thrusts inside you.

Don't Try So Hard

If nothing's working, roll over and go to sleep for a while. Your life will not be ruined if you never have an orgasm. If you search for it too diligently, it will be an elusive spirit; but if you throw yourself into lovemaking with no expectations, you may be astounded at the power of your reactions.

ANXIETY

see also Anger, page 31; Chest Pains, page 87; Escapism, page 142; Fear, page 164; Guilt, page 197 Impending Doom, feelings of, page 238; Mood Swings, page 297; Nervousness, page 304; Palpitations, page 342; Victim Mentality, page 433; Vulnerability, page 445; Worrying, page 452

Anxiety is the residue of fear—in a sense, it is the phantom ghost of something that happened, or that we think happened, and anticipate happening again.

Before we can tackle anxiety, we must know what fear is. Imagine that one rainy night you are driving down a country road. The windshield wipers are powerless to keep your range of vision clear. Sheets of rain pummel the car, and wind buffets it. Suddenly, you are blinded by the headlights of an oncoming car. You swerve and go into a skid, nearly turning the car over. Your heart is pounding, your stomach is in knots. You barely manage to get control of the wheel as you hear the whine of the other car's horn in the distance. You stop the car, thankful to be alive.

Now, we move onto anxiety. It is a month later, and you are driving down that same road. It's a sunny day; there's no other car in sight. As you approach the spot where you nearly crashed, you can feel your palms damp against the steering wheel. You find yourself struggling for breath, your stomach is tense, you can feel the pulse in your head. You are actually reliving the experience you had before and all those real physical symptoms return as you anticipate—irrational as that may be—the same thing happening again.

Anxiety is a combination of past and present experiences and appropriate and inappropriate reactions that overlap and mix together. It is a sense of dread and foreboding that is attached to an event in the past, the remnant of a former experience or set of experiences connected with current concerns as well as long-buried fears.

CASE HISTORY

On Sally's thirtieth birthday, she couldn't get out of bed. Her heart was pounding, she felt dizzy, and she had a feeling that something was terribly wrong. Thus began a series of cycles of anxiety that would last for the next five years. One of the worst symptoms was a complete inability to cook food or even go to places where she could eat. She lost her appetite, and over the next few years lost a great deal of weight.

The cycles always started in the morning—she would wake with a hot energy shooting up her back into her head. She came from a family of people with emotional problems—her father, sister, and aunt had all had shock treatment.

"I went to a psychiatrist, who put me on Prozac much against my will—I did it because I was desperate and I thought, well, my whole family's crazy, so I must have inherited it. I have to say that after three months, I felt so good I figured I didn't need it anymore and I discontinued it. But at the same time, I decided to try some preventive care. I went to an acupuncturist and herbalist and after some trial and error, found Siberian ginseng and St. John's wort. I started a total program of good health care: I eat fish and lamb now, although I used to be a vegetarian, and eat no refined sugar at all. I get a massage and craniosacral therapy once a month, and do tai chi every day. When I know I'm going to be stressed, I take my two herbs daily for a week. This program is so much better for me than the drugs. Now I think I'm in charge—I have *regular* anxiety over issues that I'm dealing with, but I haven't had an anxiety attack for a year and I don't think I ever will again."

As Sally points out, anxiety can be a normal part of everyday life—a lot of people are happily neurotic, often even proud of being a little eccentric. Perhaps they waste more time than they should fretting over topics and people that aren't worth the trouble, but they aren't harming themselves or others.

But anxiety can develop into a crippling condition, overlapping with panic attacks, phobias, and obsessive/compulsive behavior. Obviously, it's easier to treat anxiety naturally in its infancy; when it becomes ingrained and overwhelming, it's harder to manage.

The Difference Between Anxiety and Stress

Stress is physiological arousal—the body's reveille to a bad situation that has to be attended to. In calm individuals, the stress reaction vanishes as soon as the problem is taken care of. But anxious people who are highly reactive stay stressed—their stress may actually increase—after the stressor is gone.

Stress is our perception of an event as uncomfortable or tension-producing. It stimulates our body and mind to produce "fight or flight hormones" that can prepare us for the worst. Stress comes with a variety of physical symptoms, such as palpitations, shortness of breath, sweaty palms, and a knot in the stomach. We may have stress reactions to almost any event or thought of an event that is going to take place, whether it's our upcoming wedding or a tax audit.

But when we imagine everything as stressful even if it's really not, this is anxiety. With anxiety, we build up an arsenal of emotional big guns that fire at gnats as easily as at wild tigers.

It's not a bad thing to live with anxiety. It puts you in touch with what's really important to you—if you're concerned, you rally yourself to handle the problem. Rather than responding to situations by rote, you use your emotional passion and probably end up with a better solution than the laid-back individual who isn't roused to do or feel much of anything.

You don't necessarily need to eradicate all your anxiety, but rather, you want to tame it and take some of the fear and impending doom out of it. The treatments listed here have proven successful at various times for various individuals:

AROMATHERAPY

The healing benefit of plants goes beyond the use of herbs as teas, infusions, and poultices. The essential oils of plants are also medicinal and can effect extraordinary mood changes as well as relief from physical symptoms.

The concept of this therapy was formulated in 1928 by René Maurice Gattéfossé, a cosmetic chemist who discovered that he could use lavender to cure the chemical burns he had suffered in a laboratory explosion. During World War II, a disciple of Gattéfossé, Dr. Jean Valnet, treated soldiers on the battlefield with essential oils when he ran out of penicillin. He also treated psychiatric patients and discovered that different fragrances have incredible powers to affect the emotions.

When we smell something and take a deep breath, the essence is picked up by the hairs that line the nose and travel through our olfactory system on nerve impulses directly to the brain. The lungs simultaneously take in the molecules of plant essence mixed with oxygen.

The area of the brain that processes scent is located in the limbic system, the emotional house of the mind. A whiff of a particular herb can alter physiological responses because the limbic system also influences endocrine and immune system activity in the body. The scent center also happens to sit right beside the area of the brain that is responsible for memory. Many people are able to retrieve the most minute details about a past experience by walking into a strange place and smelling something that reminds them of that time long ago. (In fact, realtors suggest that you place a drop of vanilla on the light bulbs in your house when they're showing it, because that particular scent makes people think of cookies baking at Grandma's house, that is, feeling "at home.")

Oils have a variety of properties that are helpful to mind and body—some are calming, some stimulating, some promote an optimistic mood, some are aphrodisiac. Just as with herbal preparations, the oils may have anti-inflammatory or antibiotic properties as well. By inhaling the correct essential oil, you can not only change your mood, but can also heal various stress-related physical symptoms.

Essential oils can be placed in a diffuser to cleanse the air in a sick room, or they can be used in a potpourri burner that you can put on your bedside table at night so that you can derive healing benefits while you sleep. Oils can be added to your bath, or you can simply pour a few drops into a cotton ball and keep it in a plastic bag in your purse, so that you can sniff it throughout the day.

Perhaps the most effective way to use oils is in a massage, where you have the combined effect of scent and touch to heal the mind and body. The essential oils are too strong to be used full strength in massage, and so are mixed with a nonscented carrier oil, such as Sweet-Almond oil, Grapeseed, Avocado, Jojoba, or Sesame. During massage, they are absorbed through the skin. They remain in the body for several hours before being excreted through the pores.

You can use Bergamot, Geranium, and Ylang-ylang to treat depression and anxiety.

If you are agitated and need to calm down, you might try Roman chamomile, Mandarin, Neroli, or Patchouli.

If you feel hopeless, you might try Jasmine or Mandarin.

If you are fatigued and have no energy, Orange or Peppermint might be helpful.

If you are distracted and can't concentrate, try Frankincense.

If you just need to relax, the oils to use are Sandalwood or Ti-tree.

Ayurvedic (Indian) medicine employs the essential oils in various treatments in order to harmonize a personality that is in some way out of balance.

AUTOGENIC TRAINING

Johannes Schultz, a German neurologist, developed autogenics as a result of watching people under hypnosis who had been told that their limbs were warm and heavy. The type of complete relaxation they experienced, he thought, could also be taught to the waking mind.

Autogenic means "self-generating," because the suggestions for calming down and feeling relaxed come from within you. You repeat to yourself over and over the phrases that convey a feeling that your body is eminently comfortable, and the suggestion takes over. When we feel truly relaxed, the arteries in our extremities open up, bringing better blood flow to the area and a warm, heavy feeling. Since we can usually remember the sensation we had when we were completely at rest and peaceful, we can adjust our nervous system to recapture the memory of warmth and heaviness when we're in the midst of a stressful experience.

You may wish to tape record the phrases or have a friend say them to you. You may also think them silently to yourself.

Sit in a comfortable chair and put your feet flat on the floor. If the chair has arms, rest your forearms on them; if not, let your hands lie in your lap. Close your eyes and begin to breathe as you say to yourself:

I am quiet and relaxed.
My right hand feels heavy.
My right hand feels comfortable and heavy.
My right hand feels heavy and relaxed.

I am quiet and relaxed.
My left foot feels warm.
I can feel the warmth in my toes, flowing into my heel
My left foot is warm, heavy, and relaxed.

I am calm and relaxed.
I am quiet and at peace.
I feel relaxed.

When you work this exercise to the fullest, you need to inventory each body part and express the fact that it feels warm and heavy to you. When all your limbs are relaxed, you can take the feeling deeper, into your solar plexus, your heart, and your mind.

Ayurvedic Medicine

The meaning of Ayurveda in Sanskrit is "science of life." The basic principle of this type of belief is that we can avoid disease by maintaining a balanced awareness of everything in our lives. Using diet, exercise, herbal therapy, meditation, aromatherapy, primordial sounds, music therapy, and several other practices, we can achieve a feeling of peace and awareness in our lives.

Doshas Help in Diagnosis

Ayurveda believes that everyone has a basic nature or *prakriti*. Everyone on the planet is one of three types or *doshas—vata, pitta, or kapha*—and these depend on your build, your personality, your behavior, your moods, tastes, and talents. Although we all have a little of each dosha inside us, we belong to one camp more than the other two.

Vata dosha is a quick, nervous type. These individuals tend to be thin and wiry, always moving, learning, trying something new. They are often anxious and often feel cold.

Pitta dosha is the sanguine type. They are of medium build, usually very smart, with strong digestion, sharp hunger, and thirst. They are good speakers and tend to be fair-skinned. They may be aggressive and quick to anger. (They are what Western medicine would deem "Type A personalities.")

Kapha dosha is relaxed, slow, heavy. They are usually powerfully built, with great physical strength and endurance, and may have a tendency to put on weight and sleep too much. They may take their time learning new things, but generally remember well once they've mastered a skill or idea.

Each dosha corresponds to an organ system, and each is responsible for different mechanisms of the body. According to Ayurveda, you should eat, exercise, and take herbs according to your dosha. Your psychological state and the mental and emotional problems you feel will be based in and treated by the specifics for that dosha.

Vata

Your imbalances will have to do with movement. Your nervous system is highly sensitive. This means that you are generally imaginative, spontaneous, resilient, and exuberant about life. But when out of balance, you may be prone to needless worry; impatience; an overactive, anxious mind; an inability to concentrate; and depression. Your body may react with insomnia, fatigue, irritable bowel or other gastrointestinal symptoms, restlessness, poor appetite, and an inability to relax.

Pitta

Your imbalances will have to do with metabolism. You are generally confident, enterprising, and happy about life, but when out of balance, you may be prone to anger, hostility, self-criticism, and resentment. Your body may react with heartburn, ulcers, hemorrhoids, or stress-related heart attacks.

Kapha

Your imbalances will have to do with structure. You are generally a calm, sympathetic person, very courageous, forgiving, and loving. But when out of balance, you may be subject to mental inertia, depression that carries a sense of heaviness, or overattachment to those close to you. Your body may react with eating disorders, oversleeping or drowsiness, sluggishness and fatigue, congestion, and fluid retention.

This does not mean that a pitta can't have a kapha imbalance, or that because you are a vata, you might not feel fatigued sometimes. In attempting to find the right balance, you don't need to aim for a perfect symbiosis among the three, but rather, you must find what is right for your particular nature. Also, in Ayurveda, there is no real urge to cure physical symptom. The imbalance has to be adjusted in your mind first, before you can understand how it has affected your body and how to put it right again.

According to Deepak Chopra, who has been the most prominent physician to practice Ayurveda in America, there are certain key methods to restore balance. Each treatment is different, because each type or blend of person is different. However, all types are directed to make changes in diet, exercise, daily routine, and even seasonal routine. In addition to your other treatments, you will be instructed to meditate daily—no matter what your dosha. Meditation clears and purifies the mind and makes the body able to accept change and healing. (See Meditation, page 292.)

Your Ayurvedic physician will counsel you to restore balance in the following ways:

Balancing Vata

quiet/meditation	staying warm
drinking fluids	stress reduction
rest	regular habits and meals
sesame oil massage	10 P.M. bedtime
low impact exercise	

Balancing Pitta

moderation in everything	staying cool
balance of rest and activity	taking leisure time
exposure to natural beauty	avoid caffeine, tobacco, laxatives,
moderate sports	alcohol
	avoid hot, spicy foods

Balancing Kapha

stimulation	regular, physical exercise
weight-control program	staying warm and dry
avoid sweets	variety in experiences
clear sinuses with	dry massage (done with raw-silk
saltwater rinse	gloves)

Restoring the Mind and Body to Health

In addition to the foregoing recommendations, there are various foods that are either suggested or prohibited for each dosha. Certain herbs are also prescribed. Each person is given his or her own program of massage using different essential oils that will remove toxins (see Aromatherapy, page 46) and different laxatives and enemas that do the same internally. Followers of Ayurveda are also counseled in the use of primordial sounds for meditation (similar to "om," which is the universal sound and is supposed to connect the meditator to the "harmony of the spheres" described by many philosophers. Your physician will give you your own sound, which will help your brain focus and derive more healing benefit from your meditation.

In order to start a program of Ayurvedic medicine, you will have to choose a physician who can guide you on this program of healing. If you live in a community with a large Indian population, you might ask for a referral at a local community center or a health care or social services office.

If you are currently following a course of Western medicine and are taking medication, your Ayurvedic doctor will wean you off these drugs slowly as you begin your new health program.

*B*ACH *F*LOWER *R*EMEDIES

Edward Bach, a British homeopath, discovered the extraordinary subtle power inherent in the energy of flowers during the 1930s. He felt that these particular 38 remedies, derived from the essence of flowers, resonated with human emotions. It was as if the flowers themselves vibrated with a particular energy that was useful to us, giving us peace from internal torments and putting us more in harmony with nature. These remedies cure, he said, "not by attacking the disease, but by flooding our bodies with the beautiful vibrations of our Higher Nature. . . . There is no true healing unless there is a change in outlook, peace of mind, and inner happiness."

The healing power of the Bach flower remedies is based on our receptivity to a belief that the soul is in charge of whatever we do. (In this, they differ from homeopathic remedies, which resonate with particular personality traits.) Within each of us, Bach thought, are the elements of each of the 38 emotional aspects he described in his flowers. But one or the other of them may be out of balance at different times.

These remedies also differ from homeopathic treatments in that they are completely harmless (many of the homeopathics are distilled from poisons). The wild flowers used are picked at their full maturity, just before they drop. They are enhanced by earth, air, sun, and water. The flowers are distilled into an essence with pure spring water and alcohol as a preservative and can be kept indefinitely in brown-glass bottles.

Why should these essences have such a profound effect on mood? It is generally accepted that each thing in the universe has a vibration to it, and its particular frequency is what makes it blue or green, hard or soft, loud or muted. According to Bach's theory, the flowers act like a tuning fork, resetting your body's cells to their correct vibrational frequency.

Bach was certain that being emotionally upset was undoubtedly the cause of many physical ailments. The relatively new field of psychoneuroimmunology (the science of the way the brain and nervous system affect the immune system) believes the same: Mind and body are one, and by healing one cell, you can heal the whole. As you start to think, you emit nerve signals that communicate with hormones and neurotransmitters that travel throughout your body. A thought that resonates with a particular flower, then, can start to change the entire sequence of events that leads to physical or emotional illness.

Let us assume that you've been feeling very self-critical, and despite the fact that other people tell you you're good, you feel like a failure. But when you take Larch, you can open the door to many possibilities. Larch makes you more realistic in tackling problems and makes you able to assess yourself and the situations you get into more clearly. You may be able to break through a particular block that exists at a lower frequency and raise yourself to a higher, more well-balanced frequency. When you are affected by the flower, you become more aware of yourself and your abilities, and it becomes easier to change your perspective.

The most well-known of the remedies, Rescue Remedy, is almost considered an emotional emergency kit. A combination of five different flowers, Rescue Remedy is an antidote to a catastrophe (a car accident or earthquake), a big event (from a trip to the dentist to your wedding), or a stressful environment where an unexpected disaster might arise (if you work in a hospital, prison, or police station).

Bach flower remedies may be healing, just as beautiful music or an inspirational work of art are healing. This is not simply a placebo effect—when we are struck dumb with joy or delight, our breathing changes, our pupils dilate, our blood pressure drops. As our emotions become more stabilized by the flowers, we are better able to handle stress, transitions, or trauma. The flowers help us develop our potential to feel and act differently.

The remedies can be taken alone or in combination, although no more than five remedies should be used at one time. The dosages are generally four to six drops in a half-glass of water to be sipped slowly as needed, but you can also squeeze a few drops under your tongue for more immediate relief.

BEHAVIORAL THERAPY

Unlike the many psychological theories that doom us to the personality and behavior patterns we were born with or inherited, behavioral therapy says that we can change. All we have to do is want to. We have the power and ability to alter our patterns, given the right motivation and willpower.

Behavior is triggered from impulses within the brain, and the brain is stimulated by various chemicals we produce, some of which make us feel positive, enthusiastic, and energized and others of which make us feel miserable, hopeless, and desperate. By making a commitment to change and following through, we can actually alter brain chemistry just as surely as we can with a mood-altering drug. In a study on patients with obsessive-compulsive disorder, those who mastered behavioral techniques and conquered their compulsions actually showed neurological change on a PET scan (positive emission tomography, a sophisticated type of CT scan).

CASE HISTORY

Andrea couldn't remember when she and her husband stopped communicating, but it seemed as if no matter what she said, it provoked an attack. He told her she was stupid, worthless, ridiculous, and revolting often enough that she began to believe it. It became so bad that she would get knots in her stomach every time she heard his key in the door, and the only thing that would take the stomach pain away was eating.

"I went to see a behavioral therapist that someone had recommended. I was just desperate. The only thing that gave me pleasure was food, but then after I'd eaten, I felt guilty and awful because of the way I looked and felt. The first thing this doctor suggested was to move the scale from the bathroom to the kitchen. She never said I had to get on it—she just told me to put it in there, so I did, right next to the refrigerator. After my husband tripped over it a few times, he threatened to throw it at my stupid head. Something inside me clicked, and I told him I was leaving."

The therapy was designed to alter Andrea's eating habits, but it served double duty. It made her wake up to her terrible marriage that had kept her in this state of suspended animation.

She learned to weigh and measure her food, to eat six meals a day and check off her nutrients on a chart she kept in her purse. She put ten dollars in a bottle for each 5-pound loss, and when she finally lost 40 pounds, she bought herself a new, form-fitting outfit. Her therapist helped her to understand that her behavior around eating—standing at the refrigerator and eating out of containers or buying three snacks before she boarded her commuter train in the evening—were part of an unconscious self-destructive pattern. When she became aware of what she was doing around food, she was able to change it.

Now 56, seven years post-divorce, Andrea feels ready to meet someone new. Her final comment about learning new behavior is, "I have become someone I like—someone whose friend I'd like to be."

Behavioral therapy involves an understanding of the desire and reluctance we all have around behavior that has become routine and even ritualized. According to behavioral therapists James O. Prochaska and Carlo C. DiClemente, who tested their theories on long-term drug addicts, there are five stages to change:

Precontemplation: You have no idea that your behavior is destructive. You may be told by others that something is wrong, but you deny that you have a problem.

Contemplation: You see that the problem exists, and you think that you might consider changing it someday— not necessarily now.

Preparation: You have an intention to change the behavior, perhaps in the next month or so, and take certain steps (such as moving the scale into the kitchen) to prepare for the inevitable.

Action: You have been able to stick to a healing pattern of behavior (eating only at meals, sitting at a table, eliminating all snacks) for a period of one to six days. This is not necessary change, but it is a clear signal that you have met the problem head-on and intend to deal with it.

Maintenance: You have been able to keep up your new behavior for six months to a year. Maintenance is not always the end, however. It is quite likely that when you reach a plateau or encounter a new hurdle that feels overwhelming, you will flag in your efforts and spiral back to a precontemplation stage, from which you'll have to pass through all the stages again. It is not unusual to have to work your way through these five stages three or four times before maintenance really sticks.

In order to succeed at behavioral change, we must first want to quit doing whatever it is that's bad for us. We must commit to getting rid of the old familiar habits that feel so right. In order to make a commitment, we have to

- know what we want
- stop blaming others and events for the behavior
- stop procrastinating
- control our emotions
- make changes slowly, one day, one element at a time
- expect obstacles, and be prepared for setbacks
- reach a plateau without feeling we have to give up

The next stage is to chart our behavior so that we can see it up close. Let's imagine for a moment that you're married but having a torrid affair, and you want to quit. You will not just need motivation and determination, but also various interventions that will stop the unhealthy behavior.

First, you need to write down three or four driving forces that keep you doing this behavior, and three or four restraining forces that make you want to quit. On one side of your tally, you can write down that the excitement and danger make sex more enjoyable and that your lover really listens to your ideas although your spouse seems bored with them. On the other side, you might write down that you are risking everything, including your children's respect and the house you currently live in. You must carefully weigh the consequences and implications of the two sides as you prepare to take action.

After this you will observe your behavior for one week without trying to change it. You have to chart every phone call, every time you pass his or her house, every time you spend extra money on a motel room. In other words, it's not the behavior itself that you must become aware of, but the particular circumstances that make it possible for the behavior to happen.

Make yourself a graph on which you will show behavior before the change and behavior after you have put your interventions into practice. You may notice that you call each other more frequently when you haven't slept together for a week or two, or at the office, or on weekday evenings before your spouses come home. At those times, then, you will have to be particularly vigilant about not calling, since your desire to do so is generally greater when you have a routine that feels comfortable.

During your second week, you are going to start changing your behavior. This means no phone calls, no drives past your lover's house or office, no returning calls if you receive them. The interventions you might put into place would be to plan events with other people that would keep you occupied, to turn your wedding ring around each time you have the urge to see your lover, to start a new project that would keep you on the phone at times when you might call your lover, to dun yourself for additional mileage if you use the car for any trips other than errands, and to go to and from work.

At this point you will set a "quit date" and mark it on your calendar. This means that you have the commitment to finish what you've started. The change of behavior is never complete until you actually stop doing it.

The activities involved in behavior change may seem petty, but the mechanism is incredibly powerful. By breaking down our bad habits into their least common denominators, we can smash them to bits. By feeling good about how successful we've been with change, we can embark on a new program of healthful behaviors that may keep us sane for the rest of our lives.

BINGEING

see also Bulemia, page 84; Eating Disorders, page 139

Bingeing is a common eating disorder that involves a loss of control and consumption of much more food than the stomach actually wants or needs. It's estimated that bulemia (which is bingeing and purging afterward) affects 3 to 5 percent of the general population, and up to 20 percent of young women. The problem is difficult to heal because often the behavior isn't conscious. Bingers talk about "blackouts" during which they literally eat for hours and can't remember afterward what happened.

What Happens When You Binge

A binge eater usually hoards food, keeping it for some future date when she feels a need to binge. She generally waits until she can be alone, often after everyone else is in bed. At this point she may consume a day's worth of calories or more in a frantic eating frenzy. The body is severely compromised by this behavior, which causes fluid and electrolyte imbalances, gastrointestinal problems including GI bleeding, and a decrease in gut motility. Because bingers typically crave sweets, they may develop abnormal insulin secretion leading to hypoglycemic panic attacks. (See, McGown, A and Whitbread, J "Out of Control: The most effective way to help the binge-eating patient, *"Psycho-Social Nursing,"* 1996 Jan; 34 (1).

When bingeing is combined with purging, it is known as bulemia (see Bulemia, page 84). A bulemic will spend several hours after a binge eliminating or vomiting.

Because bingers are so secretive about their behavior, it is often difficult to notice that anything is wrong. Those who purge maintain an average or slightly above average weight and eat regular meals in public or with the family.

Binge eaters who don't purge become obese, and they are particularly resistant to weight management programs. The weight always comes back as soon as they start bingeing again.

Signs that you may be a binge eater or bulemic might be

- eating when you're not hungry
- losing control and eating a very large amount of food in a two-hour period
- feeling that food controls your life
- feeling disgusted or guilty about your behavior
- feeling severely depressed, even suicidal when you eat out of control

Learn Some New Eating Behavior

A particular type of meditation, known as mindfulness, offers a different approach to the behavior of eating. Jon Kabat-Zinn, who heads the Stress Reduction Clinic at the University of Massachusetts Medical Center, suggests eating one raisin very, very carefully. First you simply look at the raisin, thinking about its life as a grape and how it got to where it is. Then you pick it up and feel it, sensing its texture, its lumps and bumps, the slight stickiness on your fingers. Then put it to your nose and smell it, imagining the warm, sunny field where it ripened and dried. Then rub it against your lip, feeling yourself begin to salivate, thinking about the taste of just one raisin.

Ask yourself if you're hungry or if you are just eating for the sake of having something in your mouth. Now, you can put the raisin on your tongue. Don't suck or chew it, just let it sit there, giving your mouth the abundance of taste. Then roll it around in your mouth, feeling how it pervades each tooth, each taste bud.

Finally, you may chew it, very slowly, enjoying the ability of your jaws to work, your tongue to collect the juices, your throat to swallow them. At last, swallow the raisin, but be aware of the little bits of raisin still stuck in your teeth. This raisin may be with you for some hours, reminding you of the infinite experience of eating.

Keep an Eating Diary

Write down the time, the amount and type of food, your hunger level, the level of anxiety you felt before and after eating, whether you felt "bloated" afterward, and whether you purged. Be honest with yourself when you transcribe this information. Check back each week to see how you did.

Get Back Your Self-esteem

Go after appreciation. Even though you may not think a great deal of yourself, you'll be surprised to see how much others like and admire you. But you must be aggressive about finding out. You can ask friends to write comments about you and post them on a bulletin board where you and others can see them. You can select a task you do well and make a project of it—perhaps organizing others to serve a meal at a soup kitchen (where you will get lots of support and thanks). You might also select a day when you pamper yourself with everything but food—get a massage, a manicure, a new haircut—so that you feel and look great.

Take a Breath Before You Chew

When you breathe between bites, it forces you to contemplate what you're really doing. It brings a level of conscious awareness to eating that is often lost during bingeing. Practice when you are at the table having a regular meal. Use a signal each time you breathe, like tapping one finger on your opposite hand. Now take the breath, then chew each mouthful at least ten times.

If you find yourself starting a binge, use your tapping signal when you're eating to bring your attention quickly to what you're doing. If you can put consciousness into your actions, you will be able to stop a binge in its tracks.

Start Dancing

Whether you know your right foot from your left or not, dance can be a wonderful outlet that may assist in your process of healthier eating. When you are carried away by the music and allow your limbs and torso the freedom they crave, your craving for food diminishes. Dance, as aerobic exercise, also stimulates the production of endorphins in your brain, those natural opiates that give us a sense of well-being. Dance also makes the klutziest among us feel graceful. It can be a social outlet, whether you are hip-hopping, line-dancing, or waltzing. When you keep moving and stay actively involved with other people, you can find fulfillment in something that's not food.

Visualize Yourself in Charge

You will create a place for yourself that does not depend on stuffing yourself. Sit quietly and imagine your body as a hollow tube, filled only with energy. This energy can sustain you forever and needs no outside stimulation or nourishment. The energy inside is a pulsing, warm ball of light that fills all the corners of your mind and body. As you allow the light to illuminate the various parts of your soul, you will feel yourself filling up with competence, happiness, and unity. This balancing energy also allows you control over your impulses. You will find, even as you leave this space consciously, that the power of the energy that fills you can carry you through each day. All you have to do when you have an urge to binge is to close your eyes and recapture this special filling force inside you.

Abandon All Sugar

A nutrient rich, sugar-free diet may stop the bingeing behavior. Very often, sugar acts as a trigger to start a binge that may include all types of food.

Homeopathic Help

Try the following homeopathic remedies:

> For lack of emotional outlet: Natrum mur
> For an overweight individual with cravings: Calcarea
> For an oversensitive, physically weak person: Ferrum
> For lack of confidence: Anacardium, Silicum, Aurum, China, Kali carbonicum, Lycopodium, Natrum mur
> For feeling of disgust: Pulsatilla, Sulphur, Kali carbonicum

Supplement Your Meals

Vitamin and mineral supplementation can be extremely important to binge eaters. The amino acid tryptophan and vitamin B_6 (pyridoxine) have been shown to change eating behavior and improve mood. (Mira Metal., "Vitamin and Trace Element Status of Women with Disordered Eating. *American Journal of Clinical Nutrition* 50: 940-44, 1989). Other vitamins and minerals that might be supplemented to control bingeing are folic acid, Vitamin E, and potassium.

BIOENERGETICS

Dr. Alexander Lowen, a psychoanalyst and disciple of the controversial therapist Wilhelm Reich, developed a mind/body therapy that can be useful in the treatment of mental and emotional problems.

Lowen's belief is that energetic processes in the body must be tapped to heal trauma and release emotion. The breath and various different releasing exercises are used to guide the individual toward a new appreciation of his or her emotional potential. The most common bioenergetic exercise is bending backward over a low stool with your hands over your head, breathing fully and aggressively. Another is standing over a bed and repeatedly raising your arms high in back of you and then hitting down as you breathe out forcefully.

Bioenergetics analyzes the patient in terms of a pyramid: ego is at the top, followed by thoughts, feelings, and movements. The base of the pyramid contains the various energetic processes. Lowen feels that we all have a basic drive to live, to function, and to love, and sees bioenergetics as a way to return the frustrated, repressed individual to the joy and passion he or she knew as a child. Our childlike impulses—to run, to cry, to scream—are generally suppressed as we get older. This therapy attempts to return the body to that natural state where complete freedom (and great excitement) was allowed. Lowen's contention is that bioenergetics gets to the root of problems a lot more quickly than psychotherapy does because it offers a straight path to the patient's unconscious. The bioenergetic therapist can begin to see personality conflicts by looking at the way the patient holds tension in his body.

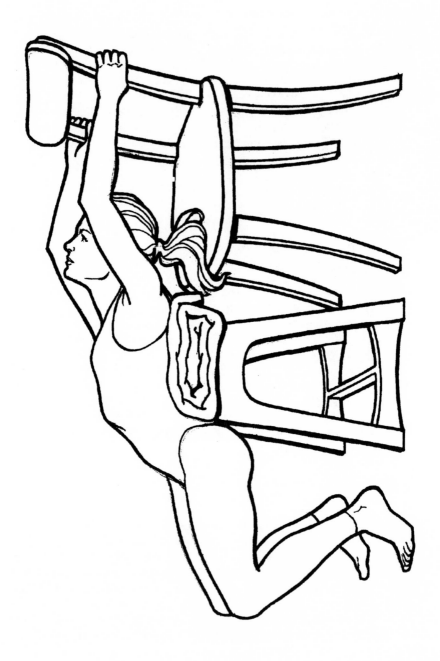

Lowen sees health, both emotional and physical, as determined by how high or low your energy is. The following are high-energy parameters.

- You sleep well and awake refreshed.
- Your eyes are bright.
- You look forward to each day and find pleasure in your normal activities.
- You enjoy being quiet.
- You move gracefully.

The following are low-energy (and poor health) indicators.

- You feel tired and have trouble getting up in the morning.
- You feel harried, driven, pressured.
- It's hard for you to relax; you're always doing something.
- You have quick, hurried movements.
- You have trouble falling asleep.

Bioenergetic therapy can be powerful and has implications for real emotional and spiritual growth if the patient is willing to read Lowen's works and learn how the physical exercises relate to the mental or emotional pain he or she is attempting to heal. In order to use bioenergetics to improve your mental and emotional state, it is essential to begin by working with a trained professional (see Resource Guide, page 475).

*B*IOFEEDBACK

Our heart beats, our muscles contract, our brain emits waves, and we don't have to lift a finger for those functions to occur. But are our internal processes really "involuntary"? The truth is that we have an enormous amount of say over what our organs and tissues do, and biofeedback is one of the best ways to learn to monitor and alter our body functions.

Norbert Weiner, a mathematician, first described feedback as "a method of controlling a system by reinserting into it the results of its past performance." If we get up from the dinner table too fast after a large meal (where a lot of blood flow is concentrating in the gut to digest our food) and are overwhelmed with dizziness, we sit down again until we have sufficient blood flow to the brain so that we can stand comfortably.

The same type of feedback can come to you from auditory and visual cues produced by the biofeedback machine. You may see flashing lights, a visual picture of a graph, or hear a set of high- and low-pitched sounds. If you are incredibly tense and you hear a beep every time you contract a muscle, you need to concentrate on turning the sound off, which you can do by relaxing and releasing the muscle.

Biofeedback is used for pain relief, internal temperature control, blood pressure and heart rate control, gastrointestinal disturbances, and many other physiological mechanisms that can cause you distress. If you suffer from stress-related problems such as heart palpitations, chronic diarrhea, breathing disorders, cold hands or feet, neck and shoulder pain, or headaches or migraines, biofeedback may provide you with a new method of alleviating pain and discomfort.

This therapy is generally taught in ten sessions by a professional biofeedback practitioner. It is almost always taught in conjunction with several relaxation techniques, such as meditation, guided imagery, progressive relaxation, or autonomic training (giving the body instructions that it is feeling warm, cold, light, heavy, and so forth.) These techniques enhance the effect you get from the machine's cues about your body's internal mechanisms.

There are a variety of machines you can use: an electromyogram (EMG), which measures muscle activity; an electroencephalogram (EEG), which measures the electrical activity of the brain; a galvanic skin response (GSR), which measures skin resistance in the hand; and a temperature gauge.

After you've learned awareness and have a sense of how your body changes when you're tense or relaxed and you understand how to use these machines effectively, you can either take a machine home to use on your own, buy one, or train yourself to do the same work without the sound or sight of feedback mechanisms. If you can "think" your hand temperature up when you hear a sound, you can train yourself to do the same mental gymnastics without that sound. Perhaps you used imagery—you thought about fur gloves or a warm bath; perhaps you simply allowed your arms and hands to relax by giving them directions such as "Your hands are warm and heavy." If you are patient and practice your relaxation techniques, you can get the same benefit off the machine as on it.

*B*IPOLAR *D*ISORDER *(Manic Depression)*

see also Depression, page 112

When you're depressed and down all the time, you have a unipolar disorder—that is, there is only one thread of disorder in your mental and emotional makeup. But if you swing radically from feeling miserable and blue to feeling high and wild, you have a double-pronged disorder. This condition, which used to be known as manic-depressive disorder, takes a person from the depths to the heights without any middle ground. The individual who suffers from bipolar disorder doesn't even sense the change: One day she is unable to get out of bed; the next day, she is impulsively racing from one activity to the next, calling friends to arrange trips abroad and talking about finishing the great American novel.

In depressive illness, there is a characteristic deficiency of neurotransmitter activity—serotonin, melatonin, and norepinephrine levels are all depressed. In bipolar disorder, however, there is an excess of neurotransmitter activity—all the neurons are firing at once.

The manic and depressive stages usually go in cycles: As one is ending, the next is beginning, with hardly any breathing space in between. The manic person may suddenly wake up and feel like conquering the world, although many new projects may go unfinished as he or she races to begin something else. Reckless behavior (fast driving, inappropriate sexual activity, spending to the limit on credit cards) is typical. The cycles may last for weeks or months or even hours, just as the depressive phase is ending. If you suffer from bipolar disorder, it may be difficult to recognize symptoms in yourself even when your friends and relatives act alarmed about the radical changes they see.

Some of the typical manifestations of bipolar disorder are

- excessively high mood
- decreased need for sleep
- increased energy and activity
- racing thoughts
- increased talking, moving, and sexual activity
- grandiose notions
- profligate spending
- being easily distracted

Bipolar disorder is difficult to treat—with or without drugs—because in the manic state, patients feel so wonderful they don't think they need help. Because of the euphoria that covers up many of the potentially dangerous aspects of mania, it is difficult to get patients to comply with medication schedules (lithium carbonate is the drug of choice with this illness). If you can use your positive mind to take care of yourself naturally, however, you can temper the hysteria. This is one reason why nutrition, exercise, body work, and other holistic therapies are recommended.

Talk to Someone

If you are prone to radical mood swings, an accurate diagnosis will get you help quickly. It is a good idea to consult a counselor, clinical social worker, or therapist who will put together the pieces of this often confusing illness and refer you to the appropriate treatment. Short-term therapy is very effective in helping a patient rebalance emotional highs and lows.

Go for D/ART

The Depression Awareness, Recognition, and Treatment Program is a public and professional education effort of the National Institute of Mental Health to reduce the prevalence of depressive disorders. For free brochures, call 1-800-421-4211.

Eat Calmly

You should add foods to your diet that will be especially beneficial, whether you are in a manic or a depressed state. The following foods contain serotonin, the neurotransmitter that gives a sense of well-being and is also a component of various mind-altering drugs: banana, mango, avocado, kiwi, plum, tomato, walnuts, and pecans.

Eat Often

It's been shown that hypoglycemia (low blood sugar) produces rapid mood swings. If you space out your food evenly into six small meals, it's easier to keep glucose and brain chemical levels in the body balanced.

Watch Your Supplements

If you feel manic a good deal of the time, you may be suffering from vitamin deficiency. You should be getting 400 mcg. folic acid daily, 1,000 mcg. of Vitamin B_{12} once a week, 40 mg. of niacin three times daily, 50 mg. of Vitamin B_6 three times daily, and 1,000 mg. of Vitamin C once a day. It's also a good idea to take an herbal stress formula that contains tryptophan twice daily.

Take a Cold Shower

The old treatment used for manic depression was to swaddle the patient in cold, wet sheets—he or she should be comfortable but immobilized. A blanket is placed over the top to keep the cold in and a hot water bottle warms the feet. Commonly used at the turn of the century for "hysterics," this treatment was found to be extremely calming. The treatment has recently come into favor again in psychiatric hospitals—the dramatic change in temperature (from cold to warm as the body's blood vessels dilate) and the tight wrapping seem to provide comfort and security for the patient.

You can use this treatment at home to center yourself and calm down, or try a cold shower, followed by wrapping securely in a large bath sheet.

Run Fast, Breathe Slowly

An exercise program is one of the best moderators of mood. When we exercise and produce natural opiates known as beta endorphins, we feel that we have accomplished something. We are also enhancing our oxygen consumption, which the brain needs for stimulation as well as relaxation.

Try a particular running technique known as *fartlek*, Swedish for "speed play." In this type of exercise, you constantly change your pace, challenging yourself to sprint, accelerating to a certain point, then slowing and stretching out the legs in longer, more measured strides and giving you some time to catch your breath. This breaks up the monotony of dull jogging and is particularly good when done on grass or trails.

You decide when you speed up and when to slow down, and this gives you a sense of mastery over your movement. The imbalance of the brain hormones that creates a manic stage can be helped by this instinctive type of training.

Manipulation for Mania

A chiropractor or osteopath will understand the correct adjustment to assist in regulation of the thyroid gland (which can be out of balance in those with bipolar disorder). The manipulation will involve work between the fifth and sixth ribs; then at various points on the lumbar, thoracic, and cervical spine.

Fall into Feldenkrais

We generally make our bodies move by directing our limbs and torso with our brain. We will raise a hand into the air or decide to bend over and touch our toes. However, Feldenkrais uses passive movement: You allow the arm to float up and the body to fall forward, for example. The use of this hands-on treatment can make you feel relaxed and joyful again. You may work in a group, where an instructor gives you exercises that challenge all muscle groups. You may also work with a private trainer, who will guide your body through gentle touch to let go of tension. The idea is to concentrate your attention on letting the movement happen rather than willing your body to do it for you.

Help with Homeopathy

The following remedies may be helpful in the healing process. Of them all, Ignatia is probably the first you should try because the description of the remedy matches bipolar disorder to a T: the person is full of contradictions.

> For chaotic, confused behavior: China, Nux vomica, Arsenicum album, Belladonna, Mercury

For impulsiveness, a sudden desire to do something: Ignatia, Pulsatilla, Argentum nitrate, Arsenicum album, Aurum

For overexcitement, sleeplessness: Valerian.

For depression alternating with bad temper: Nux vomica.

For depression with a tendency to throw things: Lilium Tig.

A Little Help from Your Friends

Support groups have been helpful in the treatment of bipolar disorder. When you are surrounded by people who understand the nature of your problem, who are not confused by the two forces that work concurrently inside you, you may feel a sense of readiness to confront both sides of your problem. It is always useful to have a buddy or mentor to call when you are feeling particularly manic and may do something rash or dangerous. Contact your local hospital or social services agency for a recommendation to a group.

Press Your Points

Pressure on the following trigger points on your body stimulates the production of endorphins, the same natural opiates you get when you exercise.

Use your right hand to squeeze your left shoulder muscle to relieve tension and anxiety. Then switch hands.

Close your eyes. Use the thumbs and index fingers of both hands to massage and press along the fleshy exterior of the ear. Start at the lower end of the ear lobes and move to the upper ear, taking about 15 seconds for the circuit. Repeat. This will clear the mind and energize the body.

Take one thumbnail and press into the skin crease of the wrist on your opposite hand (palm is facing you). Rotate the thumbnail on this point for two to three minutes to alleviate acute anxiety.

Again, using the thumbnail, press hard under the fleshy bulge of the opposite thumb right in the center. This should calm a hysterical outburst.

Blues, the

see also Depression, page 112

People sing about them all the time. That baleful, mournful sound of a voice crying the blues, with a sad guitar and harmonica backing it up, is part of the American musical legacy. But everybody's had the blues at one time or another. Being "blue," or down, is a part of being human.

There are probably dozens of derivations of this word. One that comes from sixteenth-century Europe portrays the sad, brooding individual as one who is possessed by "blue devils." Another interpretation is that it comes from "blueskin," a derogatory word for a black person. The melancholy songs of the slaves, protesting their oppression and dejection, describe loss so perfectly. We hear, in the blues, the dirge of what life is like when love is gone and times are bad.

What Happens When You Get the Blues

The world looks gray and miserable; you have difficulty believing that there's any reason to go on. You may feel annoyed with upbeat, optimistic friends, wishing only to stay in your funk and mull over the problems and hug your misery to your chest. There is an almost therapeutic nature to having the blues, as if you can't really get much farther down than this, so you might as well wallow in it.

The blues are a typical symptom of premenstrual stress, when the hormone progesterone dominates a woman's body and makes her feel bloated, fatigued, and generally miserable right before her period. The same problem occurs around menopause, when an imbalance in the hormonal cycle also affects brain chemicals. Although men don't suffer from monthly hormonal fluctuations, they, too, get the blues, although they may be more related to outside events, such as work, relationship problems, or the death of a close friend or relative.

Although it's normal and natural to have the blues, some of us get caught in the trap of enjoying feeling bad. It's at this point that it's crucial to pull ourselves up by our bootstraps and start singing another song.

Dance Your Troubles Away

It is almost impossible to feel low when you're dancing. Aside from the aerobic boost, you get a real charge when you are rhythmically keeping time with a good beat. (A musical beat, by the way, is the outward manifestation of your heartbeat. Studies have shown that even colicky babies calm down when held close to the chest and that dependable sound they heard in utero. It works the same way for an adult who is out of sorts with the world and needs a steady reminder of the permanence of life.)

You can dance alone in your own room or in a club, but be sure you get wild and improvise to a quick, incessant beat. It hardly needs mentioning that if you're going out, don't go to hear a blues band.

Play with Your Misery

Play therapy can take the sting out of the blues. A particularly good toy to use is a bubble wand—either the standard circle top or one of the newer, fancier versions. Use soapy water with glycerin or commercial bubbles and blow away to your heart's content. You can also dip your wand in the soap and run with it to produce a moving cascade of bubbles. It's best to do this in the sunlight and watch the shimmering rainbow in each unique structure. It's difficult to feel miserable when you blow bubbles.

Treat Yourself

A simple act of kindness from you to yourself can make your day. Unless your foul mood has to do with financial problems, a good therapy to break the mood is buying yourself a small gift—flowers, a new T-shirt, or a hat usually do the trick.

Drink a Flower

The Bach flower remedy for the despondent, easily discouraged, and dejected is Gentian. You might also try Heather if you are obsessed with your own troubles. Put 5 or 6 drops under your tongue, or mix in half a glass of water.

Shed Some Light on It

It's been shown that circadian rhythms can affect mood. The pineal gland in the center of the brain emits melatonin, a hormone that helps regulate our sleep-wake cycle. We produce melatonin when it's dark and stop producing it when it's light. If there's too much darkness (and too much of that hormone), other hormonal stimuli are affected, specifically, your production of serotonin, the "feel-good" hormone.

If you typically get the blues in the winter or when it's been rainy and dark for days on end, be sure you turn on some extra lights during the daytime hours. You may wish to investigate a SAD clinic (see Resource Guide, page 475) or invest in a light box, which puts out 10,000 lux of white fluorescent lights, just what you need to get you out of your mood.

Herbs to the Rescue

St. John's wort has been found to work well on mild to moderate depression. Take 300 mg. of fresh plant extract three times daily, and you should see a difference in six to eight weeks. This herb should *never* be used in combination with Prozac or any serotonin reuptake inhibitor or antidepressant.

Body Dysmorphic Disorder

see Distorted Body Image, page 118

Body-Mind Therapies

see also Alexander Technique, page 27; Bioenergetics, page 63 Feldenkrais, page 181; Tai Chi Chuan, page 417; Yoga, page 457

It has been well documented that the mind and body do not function separately but, rather, work in a complex synchrony to establish balance and harmony throughout our lives. If one is out of alignment, the other usually follows. (If you have the flu, you get depressed and fatigued; if you are overcome with grief, you very often get physical symptoms, such as gastrointestinal problems, insomnia, or headache.)

If the body/mind is diseased, everything else follows suit, beginning with the immune system. When we miss neuronal signals within the limbic system, the emotional center of the brain, we can fall prey to stress-related illnesses such as headaches, stomachaches, allergies, and more serious long-term illnesses such as heart disease and cancers. The reason is that the limbic system also houses the hypothalamus, the master gland that directs the activities of all other glands in the body and interacts with the immune system, which keeps us well.

The goal of mind/body therapies such as meditation, yoga, tai chi chuan, Feldenkrais, Alexander Technique, Trager Psychophysical Integration, Hellerwork, Mari-El, Rubenfeld Synergy, Reichian Breathwork, bioenergetics, and others are to bring the mind and body back into alignment, to harmonize the various elements that are out of balance. All these disciplines teach the practitioner, slowly and painstakingly, to concentrate, focus, and use the energy within the body/mind for practical benefits.

Bodywork aims to stimulate the nervous and lymphatic systems, to stretch and release muscles, and to improve circulation and respiration. In addition, these healing types of movement work internally as well as externally, allowing you to clear your mind and relax, devoting yourself for the time you're practicing to this and nothing else.

When you first begin to study, you naturally focus on the physical aspects, learning the choreography or exercises so that eventually you can do them with the least amount of conscious thought. Somewhere along the line, usually after you've been practicing for several months, you may notice that you are not simply doing the steps by rote, but rather, that they emanate from deep within you, a place where your concentration is focused only on the feeling you have as you perform the movement. You will find that the extraneous thoughts of work, family, tax payments, Christmas shopping, and so forth, are all filtered out as you breathe into each posture and let it fill you completely—mind and body. This is the real breakthrough, the one that starts the healing process of your mind and emotions. Those who suffer from many different conditions—depression, anxiety, agitation, fatigue, phobias, obsessive/compulsive disorders, and many others—often find that they are at peace and much more content with themselves because of their practice. Mind/body therapies teach the brain to regulate the ebb and flow of stress hormones in a balanced, even manner.

Dean Ornish and Jon Kabat-Zinn were the pioneers of yoga and meditation as therapy for heart disease, cancer, and other stress-related disorders, and their innovative programs have paved the way for others around the country. The hospital-based sessions require group participation in body/mind therapies, and comparisons between individuals who do and don't practice daily are startling. It's as if the body can't respond as well to diet and exercise if the mind isn't involved in some profound way.

You can generally find classes in the various body/mind therapies offered at local YWCAs, and you may find information about private classes on bulletin boards at health food stores, alternative bookstores, and in the Yellow Pages under "Health" or "Health Associations and Agencies."

BREATHING

We all take breathing for granted—after all, if we stop breathing, we die, so since we're alive, we must know how to breathe. Right? Wrong.

Most of us do not take full breaths—the type that affords better oxygenation to all tissues (including the brain) and at the same time removes excess carbon dioxide—a toxic gas—from the body. When we are upset or frightened, when we tighten up so that we can feel armored against the world's slings and arrows, we never get a full breath that extends right from the toes to the top of the head.

If you think about the last time you were really scared, you may remember that your breathing accelerated, perhaps so much that you started to hyperventilate. You might have felt dizzy and sick. The reason is that you were not getting rid of enough CO_2, and as you kept gasping, you were bringing oxygen into your system but not getting rid of the CO_2. (If you do this long enough, you actually black out, which allows your breathing to return to normal.)

Even those of us who don't hyperventilate may have problems with air hunger, or shortness of breath. When we take in small gulps of air, we can let only that much out. The breaths are restricted to the nose and mouth, and we end up trying to expand only our upper chest and shoulders, which leaves us huffing and puffing. Consequently, when we're upset, we end up not having enough oxygen to carry on an argument or even turn and run away from an unpleasant situation.

For better mental and emotional health, learning to breathe properly is essential. So in order to get the most benefit out of what you do every minute of every day, you are going to try to re-create what you did as an infant when your lungs and diaphragm were new and you had no idea what anxiety or fear was.

Babies breathe from the stomach, not the chest. They allow the intake of air to move oxygen from their bellies up to the solar plexus and then to the lungs and actually inflate the back and kidneys at the same time. As they exhale, the rush of air out of the body flattens the stomach area.

So now you're going to learn to breathe like a baby.

How to Breathe

Lie on your back on the floor or any hard surface. Think about melting your body down so that as many parts of you touch the floor as possible. Get your heels, backs of your legs, thighs, waist, spine, neck, and head to relax and fall away from you as you concentrate on your breath.

Place one hand on your chest and think about keeping it as still as possible. Take the other hand and place it on your belly, about three inches below your waistband. Press down gently, which will force air out of this region. Now relax your hand, inhale, and see your belly "bounce back." Watch the easy action of your hand moving up and down as you breathe in and out. Try to keep the breath rhythmic and even, and be aware of keeping it out of your chest and shoulder region (your lungs will get oxygen anyway—don't worry). You want to concentrate all the energy on that one point below your waist.

Now stand up in front of a mirror and blow into a balloon, using only your belly to do the inflating and deflating. Again, watch the action of your belly as it moves in and out, and try not to let your chest and shoulders participate at all. They should be relaxed, just going along for the ride.

When this type of belly breathing is comfortable for you, sit in a hard-backed chair or cross-legged on the floor and spend 15 minutes simply watching the process of breathing. Clear your mind of other thoughts and think "in" and "out" as you breathe. Imagine a stream of pure air entering and leaving you, like a willow tree bending this way and that with the wind. Be sure you let the air fill every corner of you—imagine it traveling up to your head, to the backs of your knees, and to your toenails.

If you experience dizziness or lightheadedness, stop and return to normal breathing. It's common for beginners to try too much too soon and overdo it. Allow several hours to pass and practice again, this time reducing the number of breaths and the fullness of the inhalation and exhalation.

As this type of relaxed breathing becomes familiar to you, you'll find that it can help you in any difficult situation. By calming your breath, you automatically lower your blood pressure and heart rate. You also trigger the "relaxation response" of your parasympathetic nervous system, your biggest ally against anxiety and tension.

Breathing is generally used in conjunction with Meditation, page 292, and Visualization, page 442, for even more effective work on mental and emotional problems.

BROKEN HEART

see also Depression, page 112

The image of the heartbroken lover, one hand to her forehead, one on her heart, is a cliché of Romantic literature and art. However, the concept of the broken heart is as legitimate as any other emotional condition, and it can be helped by natural remedies.

When we are in love, we are filled with the delight of sharing everything with another human being. The touch, the smell, the smile, the words of another become so precious to us that they actually change our perspective on life and reality. In a true love relationship, both individuals feel this jointure—they become one soul in two bodies.

When we first "fall" in love, the descent can be precipitous: We can be so overwhelmed with powerful new feelings of completeness, we may alienate ourselves from friends and family and feel distracted at work and play. As the fledgling relationship deepens and we are able to see our lover's weak as well as strong points, we can separate ourselves from the torrent of passion and gain a steadier footing along the path to lasting love.

And when the relationship ends we often have trouble separating from the experience, more so than from the other person. When we've been accustomed to doing everything together and almost thinking the other person's thoughts, it's a wrenching experience to become independent again. But there are techniques and methods of regaining balance that will mend a broken heart.

Use Your Brain Instead of Your Heart

Cognitive awareness can teach us how to think clearly about emotional problems. By writing down your negative feelings about the relationship and person you were attached to and examining them rationally, you will gain a new perspective on what really happened.

First, write a detailed account of what the affair or marriage consisted of. Were you friends as well as lovers? Did you receive emotional rewards as well as give them? What was your sexual life like? What ended the relationship? Did it taper off or end suddenly, in a stormy finale?

Now, you need to structure the information so that you can dissect it:

Irrational Belief #1

I'm a failure in love. Love is not one thing, but many overlapping feelings and qualities. Undoubtedly there are currently several people in your life who love you—not only your parents and children, but also close friends of both sexes. When you stop expecting just one person to give you everything, you will be able to accept the love that flows around you.

New belief: I'm successful in many different love relationships.

Irrational Belief #2

I can't function without my partner. You are currently getting up, feeding yourself, perhaps driving to work or taking care of a household. You will find as the days pass that you can go to movies or restaurants on your own and make decisions without consulting anyone else.

New belief: This situation has opened many opportunities for exploring my independence.

Irrational Belief #3

There will never be another person in my life that I care about so completely. This breakup and the broken heart that went with it has shown you only one thing: that you were involved with someone who could reject you and make you miserable. Your "caring" was actually overcompensating for an ungiving, unloving person. In your next relationship, you may be able to grow beyond this type of self-abuse.

New belief: I have learned a great deal about my capacity for love by having to deal with this person.

When you can change your distorted thinking, you can begin to understand yourself—and like yourself—better.

Smell the Roses

In order to lighten a depressed mood, try a massage with essential oil of Rose. You can also try Jasmine to encourage an optimistic spirit and sunny Grapefruit or Bergamot as stress reducers. You can keep a bottle of any of these in your purse to smell when you think you're about to break down and cry.

The Wonder of Touch

Get a professional massage or see your chiropractor for a gentle manipulation. Although most people think of massage as a relaxing time out of time and chiropractic as a medium for necessary adjustment of the spinal column, they can both be much more.

Touch can open up the pathways to emotion that we block in our everyday, armored existence. When we are trying to hold back certain feelings, we clench our muscles, locking in memories and thoughts we'd prefer not to deal with. When effective touch—pressure, squeezing, rotating, and so forth—is applied to certain areas, the musculature and connective tissue give way and the door is unlocked. Another factor involves lying on a massage table or chiropractic couch. When we are in a prone position, we are more vulnerable and are less likely to erect the shield to our emotion that we keep up when we're on our feet or seated.

You may not wish to pour out your heart to the person who heals with touch, but it's a good idea to mention before your session that you are under a lot of stress. This will put your practitioner on notice that you may be ready to release some buried feelings. Don't be surprised if a light brush across your neck or an intense pressure on your upper thigh starts the tears flowing.

Don't be afraid of letting go. The type of release you can get from touch can act as a trigger for deeper work on your unhappiness.

Junk the Junk Food

This is a time when you are likely to lose your appetite or put anything in your mouth that happens to be in the house. It's important for your spirits, appearance, and immune system that you eat healthfully, even if you don't want to. In a pinch, decide on a fruit fast or a vegetarian juice fast for four days. It will give you lots of energy and it's easy to prepare.

Desensitize Yourself

There are few things as difficult as going through the paraphernalia of a life together once it's been torn asunder. If your lover has cleared out, you're in luck. If you have to deal with the debris of a life together, however, it's best to do it in a calm mood. Get a cup of herb tea and sit with your old photo album. You're going to look at those lovey-dovey pictures coldly and clinically. That was one time in your life, and you learned from it, and now you can move on. Turn the page.

Rather than tearing them up or throwing them out, it's best to use them to your advantage and treat them like ordinary snapshots. You can do the same with jewelry and other gifts from the relationship if you take your time and possibly get the support of a friend or relative.

Flower Power

The Bach flower remedy for a broken heart is Hellebore. Take 5 to 6 drops under the tongue or mixed in half a glass of water as needed.

Healing from China

According to Chinese medicine, the problem of a broken heart might result in either too much anger, too much pensiveness, or too much sadness and grief. Excess pensiveness (associated with the spleen) results in "knottedness or stuckness"; too much anger (associated with the liver) makes the *chi,* or life force, move upward in the body. Sadness and grief (associated with the lungs) weaken the chi. A Chinese doctor might try to deal with the anger—and excess liver activity—that causes dizziness when you even think about the person who betrayed you. Acupuncture points might be used to cool and disperse the firy elements in the liver. An herbal formula for psychic bleeding is *yunnan paiyao,* available in Chinese pharmacies and through mail-order catalogues. Take one a day for a week.

*B*ROODING

see also Depression, page 112; Grief, page 193; Sadness/Despondency, page 375

When you can't let go of a thought and it runs through your mind over and over, you are brooding. One common symptom of depression, brooding is easy to do on a variety of subjects—from a harsh word to a lost job. We may turn the problem over in our mind a thousand different times, and each time it gets worse, the result more unfair, the consequences more difficult. We may brood when we are sad or when we crave revenge for a wrong done. Like a dog worrying a bone, we take our misery and hold onto it for dear life.

▨ *What Happens When You Brood*

You may find yourself irritable and distracted, unable to listen to others or concentrate on the regular events of your day. You may seem "not yourself," as though you had been changed by the event or slight. Things that used to console you don't work, and you find that nothing gives you any pleasure.

Brooding fosters other unproductive behavior—you may avoid other people and social events, you may not eat or eat too much, your sleep patterns may change, you may abuse substances, or take risks. You may find yourself tele-phoning the person you want to have it out with and then hanging up, or driving past his or her house or office, plan-ning to confront him or her, then chickening out at the last moment. Brooding can eventually lead to a feeling that everyone is out to get you, and to delusional behavior, where you imagine ways to get revenge.

But you can, and should, take care of brooding before it reaches that stage.

Try a Flower Remedy

The Bach flower remedies to try are

White Chestnut, for persistent, unwanted thoughts, pre-occupation with a worry or event, and mental arguments

Heather, for those who are obsessed with their own trou-bles

Holly, useful for those who want revenge

Borage to open the heart and drive away sorrow

Take 5 or 6 drops in a half glass of water or under the tongue as needed. If the first remedy you try doesn't alleviate your symptoms, try the next.

Look at Your Dreams

You can learn a lot about the problem you're holding onto by examining the way your unconscious deals with it. Keep a pad and pen by your bedside and before you go to sleep, tell yourself that you will dream about the problem. As you awake, first notice how you feel. Are you frightened? Determined? Angry? At peace with yourself?

Next, jot down any images and characters you can recall. Who do these people represent to you? Were you in your dream? What were you doing? If you represent at least part of every character in your dream, what parts of you are in oth-ers? Finally, ask yourself, what changes would you make in this dream if you could? Since brooding involves a good deal of thinking and pensiveness about a particular subject or per-son, you will undoubtedly find a lot of food for analysis. Your unconscious may open new ways of treating the issue.

Use Hypnosis to Clear Your Head

Sit in a quiet place and begin to breathe calmly and slowly. Keeping your head steady, roll your eyes up. Now close your eyes and begin to count backwards from ten. You will sense the rest of your body dissolving as you keep your gaze up and begin to suggest the following:

I am at ease; my body is heavy and warm.

I have no cares or worries—they have all been taken care of.

I can forgive and forget.

I am not afraid to let go of my anger.

As you feel these suggestions begin to take hold, root them in your mind and heart and slowly allow your eyes to relax open.

Communicate and Get Your Thoughts Out of Your Head

It's purposeless to go over the same arguments again and again when you're the only debater. Not only can't you solve the problem, you actually create more facets to the problem you began with when you have no sounding board. Although it takes nerve and persistence, you should confront the person who is responsible for the thing you've been brooding about. Call up and arrange a time to talk on neutral ground—a coffee shop or public park is best. You will want to have a list of points to discuss, but remember not to stick too closely to the script. It's vital that you remain flexible and allow the other person his or her version of the story and opinions about its outcome.

*B*ULEMIA

see Bingeing, page 59; Eating Disorders, page 139

Bulemia is a particular aspect of bingeing and is common in adolescent and young women. (It is estimated that as many as 15 percent of college women have been bulemic at one time or other.) Rather than having difficulty with the passage from childhood to adolescence, like the anorectic girl, the bulemic is having problems becoming an adult. Her attempt to control her body is a symbolic attempt at controlling the world. A thin, lean, almost masculine shape lends the authority that a girl might feel she needs when she is striving for independence but nervous about getting it. Often, bulemic young women have mothers who never worked outside the home and fathers who were always out working, rarely available for an intimate relationship.

The pattern of bulemia is to eat sparingly and then, in a feeling of despair and "falling off the wagon," to binge—usually on sweets—for hours on end. Sometimes girls will hoard candy and cakes just for the occasion. After the binge, the bulemic will induce vomiting with ipecac or by sticking a finger down her throat or will use diuretics and laxatives to induce copious and frequent bowel movements.

In addition to the physiological problems brought on by bingeing (see Bingeing, page 59), bulemia also brings with it chronic sore throat and esophageal tearing (from vomiting), and tooth decay (from stomach acids brought up while vomiting). Long-term bulemia can also result in cardiac arrhythmias and heart failure.

The same therapies useful for bingeing are helpful in the treatment of bulemia.

Chest Pains

see also Anxiety, page 43; Palpitations, page 342; Stress, page 407

If you're in an emotional uproar, it's common to find that you have symptoms very similar to those of angina. IF YOU HAVE A CRUSHING, SQUEEZING, OR STABBING PAIN IN YOUR CHEST OR DOWN ONE ARM, YOU MAY BE HAVING A HEART ATTACK—DO NOT ATTEMPT TO SELF-TREAT. Call 911 immediately, or call a neighbor and ask him or her to take you to the hospital. If you know that you have a heart condition and are being treated for it, place a nitroglycerin tablet under your tongue.

What Happens When You Have Chest Pain

If the pain comes and goes, or if it registers as a dull ache, then this could be a physical pain related to an emotional state. (You should still have it checked by a physician.) The terror of thinking that you might be seriously ill or might be about to have a heart attack can make the pain worse. In fact, if you are angry, sad, hysterical, or depressed, you may read the pain as a symbol. Your heart—the center of your body and your emotional core—is sore and needs healing.

Stand in the Sun

There is a great therapeutic effect in nature that is often discounted in our busy, work-oriented lives. The sun, the centuries-old symbol of warmth and joy, can in fact lighten your heart and take away the pain.

If the sun is out, no matter the weather, give yourself a ten-minute sun break. Stand with your face turned upward (never stare directly into the sun's rays, however) and allow the sensation of heat to penetrate your chest. Breathe slowly and deeply as you inhale the beneficial beams.

Breathe Out the Bad Emotion

Very often, chest pain is associated with poor breathing habits. If you're anxious, you tend to breathe from your upper chest rather than allowing a full, deep belly breath. You may hyperventilate—rapid, shallow breathing that doesn't rid the body of enough carbon dioxide—and this air hunger can exacerbate the pain you already feel.

If you watch a baby breathe in sleep, you'll see exactly what you should be doing, allowing the breath to come right from your center, inflating and deflating your stomach. Lie on the floor and put your hand on your belly. Then begin to inhale slowly, bringing the breath from your center. Watch your hand move up and down as you breathe, keeping your shoulders and chest still. Practice this seated and standing as well.

When you feel that you are losing control and you start to feel tightness in your chest, start the belly breathing immediately. Use the cue of putting your hand on your stomach to remind yourself of the way it's supposed to feel.

Remedies for the Pain

Homeopathic remedies can be helpful.

> For pain in the breastbone: Sulphur, Arsenicum album, Causticum, China, Phosphorus

> For heart palpitations from frustration: Aconite, Chamomilla, Natrum mur, Ignatia, Sepia

Supplemental Assistance

Take 50 mg. of Vitamin B complex daily for stress reduction and add the antioxidant protection of 500 to 1,000 mg. of Vitamin C and 400 to 800 IUs of Vitamin E.

Press a Point

For centuries, Chinese doctors have stimulated the point Pe6 (pericardium 6) for relief of chest pain. This point is an inch above the crease of the wrist in between the fourth and fifth fingers. Two needles are typically applied at this point for 30 minutes, and the doctor then twirls or jiggles the needles every five minutes. One to five treatments generally alleviates the pain for two to six months. Or, you can simply press this point with the index and third finger of your opposite hand.

Let a Flower Soothe Your Heart

When you feel anguish in your chest and are frightened, take the Bach flower remedy Rock Rose, which is good for terror, fear, or panic, as is Rescue Remedy.

Agrimony is the remedy for those who suffer inner torment but feel they have to mask their real feelings with a cheery exterior. Take 5 to 6 drops under the tongue or mixed in half a glass of water.

Visualize Your Pain

The picture of pain means different things to different people. As you close your eyes, you will draw a picture with your mind of whatever is bothering you. Is it an ice pick stabbing your heart? Is it a hole in the center of your chest? As you create an image, you can fix what is wrong—you might pull out the ice pick and sew neat stitches or even laser the wound closed. A hole might be filled in with joy and friendship. As your mind heals the wound, you will find that the physical feelings of pain begin to abate.

Feedback Information

Using biofeedback equipment, you can actually see and hear the constriction of your blood vessels when you tense up. By learning to relax and pay attention to your body's "involuntary" responses, you will be able to alter your cardiovascular and respiratory systems and reduce or eliminate pain.

CHINESE MEDICINE (Traditional)

In the West, we view health as an attempt to keep the various organs and tissues of the body from becoming diseased. In China, however, body, mind, and spirit are one intricate system that cannot be separated. Preserving that harmonious balance is the goal of Chinese medicine.

The general rules and guidelines of this medical system were set down by the Yellow Emperor, Huang Ti, in the third century B.C., and other great thinkers in the next several centuries amplified his ideas. Their treatments for wellness and illness include diet and exercise, herbalism, acupuncture, moxibustion (the burning of an herb on the skin), breathing therapy, physiotherapy, and massage.

The complexities of traditional Chinese medicine take years to unravel; however, the most basic concept is that the harmony of the body is seen as a balance of three essential elements: Blood, which governs tissue, or the corporal part of the body; Moisture, which governs the internal environment such as water, mucus, marrow, and so forth; and chi, which means "life force" and is responsible for the shape and activity of the body. *Chi* is also used to express the mixture of Blood, Moisture, and *chi*—together they represent body, mind, and spirit.

A second major principle is that of the five organ networks. Rather than discuss the body in terms of its organs, Chinese medicine breaks up the body into organ networks. The internal structures, or *yin* organs are Liver, Heart, Spleen, Lung, and Kidney. The *yang* organs, which process the external environment, are the Gallbladder, Small Intestine, Stomach, Large Intestine, and Urinary Bladder.

The theory that governs internal and external in the body is based on the Taoist philosophy of two complementary forces that govern the universe. *Yin*, the force of earth, is yielding and receptive; *yang*, the force of heaven, is strong and untiring. These two are not opposites but are, instead, flip sides of the same coin. For example, take water—it can be *yang* when it pours out of a hose, but can turn *yin* when it freezes. Although females are heavily yin, and males predominantly yang, we each contain a bit of the other inside us. The same is true for every organ and system in our bodies and for every living thing on earth. As long as we move in harmony with the Tao (the "Way"), we are healthy; if we become out of synch with it, we become ill or disturbed.

The wellness or illness of the body is an ever-changing proposition. We all go through cycles, which the Chinese refer to as the Five Phases. These phases—Wood, Fire, Earth, Water, and Metal—identify stages of transformation, contraction and expansion, growing and dying. Wood is birth when life begins and starts pushing upward and outward. It turns into Fire, which increases energy. As it degenerates or becomes dormant, it is Metal, and as it retreats, it becomes Water. Earth stabilizes us and restores our balance.

Each of us tends toward one of the five phases in personality and in health cycling. But in addition to our predilection for one phase or another, we also manifest our physical and emotional problems in terms of climates. Our illness may be one of the unpredictable *wind* (which corresponds to *wood*), the inflammation of *heat* (which corresponds to *fire*), the sinking fullness of *damp* (which corresponds to *earth*), the withering effects of *dryness* (which corresponds to *metal*), or the chilling of *cold* (which corresponds to *water*).

How a Physician of Traditional Chinese Medicine Might Diagnose a Mental Problem

The doctor would first complete a medical history unlike any you've ever had—he or she not only wants to find out what's bothering you but what kind of person you are (in order to ascertain your phase, climate, and emotional tendencies). The doctor would also note your physical appearance, your shape, your manner, your personality, and your behavior. He or she would ask questions about your *chi* (your life energy), your *jing* (the essence that guides development and reproduction—for women, this is menstrual blood and for men, semen), and your *shen,* or spirit. The *shen* gives vitality to the *chi* and *jing* in every individual.

After a physical examination, the doctor would listen to your voice, breathing, and coughing. He would also try to detect certain classic odors that might pinpoint an ailment—a "rancid," or "fishy," or "bleachlike" odor is present in sick individuals.

Next, the doctor would take a thorough history and find out what you think is wrong, when it first started, what types of symptoms you've been having, and so forth. He or she would ask about your temperature, headaches or dizziness, perspiration, thirst and appetite, sleep patterns, gynecological and urological concerns, or any pain you might have. The doctor would also want to find out about your emotions—whether you are quick to anger or whether you simply give in when demands are made on you.

The examination of the tongue can tell the physician a great deal, since changes in the color and coating of the tongue indicate complexities of sickness. If you have a very red tongue, this may mean that you are susceptible to problems of *heat,* which might show that you are deficient in Moisture. If your tongue is pale, you may have a chronic deficiency of Blood, Moisture, and *chi.*

Finally, the doctor would take your pulses to feel the movement of blood in your vessels. By noting the quality and type of pulses in your body—there are 32 subtle pulses that can be detected—the doctor can get the regulation of the blood, *chi, jing,* and *shen* throughout the body. A healthy pulse should be "lively" and "elastic" and have an even beat. The doctor will also press on various acupuncture points that might be sensitive to see if the skin feels dry or moist, cold or hot, and whether pressure or release of pressure causes pain or relief.

After this lengthy diagnosis, the doctor would be able to peg one of eight typical patterns of imbalance in yin and yang, cold and hot, interior and exterior, and deficiency and excess. Each of these patterns is treated to alleviate the disharmony inside you, which would mean that both physical and mental symptoms should start to vanish after a course of treatment.

The important difference from Western medicine is that the doctor is looking at the whole person rather than a target organ that is sick.

Treating Your Illness

A doctor of traditional Chinese medicine would use acupuncture along the various points of the meridians that had the imbalance (see Acupuncture/Acupressure, page 7).

The doctor would prescribe various herbs as well, and you would receive a personal prescription for a mix of herbs to treat the various facets—physical, mental, and emotional—of your condition. (The only Chinese herbs prescribed in this book are patent formulas that can be adapted to many individuals' needs. You must consult a Chinese physician for individualized treatment.)

Herbs are classified as to temperature, flavor, and direction. So depending on your diagnosis, you might need an herb that is cool or warm, sweet, sour, bitter or salty, and ascending or descending or floating or sinking. If you are always tired, have puffy eyes, can't concentrate, and your feet are cold at night, you would need a mixture to tonify *chi*, disperse Moisture, and strengthen the Spleen. If you are listless, have lost your sex drive, and can't sleep through the night, you may need a Kidney tonic, as well as herbs to replenish Blood of the Liver and the Heart.

In addition to acupuncture and herbs, Chinese medical therapy includes *qi gong* breathing. These therapeutic exercises are designed to move energy throughout the body from the center, or *tan tien,* a spot three inches below the belt and three inches inside. Daily practice relieves dysfunction and leaves you with a feeling of calmness, alertness, and rejuvenation. You might be instructed to stand with your feet apart and your hands in front of you as though you were holding a ball. You should imagine your head touching heaven and your feet firmly planted in earth as you begin to manipulate this imaginary ball. Bounce it from hand to hand, then move your hands very slowly in and out, capturing the magnetic feeling between them. You can hold your hands over your head and sense the healing warmth penetrating your mind. As you become more experienced in *qi gong* practice, you will be able to send healing *chi* to your mind and use it to alleviate various emotional problems. According to Chinese medicine, *qi gong* helps to relieve tension in the cerebral cortex and reduces the excitability of the sympathetic nerves. By toning down the sympathetic nervous system (which is what produces the classic stress reaction of rapid heartbeat, dilated pupils, increased respiration, and so forth) we can access the parasympathetic system, which reverses the stress reaction and calms us down.

How Traditional Chinese Medicine Treats Mental and Emotional Illness

Once your physician has established whether you are more wood, fire, earth, water, or metal, you will have a pretty good idea of what might go wrong when you feel upset. He would also strive to strike a good balance between your Blood, Moisture, and *chi*. When you aren't feeling comfortable with yourself, you will exhibit either collapsed or exaggerated patterns of your particular aspect.

For example, a Wood type is usually clear thinking and confident. But when Liver is congested, the person could be intolerant and impatient and experience vascular headaches, muscles spasms, and high blood pressure. If Liver is depleted, the person could feel ambivalent and peevish, behaving in an erratic manner and coming down with nerve inflammations or random aches and pains throughout the body.

The various organ networks would have to be adjusted, using acupressure, herbalism, nutrition, breathing, and lifestyle change. The holistic, multidirectional approach of traditional Chinese medicine will, in fact, change all of you—outside and inside—in addition to alleviating mental and emotional problems.

CHIROPRACTIC

see Manipulation, page 288

COGNITIVE AWARENESS

The goal of cognitive therapy is to help you analyze your emotional problem in light of mental awareness. If you can identify the negative thinking inherent in most depression and anxiety, and relabel it, you can eliminate it.

Many therapies employ a whole-life approach, that is, you have to know the roots of your problem and remember what happened to you as a child in order to make sense of your current dilemma. Cognitive therapy, however, ignores past and future and concentrates only on the present.

Since we typically filter our experiences through a veil of personal beliefs, it's important to examine the way we use other people's opinions of us and events themselves to make them worse than they actually are. By taking a rational look at our thought process when something difficult happens, we are better able to see the truth and therefore feel better about the outcome.

Another feature of this type of therapy is to eliminate irrational thinking and replace it with logical facts. In order to change your mind about the way you feel, you can make a diagram of your thought process. A typical set of cause-and-effect statements might go like this:

My husband always yells at me when the kids are running wild.

If I weren't such a permissive parent, my kids would toe the line and my relationship with my husband would improve.

Therefore, the only way to work on my marriage is to be a stricter parent.

You can see the lack of logic inherent in this example, but it's the kind of thinking we all do every day. First, the woman has an all-or-nothing attitude about the problems in her marriage. She thinks it's all her fault, and she pegs it on the way she handles their kids. She has not factored in her husband's lack of involvement with the children, nor has she included any other elements (friendship, sexuality, similar philosophies of life) that might influence their marital relationship. She uses emotional reasoning and magnifies the problem as she jumps to conclusions about why things are bad. Because she has lumped all the issues together with magical thinking (bad marriage, wild children, all my fault), she can't see that perhaps she's not the only one to blame and that perhaps she and her husband might work on their marriage outside the context of being parents.

Instead of reasoning that she has to "work on her kids," she can put a different label on the problem, which might be "work on having give-and-take discussions with her husband about all issues, not just the children."

A course of therapy (about 16 to 20 weekly sessions) is generally recommended in order for the new thinking to kick in, but you can certainly use the principles yourself, even if you choose not to work with a therapist. Afterward, you can use the techniques every time you find yourself unable to deal with emotional difficulties.

Use Cognitive Therapy to Alleviate Mental and Emotional Problems

You are going to become a detective and sleuth out the various clues that will lead you to a logical conclusion. The skills you will learn involve writing down what's actually occurring and adopting a positive attitude about the information you find.

- Write out the event exactly as it occurred. Your boss called you into his office to criticize your work on a project.

- Identify the element of this event that upsets you. Was it the dismissive way he talked to you and took phone calls during your meeting? The fact that you thought you did good work? The fact that he didn't criticize your co-worker?

- Identify your negative emotions—are you angry, frustrated, frightened, and so forth?

- Write down all the negative thoughts that go with these emotions. Do you assume you'll be fired? That everyone in the office will know you're a screw-up?

- Examine the irrational statements you've just made— why should a little criticism cost you your job?

- Substitute rational responses. Tell yourself how well you've done on other projects for which you've been praised and acknowledge the excellent parts of this project that are still in the works. You can also say that your boss generally likes your work and that his manner is dismissive with everyone.

- Figure out what steps you should take—if any—to deal with the original event (that scene in your boss's office).

- Think about something else—a productive way to solve the project's problem or something unconnected to work.

COMPULSIVE SEXUAL ACTIVITY

see also Sexual Dysfunction, page 387

If you *need* sexual stimulation all the time—particularly with multiple partners who may be strangers—you are suffering from a condition very much like an addiction to drugs or alcohol. The desperate need for repetitive sexual activity has been linked to childhood sexual abuse or other early unresolved traumatic events.

▓ *What Happens When You Have a Compulsive Need for Sex*

There are certain distinct patterns that outline this behavior:

- You have a trancelike preoccupation with sex that fills nearly every moment.
- You search compulsively for sexual outlets, regardless of risk or cost.
- You have special rituals that precede the sexual behavior and intensify the arousal—for example, you will put on undergarments or shoes that trigger your excitement; or you may sit in a hotel lobby watching people as you read a newspaper.
- You have a feeling of hopelessness when you think about stopping this behavior—you believe you are unable to control yourself.

Most people who practice this behavior are terribly lonely and suffer from low self-esteem. They may also use drugs and alcohol to forget or dull the ache inside as they commit acts that are devoid of love or intimacy.

Sexual addicts aren't always single people desperately seeking Mr. or Ms. Right. They may be married or partnered with people who are either unaware of their extracurricular activities or who tolerate the behavior because they themselves come from families with similar patterns. Some people who have an inordinate urge for sex have only one partner, with whom they are obsessed.

Take 12 Small Steps

Twelve-step programs, similar to AA, are available for any type of addiction, and you can usually find a group that will offer you support by looking in the Yellow Pages under "Social Service Organizations" or "Alcohol Addiction Treatment" (which includes numbers for other addictions) or by getting a referral from a local social services agency. Meetings are generally held daily, and you are matched with a mentor whom you can call at any time of day or night whenever you feel the need to go out prowling for sexual contact. By acknowledging your problem, you are taking the first step toward admitting that you have the ability to control your compulsive behavior.

Have Some Hugs Instead

Stimulation that is sensual but not sexual can teach you the value of intimacy. It is important to reconnect with the beneficial aspects of touch—hugging a friend or relative, snuggling with your partner (with no sexual contact), stroking and playing with a pet.

Abstinence is usually part of any therapeutic program, and this means you should restrict all sexual outlets. The first behavior you will have to stop is the ritual you perform before sex, whether that is masturbation, watching or reading erotica, dressing in a certain way, or having phone sex. The value of giving up all these behaviors at once is that they're all connected; the difficulty is that they take up a lot of time, which you must learn to fill in other ways. This is a good time to learn a new skill (a musical instrument, a foreign language, flying a plane) that will excite and stimulate you in other ways.

Get Together with Your Family

Family therapy is generally the best means of dealing with this problem, which at heart has more to do with a sense of loneliness and lack of contact with others than it does with sex. If your family doesn't know about this behavior, it is a hard call as to whether you can disclose everything, but it is the most effective way to work with the problem. And even if you can't discuss the issue now, it's vital that you renew your commitment to family while you're dealing with your problem. This might mean getting more involved with your local parent-teacher organization or church or community activities together.

The Aroma of Calm

The essential oil of Marjoram can be used to quench sexual desire. It is an "anaphrodisiac" as well as being a powerful sedative. Use a couple of drops in a diffuser by your bedside at night.

Homeopathic Help

The following remedies will assist you as you attempt to change your behavior:

> For excessive sexual behavior: Calcarea carbonicum, China, Lycopodium, Nux vomica, Phosphorus, Sepia, Staphisagria
>
> For sexual excitement: Natrum mur, Platina, Staphisagria
>
> To calm feelings of lust: Hyoscyamus, Lachesis, Phosphorus, Platina, Staphisagria, Aconite, China, Pulsatilla, Sepia
>
> To calm compulsion toward indecent exposure or dress: Hyoscyamus, Belladonna, Mercury, Phosphorus

Inhale the Power of a Tender Massage

Aromatherapy massage by your partner or yourself can be a healing experience. (It is best not to use a professional massage therapist because the experience will be too close to anonymous sex.)

Rub Yourself Down

Essential oil of Jasmine can lift your spirits; Clary Sage, Ylang-Ylang, and Bergamot work well with depression. If you are feeling overstimulated, Lavender, Geranium, or Sandalwood (or a combination of the three) can be relaxing.

CONFUSION, MENTAL

see also Aging, page 17; Anxiety, page 43; Stress, page 407

We can be clear-headed and rational one moment, then wandering around in a daze the next. There is nothing so frightening as feeling that we have lost control over the system that keeps everything else going. But is mental confusion a physiological or a psychological state?

▓ *What Happens When You Are Mentally Confused*

Your train of thought is constantly derailed; your ability to remember, even short-term events, seems impaired. You may feel as though you are in a stupor, dull, heavy, and without interest in anything; or you may be highly agitated, desperate to recapture the elusive thoughts that virtually seem to tease you and then jump away.

Mental confusion may be caused by stress or anxiety, by drug or alcohol abuse, by a traumatic experience such as rape or the death of a close friend or relative, or it may be a sign or symptom of middle age or old age. (This is not to say that everyone gets confused when they age; unless it is disease-based, loss of short-term memory is a passing problem for which there are many good treatments.)

Obviously, it is important to make a distinction between forgetfulness and confusion and dementia. IF YOU ARE SERIOUSLY IMPAIRED MENTALLY, YOU NEED TO BE UNDER A DOCTOR'S CARE. The characteristics of dementia are being unable to function in a work or social setting; inability to reason; inability to recognize time, date, or the people around you; inability to perform simple mathematical calculations; and a disintegration of your emotional state.

If you have been misplacing your keys a lot lately, but you have also been busy thinking "big" thoughts about the meaning of life and death, you are fortunate to be in a period of transition—common at various life stages such as midlife and old age. Because you are looking at the wider screen, you don't see the tiny details as well. But maybe that's all right—just relax.

Lower Your Stress

If you are overwhelmed with responsibilities and things to do, you may be blanking out because your brain can't take any more. Give yourself one rest period a day to meditate, read a book, listen to music, or sit in the sun with your cat. You may find that these breaks allow your mind to calm down and straighten out.

Eat Some Fish

Omega-3 fatty acids, found in oily fishes such as mackerel, carp, herring, sardines, and bluefish, have been found to prevent blood platelet aggregation, which helps to accumulate plaque in the arteries. They also lower serum triglyceride levels and elevate HDL (good) cholesterol. By keeping good blood flow and oxidation in the brain, we can think more clearly.

Check Your Prescriptions

Many people are not aware that their over-the-counter and prescription medicines may not mix well. Very often, elderly people are overmedicated, and their combination of drugs may produce vagueness, irritability, or bizarre behavior. You should always tell your physician which drugs you're taking, and if you have no more need for that medication, you should throw the bottles away.

No More Substance Abuse

It's common for people who are depressed, bored, or lonely to abuse drugs and alcohol, and these will definitely affect memory and mental functioning. If necessary, get into a substance-abuse program and stick with it; otherwise, wean yourself off the drugs and alcohol.

Focus Your Mind

A good technique for better awareness is mindfulness meditation, which will allow you to focus on one subject at a time. Select a routine activity you do every day—you might pick writing your signature, which is a trademark of your personality. First, pick the pen you're going to use and examine it carefully. Look at the color, the shape, the way it fits in your fingers. See how the cap opens and closes, or the top clicks on and off. Now examine the paper you'll be writing on. Feel its smooth texture on your cheek and smell the clean paper pulp. Experiment with nonsense drawing—circles and lines—until you are ready to form letters. Draw your name slowly, then quickly. You will find that this type of exercise directs your mind and gives it an anchor, which will be helpful throughout the rest of the day when you are bombarded with many subjects and ideas.

Make Lists

If you forget things, write them down. Keep a pad and pen with you at all times and list exactly what you have to do in order of importance. Check them off as you complete them. Getting your priorities straight will make you feel more comfortable and competent.

Suck on a Lifesaver

Wintergreen lifesavers may improve memory and clarify your thinking. The scent of wintergreen goes directly to the brain through the nasal passages and stimulates the area in the cerebral cortex that deals with recollection.

Challenge Your Brain with Play

One wonderful game to play with friends that will encourage your memory to function better is called "I packed my suitcase." The first person in line says, "I packed my suitcase and into it I put a toothbrush (or any other item)." The second person repeats the sentence and adds an item, the third repeats what the first two have said, and adds an item. By the time you have ten items in the case, ranging from toothbrushes to armadillos, it's a real challenge to repeat the whole list in order. The secret is to create a visual link between the person and his or her item. For example, if a person suggests a pair of shoes, take note of the particular shoes he's wearing; if a person suggests a computer, create a mental picture of that individual with a video monitor instead of a face, and so on.

Focus on Chinese Herbs

The Chinese prescription for senile dementia (which may also be applicable to general mental confusion) is *gui pi tang,* or Spleen restoration decoction. This formula was established in the sixteenth century and is still used successfully today to alleviate forgetfulness, irritability, confusion, insecurity, fatigue, and loss of physical control.

The analysis of a loss of mental powers is seen as a disharmony between the Spleen, which governs thought, and the Heart, which is in charge of the spirit and emotional control. This patent medicine, two doses of which should be taken daily on an empty stomach, is intended to strengthen and stabilize Spleen energy, tonify the Heart and Blood, and reestablish harmony between the two organ networks.

Energize Your Brain with Exercise

Studies with several groups—one performing aerobic exercise, one performing flexibility exercise, one sedentary—three hours a week for four months showed that cognitive ability improved dramatically in the aerobic exercise group. The stress hormone noradrenaline, secreted during exercise, is also responsible for increased brain stimulation. In addition, a nerve growth hormone is also secreted when we're physically active. Although we lose neurons daily, this hormone can influence further dendritic branching (the connections made between nerve cells). Since mind and body are one, the more you get the cells in your body moving, the more you get the cells in your mind moving as well.

Herbs for the Mind

Gingko biloba has been shown to increase alertness and reverse various types of mental problems resulting from stroke or cerebral impairment due to vascular changes. It has been shown to be effective in alleviating memory loss, confusion, dizziness, headache, ringing in the ears, and mood disturbances. Take 120 to 360 mg. of ginkgo leaf extract daily.

Gotu kola also increases intelligence and rejuvenates the nervous system. Take 100 mg. daily for several weeks, then pause for a week or two before repeating, if necessary.

Supplement Your Psyche

Zinc (30 to 50 mg. daily) supplements can be extremely helpful for memory and depression.

Practice Yoga

Standing on your head, or reversing your head-to-foot posture in the shoulder stand (lie on the floor and raise your legs, supporting your hips with your hands), is a great way to get the blood flowing where you need it.

CRANIOSACRAL THERAPY

see also Manipulation, page 288

This gentle, noninvasive form of bodywork grew out of the practice of osteopathy and became popular in the 1970s and 1980s. There are currently 26,000 physicians, massage therapists, physical therapists, and chiropractors who use this technique, which has been proven effective for depression, anxiety, dizziness, headaches of all varieties, and ADD and ADHD.

The craniosacral system consists of the membranes and cerebrospinal fluid that protect the brain and spinal cord. It starts at the top of the head and extends to the end of the tailbone. The membranes are moved by the gentle ebb and flow of the fluid, which, in optimum health, moves freely within a closed hydraulic system.

The point of this therapy is to release restrictions in the body by listening to the subtle rhythm of fluids in the cranium and soft tissue. The craniosacral system consists of the head and spinal cord; however, it is influenced by tissues, structures, and organs outside the system. A trained therapist can palpate the feet or shoulders and sense the ebb and flow of the bodily fluids. Although most individuals have ten cycles per minute during which the cranium fills with and empties of cerebrospinal fluid, there can be restrictions that block this rhythm. By using only five grams of force on various structures—from the cranial cavities to the fascia or connective tissue beneath the skin all over the body—the therapist can release the problem and reestablish a rhythmic pattern.

How Craniosacral Therapy Works on Emotional Problems

If we were punished at five by a bully who beat our back and shoulders, we may still hold tension there. Stubborn problems that may cause somatic dysfunction are known as "emotional encapsulations," or restrictions of energy that have been held since some particular trauma occurred, months or years ago. If we're walking around with hunched shoulders or a churning gut because we're sad or mad, our sympathetic nervous system is pitched high—we're always ready to combat stress. But with this type of therapy, we are aided in using our craniosacral rhythm to lock on to the parasympathetic nervous system, which calms and relaxes us.

Arcing is the process by which the therapist listens carefully to the body to pick up its ebb and flow and also to see where the rhythm comes to a halt—a moment when the central nervous system actually relaxes. This "still point," when the craniosacral rhythm briefly stops, is the body's natural way of processing conflict. It facilitates the release of transient anxieties and makes change, both physical and emotional, occur. A patient may come to a still point naturally, or the therapist can induce it by manipulating the various points on the cranium or spinal column.

This type of therapy can be used in conjunction with acupuncture, chiropractic, or bodywork like bioenergetics or Alexander technique.

DANCING

There's a line from a 1930s musical comedy that celebrates the notion of "dancin' your cares away," and this is one of the best explanations for the power of dance in mental health. Early man used dance, one of the oldest "therapies" in existence, as a cathartic ritual to purge his body and soul of evil demons. Up to the present day, shamans or wise men and women of native tribes use this technique to excise bad spirits from those who suffer pain and depression.

When you dance, you free yourself in time and space. Think of the whirling dervishes, the Hindu temple dancers, the spinning wonders of Scheherazade and Salome. The alternating states of calm and frenzy that can be achieved in a dance are a suitable palliative for a tortured mind. And as the mind latches on to the rhythmic beat of the music and the body heats up in an aerobic sweat, the brain starts sending healing endorphins throughout your system to make you feel better.

Dance therapy is a relatively new therapeutic field in mental health; however, there are a considerable number of practitioners who work with patients one on one and in group settings. This treatment has been very successful in mental hospitals, where patients may be on medication that has robbed them of the will to express themselves. Because dance often creates an altered state of consciousness, we can banish pain and stress within movement. Dance can lift these drugged, dulled patients out of their everyday tedium so that they can throw off their inhibitions and get to the heart of what's bothering them. Dance therapy is also wonderful for elderly individuals. It allows them to feel competent and beautiful as they stretch and breathe and clap in time to the music. It allows many alienated people to come together, since dance is often a social outlet.

On a far more basic scale, you can use dance as a therapeutic tool. It is excellent therapy for the blues, feeling sad and hopeless, and interestingly enough, it can be a real jolt to your system when you are feeling so fatigued you think you can't move. Like exercise, it triggers an exuberant rush of feelings that jogs you out of your black mood. You can be anything you want to be as you master movement—a wild pirate, a delicate princess, a hip street kid who has all the right "moves." Dance allows you to play with the elements of your problem as you stand at a distance from real life, whirling your head around, for example, to get rid of the tension of anxiety-provoking thoughts. The continual circles present in most dance forms are the most comforting structures in human architecture: There is never a beginning and end, but always an uptake as the circle widens, contracts, or turns back on itself.

You can dance alone or with a partner. If you're by yourself, select some music with a good range of dynamics, something that starts slowly and builds to a crescendo. Move the furniture out of the way and allow your body, hands, and feet to take over. To get rid of self-consciousness, you can imagine that you are being moved by a spirit inside you and that you have no control over your actions. Use your natural rhythms and let your body tell you what it wants to do. Don't try to think about steps or looking graceful or where you're going to go next. The framework of the piece of music you've picked will give you a starting and ending point.

If you decide to use dance therapy with a friend, you have a good range of possibilities: There are usually local clubs where you can folk dance, square dance, line dance, do hip-hop or more traditional ballroom dance. Dancing, a supremely social activity, is also a great way to meet people and interact with them intimately even when you don't know them.

Dance is a boon to the heart as well as the body and spirit. It allows us quite literally to be moved and to move others. It can restore the soul and lighten the burden of whatever unpleasantness you've been dealing with.

DEATH, THOUGHTS OF

see also Depression, page 112 Hopelessness, page 226

If you are in a serious depression, it is not uncommon to feel that you have nothing left to live for. It is also typical for old people who have lived a full life but are suffering with a terminal illness or a debilitating physical or mental dysfunction to dwell on thoughts of death. IF YOU ARE CONTEMPLATING SUICIDE, YOU SHOULD TALK TO A PROFESSIONAL BEFORE YOU DO ANYTHING.

What Happens When You Have Recurrent Thoughts of Death

You feel detached from everything and everyone around you, you give away possessions that no longer have meaning to you, you make plans for killing yourself or for writing suicide notes, you lose your desire to take part in any activity, you lose your fear of death and enjoy the idea of death or dying.

There is another manifestation of this symptom that seems to combine depression with impulse control. If your mind is filled with images of death—violent accidents or dead people or decomposing bodies—you may be "hooked" on death in the way that an obsessive person is driven to hand-washing. In one way, this type of death wish is a resolution—you may see yourself calmly lying in a casket with all troubles at an end. But even if you don't *feel* depressed, the repetitive thoughts about death should be dealt with and examined.

Talk to a Professional

If you have repeated fantasies about dying or being killed or killing yourself, it's imperative that you talk to a professional about your feelings. Generally in therapy it's easier to see that you are not really set on killing yourself, but rather, that your life has become intolerable and you feel powerless to fix it yourself.

Thinking and talking repeatedly about death is one way of saying to others that you want them to make your life better. Depending on the type of therapy you're in, the professional will counsel you to do certain daily exercises, perhaps to make appointments you must keep, perhaps to volunteer at a hospital or take up a partnered sport where you owe something to someone else.

Quiet Your Soul with Meditation

Until you can find the depths of the problems that haunt you, it is impossible to live with yourself. Sometimes only in the silence of a meditative session is it possible to turn off the cacophony of life and just *be* with yourself. There is no goal to meditation, nor should you be thinking about any particular topics. Rather, as you relax into deeper levels of feeling, you will be able gradually to make peace with yourself.

Life-Affirming Food

It's enormously important that you maintain excellent nutrition, although you will probably have lost all interest in eating and have little appetite for any particular foods. Stick with a natural diet high in carbohydrates for extra energy. The best combination of foods for you right now is vegetables, fruits, and grains, with plenty of pure spring water. Keep your protein and dairy low and avoid all junk food, caffeine, tobacco, and alcohol.

Get Up and Move

Some form of daily aerobic exercise is essential, even if you are chronically exhausted. The easiest and cheapest form of exercise is walking. Get up at the same time each day and do two brisk miles, which should take you about 25 or 30 minutes. (In areas where the weather is inclement, you can do your stint around a mall.) Make sure you pay attention to everything around you—houses, people, birds, signs—the evidence of life can give you back your will to live.

Take Melatonin Supplements

This supplemental dose of the neurotransmitter that defines light and dark in the human brain will help you sleep more soundly, which will help you wake in the morning feeling refreshed. It also triggers the increased production of serotonin, a companion neurotransmitter that gives us a sense of well-being. Take no more than 1 to 3 mg. daily.

Come Alive in Bed

Our sex drive is an instinctive motivation to keep us going, keep us vital, just like hunger, thirst, and avoidance of pain. If you have a partner and have been avoiding intimacy during your depression, have a talk with him or her about simple, noninvasive ways to return to some kind of touching. You don't have to have intercourse to be sexual, and at this time, a comforting back rub and gentle kisses are probably all you can tolerate.

If you don't have a partner, this is a good time to experiment with new ways to love yourself. Masturbation and treating your body well—with bubble baths, oils, creams, and different scents—can get you back to a good sense of yourself.

The Paws That Refreshes

Living with a pet can revive your spirits. In fact, it has been clinically proven that individuals who have the responsibility of taking care of an animal tend to take better care of themselves. In studies done in nursing homes and hospitals where pets are brought in once a week, it was found that the patients looked forward to that day and prepared for it, regardless of how sick or hopeless they felt. The effect is magnified, of course, if you have an ongoing relationship with the pet. The unconditional love you get from an animal and the stimulation you receive by stroking its fur is a calmant and actually lowers blood pressure and heart rate. Then there are the practical caretaking duties—you can't think about killing yourself if you have responsibility for a dog or cat.

If you currently live with an animal and are in a chronic depression, this is the time to spend more hours of the day grooming, walking, and talking to your pet.

Surround Yourself with Life-Loving People

Other people have felt the way you do, and other people may be the best spur to getting you back to life again. The best thing about joining a group is that you will have to give as well as receive. The affection, challenge, and sometimes the needling annoyances of others who will not simply let you lie down and die is not replicated in any other form of therapy. Call your local hospital or medical center for a suicide survivors' group or a general mental health group. You may also find help from regular groups of people with cancer or AIDS who may have considered suicide.

Depression

see also Bipolar Disorder, page 67; Blues, page 72; Broken Heart, page 78; Brooding, page 82; Death, thoughts of, page 109; Distraction, page 121; Eating Disorders, page 139; Escapism, page 142; Exhaustion, page 149; Fatigue, page 158; Gastrointestinal Disorders, page 189; Hopelessness, page 226; Impending Doom, feelings of, page 238; Lack of Self-confidence, page 268; Loneliness, page 277; Loss of Libido, page 280; Mood Swings, page 297; Numbness, page 313; Palpitations, page 342; Postpartum Depression, page 350; Sadness/Despondency, page 375; Sexual Dysfunctions, page 387; Sleep Disorders, page 404; Tearfulness, page 421

It's the rare individual who has never been depressed. Depression, whether acute or chronic, is a common twentieth-century phenomenon. Whether we say we feel down, blue, lonely, or just rotten, we've all experienced some form of depression at one time or another.

But there are those who have a great deal more than a few bad days a month. These people never see the glass as half full because they are miserable all the time. Never being able to have hope means that you have no reprieve, nothing to look forward to. This is chronic depression.

But short of misery lies a huge emotional terrain that is eminently treatable by natural therapies. One of the problems with using the treatments in this book is that you must have a will and desire to make them work, and one of the classic symptoms of depression is lack of will and desire. It is therefore a good idea to enlist the aid of a partner, friend, or relative who will participate in this program with you.

CASE HISTORY

Jennifer, now 41, was the oldest of seven children and always expected to do more and be more competent than her brothers and sisters. When she tried hardest, she was told she was good for nothing, and her father beat her often to show her how worthless she was.

She married a man who abused her mentally and physically. "I didn't care about myself—I helped him to get his drugs, allowing him to beat me even when I was six months pregnant. I was at the bottom, so depressed I didn't even think about my baby when I tried to commit suicide.

"Thank God, my best friend got me committed to a psychiatric ward in a local hospital. They medicated me, but the Xanax did nothing. I was still hooked on the man I'd married, still crying for him every night. I was so worried that he and the kids couldn't function without me.

"It was at some point after I got out of the hospital that I realized what an enabler I was, how much I needed to help people, because I was too depressed to help myself, I guess. About that time I met my Reiki teacher and learned how vital this power I held in my hands was, and how great it was that I could give it to others. So when my son started college, I went back to school; I signed up for a Medlab tech program. As I studied and met new people at school, I saw myself in a different light. I finally realized that there was plenty of joy around— I simply had to recognize it. I guess you'd call it a kind of spiritual rebirth, but it made me see that there are many alternatives to saying, I'm depressed, I want to kill myself. I think my feelings are totally different now from what they used to be—I see my life as pleasure seeking; and this pleasure touches not just me but everyone I'm around."

What is depression? It is a sense that the world is out of joint, and you yourself have lost all sense of balance and harmony. Like a massive dark haze that descends on your life, it distorts your impressions of events and people and makes body, mind, and soul numb and cold. You may feel dejected and sad most of the time, or you may swear that nothing is wrong. Some depressions manifest themselves in emotional despair, while others are masked in physical symptoms similar to those we get when very stressed out: Stomach aches, headaches, palpitations, and dizziness may all be signs of depression.

Approximately 15 million Americans feel depressed each year, although only 1.5 million seek treatment. The majority of depressions clear up by themselves within six to nine months with or without treatment. As time passes, it also heals.

It's important to diagnose depression accurately. If you are experiencing a variety of the following symptoms *on a regular basis,* you are depressed:

- lack of interest in activities and people
- sadness and pessimism about everything
- inability to enjoy yourself
- irritability
- difficulty concentrating
- changes in appetite, weight, and sleep patterns
- loss of libido
- indecisiveness

If the depression continues and worsens, the following symptoms may appear:

- lack of self-esteem, feeling unworthy
- exhaustion
- abandoning work and home responsibilities
- abandoning personal hygiene
- inability to communicate with others
- feelings of impending doom, utter hopelessness
- thoughts of death

Where Does Depression Come From?

There are a variety of causes, some physiological, some psychological, some social. There is a great deal of interesting speculation about the genetic causes of various psychiatric problems, depression being one of them; however, the research is still too young to credit as gospel.

PHYSIOLOGICAL CAUSES: Certain brain neurotransmitters may not be secreted in sufficient amounts to alleviate mood disorders. The chemicals serotonin, melatonin, and dopamine are the most important to our sense of well-being. When the nerves are robbed of these neurotransmitters, they can't send messages to other nerves, and depression results. (The opposite problem, having an abundance of neurotransmitter production, can cause hyperactivity and a manic state.)

It is well documented that neurochemical imbalances can occur in several members of the same family, which means that if your parent was severely depressed, you may be predisposed to develop a mood disorder. This does not mean that you are destined to inherit a mental illness; however, it does mean that you can take extra precautions—as you might eat and exercise more prudently if your father had died at a young age of a heart attack.

PSYCHOLOGICAL CAUSES: Our personalities greatly determine who we are and what we will make of the raw ingredients bequeathed to us through our DNA. A resilient individual who is abused in childhood may still grow up unscathed by depression, whereas a chronic worrier or dependent person may succumb to the smallest incidents that trigger a bout of feeling miserable and hopeless. The more often these bouts occur, the more likely a person is to believe he or she is unlucky or deserving of pain. If you think you should be depressed, chances are you will be.

SOCIAL CAUSES: An individual who may be predisposed to be depressed can sometimes rise above it. But it is far more likely that being abused, poor, neglected, or separated from loved ones will encourage an already burgeoning depression. It has been found, for example, that older women whose spouses have died and whose family has moved away often develop what is known as a "failure to thrive." When no one needs you and you have no one to nag you about your health or call you to see what your opinion of the weather is, you may, in fact, fall prey to depression, which can, in turn, exacerbate physical symptoms that can lead to illness or death.

There are several types of depression that may stem from either psychological or physiological causes or both. Depression can be unipolar, showing all the above-mentioned symptoms; or it can be bipolar, where the individual shows first a hopeless, helpless state and then one that is just the opposite. (See Bipolar Disorder, page 67.) Or a depression may be triggered by external circumstances, such as a change of seasons (see SAD, Seasonal Affective Disorder, page 373). Although the traditional treatments for depression involve medication, all of the manifestations of this syndrome can respond well to natural therapies if you are persistent and motivated to let them work.

Depression in children can be even more difficult to recognize and treat than in adults because it is often masked as difficult childhood behavior that falls within the acceptable range—having tantrums or crying jags, for example. A hyperactive or attention deficit problem may be a symptom of depression. If your child is persistently withdrawn, lacking confidence, not eating or sleeping or socializing properly, it may be a good idea to consult a professional for an evaluation.

Following are some of the most successful treatments for depression. Depending on your particular symptoms (see above), you'll want to turn to the following pages and consider implementing some of these natural therapies.

Treatments to try: Bach Flower Remedies, page 53; Breathing, page 76; Herbs, page 216; Homeopathy, page 221; Exercise, page 145; Nutrition, page 316; Supplementation, page 409; Meditation, page 292; Melatonin, page 294; Mindfulness, page 296; Prayer, page 358; Light Therapy, page 273; Cognitive Therapy, page 94; Self-hypnosis, page 383; Tai Chi Chuan, page 417; Visualization, page 442; Yoga, page 457

DESENSITIZATION

This behavioral approach is considered the gold standard of treatment for obsessive-compulsive behavior and phobias. There's a wonderful success rate; as many as 60 to 80 percent of patients recover or see great improvement five years after diagnosis. Early diagnosis is the key—many individuals are simply branded as "depressed," and appropriate therapy is delayed.

The focus of the therapy is to bombard the mind and emotions with the very object of hatred, fear, or revulsion they have been trying to avoid. It is, in a sense, "repetition" therapy. If you're terrified of dogs, for example, you must sensitize yourself to photos of dogs, sounds of dogs barking, a trip to someone's house where you can see a dog through a window, and so forth, using more potent stimuli as the lesser ones become tolerable.

Using your powers of visualization, you will mentally bring the dog closer and closer until you are finally standing beside him, about to pet his head. You must not only think about the animal, but at the same time practice relaxing your body as you focus on the object of your fear. Keep checking back to be sure you aren't holding your breath, clenching your jaw, or tightening your stomach or shoulders. You can do a quick body scan every few minutes, telling yourself, "Breathe! Relax your feet, relax your calves, relax your thighs," and so on, up to your head.

When you are able to accomplish the mental exercises without feeling very anxious, you can proceed to an actual exposure to the object of your fear. You would first visit a dog who is crated in someone's home, then, when you found that tolerable, you might visit a dog who is leashed and kept far from you.

The key to success is constant repetition, overcoming the anxiety and working in stepwise order from least offensive to more offensive stimuli. You wouldn't have to touch a dog or play with him, for example, if you couldn't tolerate the picture of the dog.

It's a good idea to make yourself a personal chart during or after each session, to get a sense of your progress. The first time you are confronted with pictures of dogs, your anxiety level might be up at 10, the most uncomfortable level. After your session, when you are lying comfortably on your back, just breathing and relaxing, your anxiety level might be down to 0. Grade yourself from 0 to 10 each time you tackle your phobia and see how you progress from month to month. It's also a good idea to keep a diary about ways in which you see your feelings changing over time. What were the triggers for your fear originally and how are you managing them differently now?

A behavioral therapist should be consulted as to the course of action in very severe cases, particularly if the phobic or obsessive-compulsive behavior has been going on unchecked for a period of years.

DISTORTED BODY IMAGE

see also Body Dysmorphic Disorder, page 74; Obsessive/Compulsive Disorder, page 329

There are people who are convinced that they are too repulsive to be looked at by anyone else. They are sure that the hairs in their nose, the shape of their hands, or some other feature is so distorted out of proportion that they would be judged as freaks. According to research by Dr. Katherine Phillips, a psychiatrist at Harvard Medical School, the number of sufferers is small (roughly 2 to 10 percent of the population). But as Dr. Phillips reported in the September, 1991 issue of the *American Journal of Psychiatry*, the effects on those who do consider themselves deformed is devastating.

What Happens When You Have a Distorted Body Image

You feel excessive distress over the way you look, you have a compulsion to check or correct the feature that disturbs you, you are unable to engage in regular social events—even go to work—because of your perceived ugliness. You may develop ornate rituals in order to cope with this problem. If your obsession escalates, you may feel that the only option is suicide.

Those who suffer from this disorder will do anything to "fix" the problem, including pulling out facial hairs that they feel are unsightly, wearing uncomfortable belts to cinch in what they feel is a huge waistline, wearing plastic bags on their thighs as they exercise to exhaustion to diminish what they see as grotesque thighs or having cosmetic surgery to correct what they see as a gigantic nose or ugly cheekbones.

Depression usually accompanies BDD (body dysmorphic disorder), as does a disruption of serotonin production in the brain. Many sufferers were sexually or physically abused as children and are stuck with an old belief system about the way they look.

Counseling, Not Coddling

It is important to get into therapy with a professional who understands this disorder, which is very often misdiagnosed.

It's not useful to spend many sessions trying to cure you of your acute dissatisfaction with your body, when in fact the goal of therapy should be to help you adjust your view about what your body really looks like. Photography can often be helpful here—the therapist might spend some time taking pictures and having you compare them to photos of other people who have what you consider "normal" bodies.

Cognitive therapy is not necessarily helpful (although it is for many other types of obsessive/compulsive behavior) if you truly believe that your nose, hair, thighs, body, and so forth, are deformed. However, behavioral therapy might be a way to deal with getting out of rituals and getting back to real life.

Switching Behavior

Let us assume that the feature you fear is your nose. A behavioral technique for working on BDD might include removing or covering all mirrors in your house and office so that you can't examine the offending feature. Give yourself a reward each time you go out into the world to deal with a social event and an additional reward if you manage to avoid mirrors for the time that you're out and about. If you routinely try to cover your face with your hair, you might experiment with wearing a hat or wearing your hair back for increasing lengths of time, working up from one hour to several hours a day.

Relax Progressively

The dread and anxiety of confronting people in a body you consider to be grotesque can be reduced and even obliterated if you use progressive relaxation.

Lie on the floor in a quiet, dimly lit room and allow your arms and legs to fall loosely open. Beginning with your toes, give your body parts in turn the order to first tense and then relax. Work very slowly, and be sure you cover the toes, feet, calves, thighs, pelvis, hips, lower spine, ribs, middle spine, shoulders, upper arms, forearms, hands, wrists, fingers, neck, ears, top of the spine, and head.

As you feel the tension drain from one body part, congratulate yourself and repeat, "I am comfortable in my body. My body is the source of these good feelings." By the time you have completed the entire toe-to-head adjustment, your breathing should be relaxed and your attitude uplifted.

Remedy the Situation

Homeopathic help for BDD would include

> For tormenting thoughts: Natrum mur, Arsenicum alcum, Causticum, Lachesis, Sulphur

> For lack of confidence: Anacardium, Aurum, China, Kali carbonicum, Lycopodium, Natrum mur, Pulsatilla

Flower Power

The Bach flower remedy for those who are hard on themselves and completely self-denying is Rock Water.

Pray for a Change

There is nothing you can do about the body you were given, and it's clear from many case histories that people with BDD are dissatisfied with plastic surgery. It is only when you can put yourself in the hands of a higher power and understand that you are accepted for who and what you are no matter what you look like that you can accept yourself. You don't have to be religious or observant to abolish feelings of rejection by concentrating in prayer on everything that's inside you, rather than what shows to the outside world. After all, when we give ourselves up to a spirit or force that is beyond our knowing, we do not go as bodies but as souls. This awareness can provide a surety and self-confidence unavailable anywhere else.

Find a New Image in Feldenkrais

This nonjudgemental body therapy is used to give people a sense of their own structure and movement. It is often used for individuals who have trouble perceiving what they really look like. A Feldenkrais practitioner would have you lie on the floor and direct you to use one body part—for example, the leg and hip—in a variety of different movements. You are never told that what you are doing is wrong or right, and only you can determine when you feel comfortable in the movement.

By learning what you do to hold tension and how you can release it, you gain a different and much more positive regard for your body.

Distraction

see also Confusion, mental, page 100; Lack of concentration, page 265

If you're unable to think about any one thing because you keep being redirected by something—anything—that attracts your attention, you are distracted. Typically, distraction comes from outside stimulation, whereas lack of concentration is an internal problem and stems from an inability to keep on track with one thought among many.

▧ What Happens When You're Distracted

You appear to be elsewhere; your focus and attention level are worse than that of a two-year-old. You sit down to read a book, and your eyes flutter up if you hear a song you like on the radio. You may be sitting and talking to a dear friend, but then the door opens and your gaze is suddenly riveted on the person who just walked in. You may tap a pencil or your foot. You may find it hard to complete any one chore and have difficulty falling asleep, because thoughts float in and out of your head like butterflies you can't catch. You may feel bored a good deal of the time, because everything and nothing grab your attention at the same time. You are guilty of polyphasic thinking, or "monkey mind," when you attempt to juggle dozens of thoughts at the same time and manage to drop all of them at once.

Distraction is a key symptom of stress. It's generally an emotional reaction to overload, which is why one of the best ways to beat distraction is to learn to calm down and concentrate on one thing at a time. When the emotions race, the body tries to keep up, and this can lead to an uncomfortable jittery feeling.

Very often, depressed people are distracted as well. It's as if concentrating on the problem is too difficult, so the mind jumps around like a monkey, attempting to light on a viable surface but finding something a little off in each one. When you are always distracted, you are always on the go, hard to pin down, a moving target for grief, fear, or depression. But when you finally persevere and settle down so that the outside world can't disturb your inner peace, you can hold onto one thought, and the clarity and vision that you let in can be truly revelatory.

Focus Your Mind

The best way to calm distraction is to concentrate on one thing—your breath or a sound such as "om" or "peace." Sit quietly and begin to pay more attention to your breath. Other thoughts and feelings will crowd inside your mind; just allow them to pass through, as though you were on a train, watching the scenery go by. Breathe fully from your belly, imagining the breath coursing through you, up your back and down your front. Take air in, let air out—these necessities are all you need as you meditate.

Mindful Practice Will Restore You

Mindfulness meditation uses the everyday world to keep you on track. Select one activity, for example, putting on your gloves. Don't do this in the privacy of your bedroom; rather, select a crowded busy setting where you are likely to be distracted. Take one glove at a time from your pocket; compare the two. Look at the arrangement of fingers, turn the glove over and inside out to see how it changes. Rub the fabric on your hand or face and close your eyes to imagine the sensation of this cloth over your fingers. Now gently insert one finger at a time into the first glove. You may need to back out a few times so as to line up the angle of the finger and the fabric. Once the fingers are in place, pull the glove down over your palm, watching the distinct lines in your hand vanish as you cover them slowly. Bring the glove down over your wrist and notice the line of demarcation, where skin meets glove. Repeat the exercise on the other hand.

You will find that the sounds and sights of other people will interrupt the progress of mindfulness. Don't worry about it. Just keep drawing your mind back to the gloves. The more often you do this, the easier it will be to complete the task without being distracted.

A Calming Cup of Tea

Herbs in the form of an infusion can be used as a tonic that will nourish and support every system in the body including the brain and nervous system. You can also use a prepared tincture or take a soothing bath with a handful of herbs thrown in. The following herbs will help to alleviate distraction: betony, California poppy, cowslip, ladyslipper, lobelia, and scullcap. Take 2 to 4 teaspoons dried herb infused in a cup of water three times daily, or $1/2$ teaspoon of tincture.

Homeopathic Help

Homeopathic remedies for distraction are

For restlessness: Arsenicum album

If you jump from one topic to another, and it's hard to concentrate: Ambra grisea

For rushing thoughts: Belladonna, Lachesis, Phosphorus, Arsenicum album, Ignatia, Kali carbonicum, Nux vomica

North Pole Now

Magnetism normalizes the balance between acidic and alkaline conditions of your body fluids. North pole magnetic energy reduces hydrogenion concentration and helps with maladaptive states. A half hour with a 2,000–gauss strip magnet at your head will relax muscles and calm you down, making it easier for you to concentrate. (See Resource Guide, page 475, for access to magnetic therapy.)

Learn From the Wisdom of the East

The Indian system of traditional medicine, Ayurveda, would see distraction as a *vata* imbalance. Vata dosha affects the nervous system, and since it is governed by the elements of air and space, it lends a feeling of ungroundedness. If you have a problem with vata, you may be unable to stick with one thing at a time.

In order to balance vata, it is important to adhere to a regular schedule for eating, exercising, and sleeping. Starting the day with a warm meal, such as hot cereal, accompanied by warm herb tea will calm you but give you the strength you need for later. A good diet for this type of problem should include warm foods, salt, sour, and sweet tastes, and added butter or fat. You can include lots of hearty soups and stews, seven-grain breads, and fruit pies. Remember that you need to eat this food in a setting that will comfort and support you—never eat on the run or standing up.

Avoid all stimulants, such as alcohol, caffeine, and nicotine. Don't eat cold foods, such as salads and raw fruits, which tend to aggravate vata. If you feel a craving for sugar, make sure you combine the sweet with a glass of milk or herb tea. A wonderful drink to balance vata is called *lassi*. Whip together half a cup of plain yogurt and half a cup of water. Add a pinch of powdered ginger, salt, or cumin. You can sweeten it by adding half again as much mango pulp.

Try not to get overstimulated. Television is one of the banes of a vata existence, as are violent movies. Long, hot baths and a sesame-oil massage are particularly beneficial for the vata dosha.

Loving Touch Can Focus You

Your sexuality is a precious asset that can block external distractions. When we feel the pull of desire for another person, we are often able to zero in on what's really important and make the rest of the world go away. If you have a partner with whom you share intimate moments, explain that you would like to experiment with sexuality as a therapeutic tool. You can create any distractions you'd like—an overhead fan whirring, a TV show blaring, a radio talk show taking calls. You will allow your partner to stimulate you as you absorb the loving touch without having to respond. (Later, you'll switch so that you give attention and your partner receives.)

Every time you feel your focus leaving your partner, raise your hand or give some other sign that you need extra attention. As you become more wrapped up in the experience, completely present with the person who is attending to you, you'll find that it's easier to stay in the moment and not be distracted.

DIZZINESS

see also Anxiety, page 43; Stress, page 407

There are dozens of possible explanations for feeling dizzy. Sometimes we get up too fast and feel as if the bottom is dropping out of the world; sometimes we stand at the top of a tall mountain and look down and feel everything spinning; sometimes we see a person we are crazy about or can't stand and think we're going to pass out.

Dizziness, or vertigo, may have physical or emotional causes. You can get dizzy if you haven't eaten in a few hours, or if you've taken cold medication, or if you have a sluggish thyroid gland. Dizziness is often related to the onset of a migraine headache; it's also a sign of an ear infection or an inner-ear fluid imbalance. If you have taken antidepressant medications, you may recognize dizziness as a typical side-effect. It's also a response of the vagus nerve, which connects the brain and the heart; this is the cause of orthostatic hypotension, or that feeling that you're about to black out when you get up too quickly.

But when coupled with a particularly stressful or exciting event, dizziness is probably due to stress, which produces physical symptoms. When our sympathetic nervous system gives a message to the adrenals to pour out the stress hormones adrenaline, noradrenaline, and cortisol, we are flooded with endocrine messages that often send the body into a tailspin.

▤ *What Happens When You Get Dizzy*

You feel out of control, swept away, as though you no longer connect with gravity. Instead of seeing the world as having vertical and horizontal axes, you have a feeling that everything is going around. There's a certain vulnerability about dizziness (the delicate ladies in old novels are always swooning) and a sense that you've given yourself to forces beyond your control. You may feel as if you're going to fall down, or you may feel that you're about to lose consciousness. Dizziness doesn't always lead to fainting, however.

When dizziness has no somatic cause, it is almost always a symptom of some anxiety disorder. You become upset or distressed, your breathing becomes shallow, and you aren't getting enough oxygen to your brain. As your stress hormone level rises, your body is unable to compensate. You feel fearful and nervous and develop sweaty palms, a racing heartbeat, a knot in your stomach, and often the sense that you have lost touch with the ground you stand on. To be dizzy is to be uncentered, no longer grounded.

Take a Breath

One reason you're dizzy is because you aren't taking full breaths. This is the first thing you should correct when you sense a wave of vertigo coming on.

Herbal Tonics Will Fix You Up

A variety of nervine tonics are recommended to alleviate dizziness and to nourish your system. In order to calm down and relax, you can take motherwort, pasque flower, or St. John's wort. You might also try the antispasmodics scullcap or valerian. Gingko biloba improves blood flow to the brain and is an excellent remedy for vertigo. Take 1/2 to 1 teaspoon dried herb infused in water three times daily, or 1/2 teaspoon of tincture three times daily.

Close Your Eyes

Although the conventional wisdom for dizziness is to sit down and put your head between your legs, it's more important to close your eyes. If you continue to look at the world around you, the distraction of seeing it turn will increase your anxiety. Better to sit or lie down with your eyes shut so as to keep your focus inside instead of outside.

Hold Onto Your Hat

Sometimes just holding onto something—a piece of your clothing, a chair back, or a friend's hand—will restore your feeling of security and calm. Touching something else is important because it reminds us that we are not alone, not floating in some void, but rather, connected to others and to the universe itself.

A Chinese Fainting Remedy

If you think you're going to pass out, press G.V. 26, the point right below the center of your nose, in between the nostrils.

Practice Tai Chi

The ancient Chinese martial art is also a healthful moving meditation that can get you back on your feet. Tai chi encourages you to root in the ground like a tree. Your legs are bent, your posture is upright, and you cannot fall down because, as the Chinese classics say, "You are suspended from above." You should have the feeling of a marionette anchored by the string on top of its head.

In a recent NIH study designed to figure out the best way to improve the degree of movement in frail elderly individuals (the FICSIT study), tai chi was deemed an effective therapy. It increases the limits of stability and balance, boosts self-confidence, and increases both physical and mental awareness.

When a wave of dizziness hits you, place your feet shoulder width apart and hold your arms in front of you as though you were holding a big beach ball. Release your legs so that the knees are slightly bent. Inhale and exhale, imagining your feet growing larger and sinking into the earth. Focus your eyes directly in front of you on one unmoving spot. This "tree" pose will give you back your composure as well as your sense of balance.

DREAM ANALYSIS

For centuries, we have looked to the unconscious mind for the key to what ails us. When we're awake, we often block out the causes of our depression or anxiety because they're too painful, but in sleep, we allow ourselves the freedom to investigate what's really going on inside.

Dreams and nightmares occur during REM (rapid eye movement) sleep, the active stage of sleep following the deepest periods (Stage III and Stage IV) of non-REM sleep. When we dream, the body uses more oxygen, there is more blood flow to the brain, and body temperature rises. Brain waves are busy doing a combination of waking and sleeping patterns. In REM states, your eyes dance from side to side, either "watching" what's going on in the dream or simply moving as the brain becomes active. During this stage, the mind indulges in irrational, disconnected thinking, and the dreamer is able to create his or her own reality without being concerned about whether it "makes sense."

If we think back to childhood and our reluctance to go to sleep until our parents had checked for monsters under the bed, we can see potent symbols emerging. Our adult mon-sters—the feelings we've hidden inside us—don't reside only in our imagination. In fact, the closer we get to our dream state, the more real we can make the obsessions, worries, compulsions, and fears that may bother us.

Nightmares permit us to take that terrifying voyage into the realm of darkness we dare not penetrate when we're awake. A nightmare reflects the internal conflicts we are try-ing to work out and so provides the code to our mental and emotional problems. All we have to do is crack the code, and we open ourselves up to a new type of self-awareness that can be extremely useful in therapy, but also in everyday life, even if we're not talking to a professional about our problems.

It's important to remember that although symbols are con-venient messages we can easily interpret, they vary from person to person. One woman may dream about a tall, bare mountain-top because she's overwhelmed with sexual desire; another may dream about the same image because of a trip she took last fall. So be careful when you start to interpret your dreams that you make sense of them for yourself and for no one else.

■ *How to Remember Your Dreams*

Before you go to sleep at night, put a pad and pen on your bedside table. Tell yourself you are going to remember your dreams. (This suggestion may take a few nights to penetrate.) As you relax in bed, give yourself permission to explore all the areas of your mind that you don't pay enough attention to during the day.

We tend to be in REM sleep just before waking, so it's best to set your radio alarm to a soft music station rather than to the news or hard rock. This way, you can wake slowly and take stock of what's going on in your mind.

How to Interpret Your Dreams

First, begin to collect the images and characters you remember. Some experts feel that we represent every person we see in our dreams. Even if we populate our dreams with people we know, the fact that we're thinking about them means that they represent a part of us. If you have just a piece of a scene that's remained in your mind, write it down. Just the suggestion of "staircase in a theater," for example, may jog other pieces of your memory—who was coming down the staircase and what that person was doing there.

Next, try to recapture the activities that went on in your dream—building a house, taking a trip, falling down a hole, and so forth.

Finally, what feeling does this dream give you? Are you happy, scared, frustrated, rushed? Is this feeling similar to a feeling you've had when you're awake? What would you like to change about the dream? Can you go back and have a dialogue with one of the characters to alter his or her role slightly? Can you ask the person questions about events or images that are still cloudy for you? Ask yourself what waking event most closely resembles something in this dream. Sometimes, by consciously delving deeper into the material you have laid down in your unconscious, you can get a handle on problems that have eluded you until now.

Using Dream Analysis as Therapy

In therapeutic settings, there are proven ways to use dream material to open new avenues of healing. Here's an example of how this type of analysis can help:

CASE HISTORY

James had never had a problem with a supervisor until Nancy took over his division and he was put on a new project he didn't know much about. Nancy was a domineering boss who made him feel inadequate and insecure. He was always certain he was being watched, that he was about to lose his job. His hostility toward Nancy spilled out onto his home life, and he withdrew from his wife and kids. James began having a series of dreams that pinpointed where he was going with his personal problems.

"One night I dreamed that I was staying at a motel and the manager asked since I was alone if I'd mind if he put a big double bass that he was storing for some musician in the room. I had to climb over the thing to get to the bathroom, and in the middle of the night, it fell down next to me in bed, nearly chopping my head off.

"I realized as I woke up how much bigger Nancy seems than she really is— I must be four inches taller, but she makes me feel like a dwarf. She is pretty voluptuous, though. I guess you could say the shape of the double bass is like a woman, so that must be Nancy. Also, the idea of music is supposed to be harmonious. But here, the instrument didn't play—as a matter of fact, it nearly killed me.

"I couldn't figure out the motel at first, but then it occurred to me that a motel is really a transitional home—and ever since I started this project, I've felt as if I'm going to have to move on if I fail. Maybe the double bass isn't my boss; maybe it's the obstacles I put in my path as I'm trying to deal with her. I guess it's up to me to stop imagining the worst and just deal with what's there. The dream helped me to see that."

DROWSINESS/EXCESSIVE SLEEPING

see also Depression, page 112; Sleep Disorders, page 404

If you find yourself nodding off during the day, or you cannot wake up in the morning, you are having some imbalance in your sleep/wake cycle that may have physiological or emotional causes or both. Narcolepsy, the condition where you may drop off at any time—behind the wheel of your car or even while you're having a conversation—is an extreme disruption of brain wave patterns that must be observed and treated in a sleep laboratory.

But most people who feel drowsy much of the time are fighting an emotional problem. One classic way to escape fears or unpleasantness is to "close our eyes" to reality. In other words, sleep can be a way out of dealing with the difficulties around us. But we may not be getting the type of sleep—the deeper levels of Stage III and Stage IV sleep that revive and restore us. And this is why daytime drowsiness can become a problem.

Since, typically, we sleep less the older we get, hypersomnia, or sleeping too much, is usually an indication that something is eating at us that we don't want to acknowledge.

What Happens When You're Frequently Drowsy or Sleeping Too Much

It's difficult to rouse yourself to do any activity, even your work, or to mix well with others. Your intellectual and sex lives suffer because you can't muster the energy for either. You don't confront problems you might have in your relationships or personal life because it's too exhausting. Consequently, you sleepwalk through life, not really letting it touch you.

You should see a physician to rule out somatic problems such as thyroid disorders or epilepsy before you decide that your drowsiness is connected to emotional disorders. You should also investigate the possibility that you are sleeping a lot because you are depressed, and therefore you should treat the depression (see Depression, page 112). If you are fairly certain, however, that you have no physical illness that is causing the symptom, you may try the therapies listed below.

Talk to Yourself

Tape recording messages to yourself can be a way of working with this problem. Write a dialogue in which you ask yourself questions about your sleep/wake habits and leave spaces so that you have to answer them on the spot. The questions should be provocative, giving you no avenue for escape. Each time you do the exercise, you'll have to come up with new answers to your taped questions. And dealing with that probing voice (your own) and significant questions may wake you up to the truth.

Try a Little Eye Pressure

Acupressure points on the eyes and neck are good stimulis for staying awake. Do the following exercise when you feel drowsy:

- Overlap the second and third fingers of each hand on two points on the inner upper edge of the eye socket. Hold for three seconds, let go, and then repeat.

- Using all four fingers of each hand, circle the eye sockets on the upper and lower lids. Press top and bottom for three seconds each, let go, and then repeat.

- Place your index fingers on your temple at the joint that moves when you press your teeth together. Line up your other fingers next to it (going toward the eye socket). Press hardest on the point next to your eye for three seconds, let go, then repeat.

- Apply pressure to the point behind the earlobe and just below the part of the skull that projects behind the ear. Repeat twice.

- Place both palms over the eyes for ten seconds, feeling the warmth penetrate. Remove hands quickly.

You can also press the acupoint known as L.I. 10, (see acupressure chart, p. 10), on the top of the forearm, on the thumb side. Cross your arms and put your thumbs in the hollow formed by the two muscles, about two inches down from the crease of the elbow.

Yoga Will Stimulate Your Senses

Various yoga exercises will wake you up. Do these first thing in the morning as you get out of bed.

Lie down and bend your right knee, placing the foot beside your outstretched left leg. Slowly raise the left leg with the foot flexed until it is perpendicular to the floor, then slowly lower it on a count of four, but don't let it touch the floor. Repeat four times, touching down the last time. Then place the toes of your right foot under the left knee and allow the bent right leg to cross over the left. Try to touch the floor with it. Switch legs and repeat on the other side.

Then sit up and cross your legs in front of you. Stretch your arms up to heaven, extending your fingers. Open your mouth like a lion and stick your tongue out (this may make you yawn). Repeat three times.

Turn on the Lights

If you're constantly in danger of dropping off, be sure you work and play in a well-lit place. Keep all the lights on until you're really ready for sleep.

Keep your window shades up so that the morning light can wake you naturally.

Make a Sleep Schedule

All experts agree that many sleep problems are caused by poor sleep hygiene. You should make every attempt to keep your bedtime and wake time hours regular, even on weekends. Set yourself a limit of eight hours sleep each night. Get into bed about ten or ten-thirty and set your alarm for no later than seven A.M. Don't nap, even if you're exhausted. Instead, drink a glass of water or take a walk around the block. You want to be awake when it's daylight and sleeping at night.

Get Your Body Working

Exercise improves sleep patterns whether you sleep too much or too little. When you work out daily, you produce neuro-transmitters that bathe the brain with chemicals that make you feel alert and refreshed.

Don't start training for a marathon or working out on the Nautilus for three hours at a stretch—that type of killer program will knock you out, and may make you feel as though your sleep is never sufficient to restore you for the next day's work. But moderate exercise will do just the opposite. A brisk walk or a half hour of tai chi or dancing a couple of hours before bed or right after you get up in the morning will give you an appropriate mix of stimulation and relaxation.

Check Out Your Medicine Cabinet

Be aware that over-the-counter medicines for colds and flu or those you might take if you were stung by an insect contain ingredients that make you sleepy. Read all prescription labels and particularly avoid those that caution you not to work with heavy machinery.

Wash Your Face

Splashing your face with cold water or taking a shower and then switching the water to cold to rinse your hair is a sure-fire way to wake up.

Watch Out for Stimulants

Although coffee, caffeinic teas, and cocoa are stimulating, they may make you jumpy and on edge. You might want to try panax ginseng or gotu kola, stimulant teas that do not contain caffeine.

Good Indian Medicine

Ayurvedic principles say that you may have a kapha disorder—this particular dosha or personality type is often heavy and sleepy. You may also find that you are depressed and feel logy, almost in a stupor. It's hard for you to change your habits, and you procrastinate about doing both essential and inconsequential things.

An overabundance of kapha can be helped by getting more stimulation in every part of your life. You can use more exercise (which will help you with weight control), and more of a meditative practice that will engage you and draw you into life instead of away from it. You should make sure you don't overeat (kaphas tend to be heavy), and to take your evening meal early, which will give you plenty of time to digest it before bed. Cut down on all refined sugars and fats in the diet. Foods should be light but stimulating—the spicier the better. You should eat hot rather than cold foods. Hot ginger tea will clean out your system and make you less sluggish. Dry massage (without oil, using raw silk gloves or a loofah sponge) is a good way to wake up your system.

DRUG REHABILITATION

If you are taking mind-altering substances on a regular basis, you are "out of your mind." There is no possible way that you can face your problems head-on when your brain isn't functioning normally. This goes for any and all medications—you can find yourself disoriented and irritable from taking over-the-counter antihistamines, prescription antidepressants, or recreational marijuana and cocaine.

Drugs are not all bad, and not all drugs are bad all the time. Obviously, when you need medication to alleviate symptoms of a disease it's crucial that you take your pills. But then, once the physical problem has been taken care of, you should eliminate the drugs. Pain killers, for example, are very useful after you've broken your leg and can't function because of the throbbing and agony, but after several days it's better to eliminate the haze and confusion codeine may cause. It's actually dangerous to feel a little bit well, hobbling around in a pharmaceutical fog. You could easily reinjure yourself.

The most beneficial drugs can poison in the wrong amount or in the wrong administration. And nearly every medication has side-effects, from dizziness and palpitations to dry mouth to constipation or diarrhea (or both) to sexual dysfunction to mood changes. Often, if you take a drug beyond the period of time when you need it, it may cause the very symptoms you've been trying to eliminate or may bring on new ones. Beware of the renewable prescription—you may have been prescribed Valium when your father died, and you renewed the prescription, thinking the grief still needed to be anesthetized. But if you didn't use the whole bottle and it sat in your medicine chest for a year, it can be a ticking time bomb. If you run into a crisis, you may feel the need to drug yourself to "get through" it.

It is always easier to take an aspirin than to sit and meditate on the cause of your tension headache (even sinus headaches can be helped with meditation in addition to medication). Until we decide that we aren't going to try a quick fix for our emotional pain, we will continue to drink alcohol, smoke a cigarette or a joint, or pop a Prozac.

How do you know you're addicted? If you cannot get through an hour without a cigarette, if you have more than five drinks on five occasions over a 30-day period, if you consume some type of legal prescription drug when you have no medical reason for taking it, if you consume an illegal, recreational drug three times a week, then you have a problem.

▓ How Rehabilitation Works

Evidently, there are different strategies that must be used for different dependencies: A heroin addict needs methadone and counseling and probably a restricted environment in which to recover; an alcoholic may need daily meetings, a counselor he can always contact by phone, and a change of friends and environment (not hanging out in smoky bars).

Rehabilitation starts in the mind, with a commitment to change (see Behavioral therapy, page 55). If you are getting off drugs because others have begged you to get rid of your bad habit, it most certainly won't take. You have to want to stop, or in the case of hard-core addicts who may be robbing or even killing to get their drugs, you have to be coerced into a setting where you will be unable to obtain drugs long enough to develop a motivation of your own.

Different interventions are needed to keep the commitment fresh. Think about the rewards a cigarette brings a smoker: You have something to hold in your hand (like a security blanket); you have a strong stimulus in your nose, mouth, and lungs; and you have an instant stress reduction when the nicotine hits your brain. If you are trying to quit smoking, you have to compensate for the loss of all those pleasant experiences. When you're attempting to cut out cigarettes, you need something good for your hands, for your respiratory system, and for your brain. You also need a lot of emotional support—from a therapist, friend, or family member—to remind you that what you're doing isn't easy, but you have to do it, period.

There are several approaches to drug rehabilitation. The first is stopping cold turkey. These addicts are put on notice that the substance is killing them and they have to stop at once to save their life. This technique is used with drug addicts in prisons and institutions and with alcoholics and other substance abusers in the various 12-step programs, like Alcoholics Anonymous. The second approach, generally used in smoking-cessation programs, weans the addict off the substance slowly, substituting different interventions and setting a "quit date" at some point in the future. A third approach, used with programs for overeaters—since you can't stop eating food—takes the perspective that you must learn to handle the addiction, not the substance you're addicted to.

Any of these approaches works if you work them. Constant vigilance and attention to relapse is needed if you're going to rehabilitate yourself. But using various natural therapies such as meditation, exercise, and nutritional support can keep you on track as you learn to live clean and sober.

EATING DISORDERS

see also Anorexia Nervosa, page 34; Bingeing, page 59; Bulemia, page 84;
Overeating, page 331; and Weight Gain or Loss, page 449

There *are* societies where individuals aren't worried about their weight, but they are few and far between. Typically, in countries where there is abundance, the ideal is to be incredibly thin; in countries where people have little to eat, the ideal is to be big and fat. Why can't we all have an ideal that falls somewhere in the middle?

The American fixation with looks and weight is pathological. Girls as young as seven or eight worry that their bodies are ugly, and fat children are teased more unmercifully than handicapped kids. By the time girls reach puberty, up to 75 percent admit having gone on diets to lose weight.

Eating disorders take several forms: Some individuals consume huge amounts of food without a thought to whether they are stuffed; others eat to the point of bursting—sometimes of one particular food and sometimes of all foods—and then purge themselves of it by vomiting or using laxatives; some eat next to nothing. All of these patterns are terribly dangerous to the fluid and electrolyte balance of the body and can compromise the bones, liver, kidneys, and heart.

One urgent question to ask is why girls are affected by this illness so much more frequently than boys. We go back to the old gender stereotypes: Little boys are encouraged to be active and seek out the world; little girls are supported for being "pretty" and compliant. There are increasing numbers of male cases of eating disorders, but the incidence of this problem in girls is ten times that of their male counterparts.

But what is the real reason that girls behave so bizarrely around the issue of eating and food? Food is often a substitute for love, and nourishment is something we can deny ourselves if we feel unlovable. Many girls are convinced that they can do well in school, please their parents, attract a boy, and be socially acceptable only if they are "perfect." The two most typical ages for the onset of eating disorders are 14 and 18—when a girl first enters high school and when she goes out on her own to college or a job. But herein lies the biggest problem with eating disorders—dieting, purging, and wearing plastic bags on your thighs while you jog do not guarantee happiness. They cannot make you or your life perfect. Girls with eating disorders typically have very low self-esteem and feel ineffective and impotent in the world. They have a hard time with criticism and, in fact, read almost every comment as an intentional slap in the face. They generally come from close families who may be very overprotective although uninvolved in their daughter's day-to-day life. Often these families are quite dysfunctional, codependent on one another to maintain certain abnormal or harmful practices and denying that anything is wrong. Sexual abuse is often a concurrent problem, particularly with bulimics (who eat massive quantities of food and then purge). In such a restricted environment, normal adolescent rebellion can't take place. Many girls in this type of setting figure the only thing they can control is their own body—and control it they do, right down to starvation or obesity.

Many girls with eating disorders have mothers or sisters with the same problem. Families who are preoccupied with weight and dieting tend to support unhealthful eating patterns and ideas about food.

Fully half to three quarters of girls with eating disorders also suffer from depression because they feel hopeless to be able to change their situation. Many anorectics literally starve themselves to death; many bulimics are also at risk for suicide.

> # CASE HISTORY

Perri was fat when she was little. Unhappy as a child and distressed by her parents' divorce, she ate to soothe her woes. By the time she graduated high school, she wore a size 16. Barely 4 feet 9 inches tall, she weighed 151 pounds.

"I dieted all the time, then I'd have a bite of cake and I'd be gone on an eating frenzy. I got crazy about it—once when I was 12, I sent my mother out at midnight to get me cheesecake. If my sister took my sweets, I'd have a screaming fit. I really thought sometimes that I might eat myself to death. And I grew up totally miserable—I was unhappy with my life, my job, just about everything. I felt I was a loser, and my glass was always half empty. I was a classic bitch; I can't believe people put up with me. Me and my addiction to food, which is exactly what it was.

"One day a friend took me down to Little Portugal in Newark, and I ate throughout an entire day—beef, sausage, pastries, chocolate, cheese—you name it, I ate it. It was that night, feeling queasy and disgusted with myself, that I ran into someone I knew who was in AA. We talked about her 12-step program, and I thought, well, maybe . . .

"I have to say that I'm a dedicated atheist, so the religious stuff was hard for me. But I liked the Overeaters Anonymous meeting I went to. Then I read the book that talked about having a willingness to believe in something bigger and stronger than myself. Okay, I thought. The measuring cup is gonna be my higher power. And for the past two years, it has been.

"Today I weigh 100 pounds and I exercise three to six times a week, depending on my schedule. I weigh everything I eat and carry my own food everywhere, even to restaurants (I call in advance to find out if it's okay). I eat four meals a day. I'm on a strict no flour, sugar, or wheat diet. Overeaters Anonymous has no eating program, but this is the one that has worked for me.

"I pray before each meal, and I thank God for today's abstinence. I don't know that I'll be abstinent tomorrow—I can only hope. And I call my sponsor every day and commit to exactly what I'm going to eat the next day.

"I like myself now. I'm more calm and serene. Although I still have my bitchy moments, they don't last as long. I feel so much more positive about everything, and dealing with my addiction to food is what triggered the change in me."

EATING DISORDERS CAN BE LIFE-THREATENING. HOSPITALIZATION MAY BE REQUIRED, AND YOU CANNOT ALWAYS RELY ON ALTERNATIVE THERAPIES ALONE TO HEAL.

Treatments to try: Ayurveda, page 49; Bach Flower Remedies, page 53; Cognitive Awareness, page 94; Herbalism, page 216; Homeopathy, page 221; Mindfulness, page 296; Nutrition Rehabilitation; page 316; Prayer, page 358; Self-esteem, page 380; Support Groups, page 414.

ERECTILE DYSFUNCTION

see Impotence, page 241

ESCAPISM

see also Anxiety, page 43

There are times when we can't face difficult or terrible things head-on. And because the mind is capable of forgetting at will, it's easy to block out painful thoughts and use various maladaptive coping mechanisms to escape reality and forestall having to deal with the problem.

■ *What Happens When You Escape*

You deny that anything is wrong and actually appear cheerier and more in control than usual. You may fabricate elaborate schemes or fantasies that appear to work well with your version of reality. You may also insist that others comply with your way of thinking and banish anyone from your circle of friends who tries to tell you the truth.

CASE HISTORY

Elizabeth had suffered from bipolar disorder for years, but at 66 she was in good health and happy living on her own in Los Angeles. Five years earlier, in her depressed state, she had tried to take her own life and had been hospitalized for several months. When she got out she was stabilized and incredibly productive. She wrote a screenplay (although it was never produced), took a lover 30 years her junior, painted her apartment, and cared for a 90-year-old neighbor.

But in her manic state, she suddenly started spending money she didn't have and making up wild excuses for her extravagance. She checked in at a fancy hotel and lived on room service for a week, then called a friend and told her to pay the bill. She claimed that she and her lover had recently married (so that he could inherit her rent-controlled apartment at her death) and that they were about to go on a honeymoon around the country. She cashed in part of her savings account to pay for it. Her extraordinary stories, about a well-known television personality who was producing her script and a huge inheritance from a cousin she never knew she had proved to be false.

Her friend attempted to get her to commit herself for care, but Elizabeth refused and told the friend never to call her again. It was, oddly enough, the death of her dog that brought her back to reality.

"I had to deal with all the arrangements, taking him to the vet, getting rid of his bowls and bed, and it sobered me up," Elizabeth said. "I hadn't been eating much at all, and I got myself on an organic-foods diet, with plenty of whole grains. I took lots of vitamins and minerals and made sure I got in a two-mile walk every day. I think walking around the park, seeing the kids on roller blades, seeing the sunshine and trees that were really there, was what cured me of the escapism."

You don't have to suffer from bipolar disorder to find yourself flitting off into a world of your own creation. Although it is beneficial and healing to dream and challenge yourself with goals that you may not be able to realize right now, it can be destructive to let your imagination run away with you.

How do you make the distinction? If you are able to understand that what you'd like to have happen is different from what is actually occurring, then you're still based in reality. You should also be aware of what it is you're trying to escape from. It may take a friend or relative to cue you into your distortions.

Flower Power

Escapist tendencies respond well to the Bach flower remedy, Agrimony. This flower is appropriate for someone who conceals tortured thoughts behind a facade of cheerfulness and freedom from worry. Take 5 or 6 drops under the tongue or mixed with half a glass of water, as needed.

Let a Healing Touch Change Your Perspective

Manipulation of various types—chiropractic, Network chiropractic, rolfing, bioenergetics, shiatsu, and massage—can be grounding for someone who is lost in revery.

According to the theories of Wilhelm Reich, a controversial psychoanalyst who practiced in the 1920s, the body builds up "character armor" to protect it from harm. In order to get inside the feelings, bodywork can work dramatic results. The holding patterns we have in our muscles aren't conscious—that's why this particular form of therapy works well with people who can't own up to their problems. Instead, by giving the body over to a touch that goes deeper than the surface, we can break through barriers our mind refuses to acknowledge.

The very act of lying down—and therefore letting the body be supported on a massage table—is influential in releasing old memories and allowing feelings to flow.

Take a Homeopathic Break

Try the following homeopathic remedies:

> For cheerfulness not related to actual events: Cannabis indica, Hyoscyamus, Lachesis.
>
> For idealism not grounded in reality: Causticum, Ignatia, Lycopodium, Platina.

Meditate Your Way Back to Reality

If you begin to sit daily and close out the distractions of everyday life, it is almost a given that you will have to deal with yourself on a different level. Sitting and doing nothing is difficult for many Westerners to do; however, if you enter into this practice in the spirit of healing, you will find that your mind and feelings can change.

When you meditate, you allow yourself to be whatever you are in that particular moment. You may concentrate on your breathing, or on one sound, such as "om," or on the sensation in one fingertip as it lies in your lap. As thoughts enter your mind, allow them free passage through, as though they were scenery you were glimpsing from a car window. Look at them, then let them go.

If you sit for 20 minutes a day, you will find that the energy you were taking up creating fantasies or redesigning an imaginary life for yourself begin to fade out. Meditation will allow spirit to flow inside you—and so will take away the need to escape.

Visualize the Problem

You may wish to use your creative talents to visualize exactly what you are doing when you escape from reality. Sit quietly in a comfortable spot and close your eyes. Begin to see your whole body as though you were standing apart from it. Examine every inch of yourself: See your good features, your flaws, your strengths and weaknesses. Look at your hair—is it thinning and dirty, or lustrous and shining? What about your face—does it contain the woes of the world, or do you see active intelligence shining from your eyes? Examine your hands—are they nurturing and strong, or are they feeble and limp? Make sure you are honest about your body; if you can do this therapeutic exercise, you can begin to be honest about your feelings.

EXERCISE

The human body was built for movement. The structure of the torso and limbs, with the base of flexible feet beneath, shows the evolutionary potential we sometimes forget we've got. We aren't built for speed like a panther, or for elevation like a sparrow, but rather for continual activity that gives us a variety of possibilities up and down and in three dimensions. We are capable of walking, crawling, running, stooping, turning, jumping, hopping, leaping, dancing, falling, swimming, and gliding.

Why should physical movement effect a change in our mental or emotional state? The subtle connection of mind and body dictates that we expand our lungs to get more oxygen, which in turn can flow to the brain so that we can think more clearly. In addition, the aerobic movement triggers the production of neurotransmitters in the brain that make us feel good and beta endorphins that act as natural opiates, killing pain.

Probably no other natural remedy shows the alignment of physical and mental health as well as exercise. Because moving around affords such good benefits to the cardiovascular system, and oxygenated blood flow is essential to good brain function, you can increase your mental and emotional stability with exercise. A regular daily workout lowers LDL cholesterol and raises HDL cholesterol and triglycerides, lowers blood pressure, decreases the stickiness of blood platelets and thins the blood so that it can move through arteries more easily, strengthens the heart muscle, gives you motivation to stick to a good nutritional program, and alleviates tension and elevates your mood as you see the progress you make, little by little, step by step. You feel so good you want to keep feeling better, and this positive addiction moves you to make other life changes such as quitting smoking, getting more sleep, and being more sexually active.

You don't need to knock yourself out to get great benefits. Moderate daily exercise (a brisk 2-mile walk, a 5-mile bike ride, a 20-minute set of laps in the pool) will keep your system toned and fit. Exercise relaxes you, and the more relaxed you are, the harder it will be for you to allow emotional or mental problems to get to you. As you learn to use the calming benefits of exercise in your life, you'll be better able to roll with the punches, take a deep breath, and carry on.

But for many individuals, a daily session of movement is a difficult habit to form. It is common to start an exercise program with a can-do, gung-ho attitude, and then find that life intervenes. Suddenly, there's an appointment during your regular walk time that you must attend, or you wake up one morning feeling under the weather and you don't get out, or the holiday rush seems more important than your daily swim. Of course, sloughing off once or twice doesn't matter to your mind or body; however, it's much easier *not* to exercise the next day.

■ Sticking to Your Exercise Goals

If you make yourself a commitment, you should keep it. Write yourself an exercise contract, stating that you vow to begin, on X date for an indefinite period—possibly a lifetime—a program that combines aerobic and anaerobic activity. You may want to ask a friend or relative to witness your signature on this one or to sign along with you. Support in starting an exercise program is sometimes the key to continuing. If you have to meet a partner for a tennis date or get to a martial arts class on time, you are more likely to stick to your promise.

Be sure you have your doctor's okay before beginning any exercise program. Your goals may be too lofty for your current state of health. Remember, an injury can set you back emotionally as well as physically: You may feel like a failure if you try too much and can't accomplish it. The idea is to have this therapy change your expectations about what you can and can't do. Many novice exercisers claim that the most exciting part of getting fit was the day they were finally able to run a whole mile, stand on their head, or touch their toes—things they never dreamed possible when they began.

What Kind of Exercise Improves the Mind?

There are four types of exercise, and one or all may be right for you.

FLEXIBILITY EXERCISE: This is the basic preparation for all other types. You must warm up and cool down no matter what your daily regimen. Stretching ensures that the tendons and ligaments around your bones are kept elastic, which means they will be less prone to injury. You should make sure that your stretches work the entire body—starting with the head and neck, work your way down to the shoulders and torso, the waist and hips, legs, ankles, and feet. Be sure you include movements that pull you up, turn you side to side, and work the big muscles of the legs to support your weight.

AEROBIC EXERCISE: The vital one for your circulatory system, this gets your heart rate up to 60 or 70 percent of your maximum rate. Take your pulse before you begin exercising (the carotid artery in your neck is the easiest to feel), then stop halfway through your routine to see if you have reached your ideal rate. The ideal goal is to keep your level of activity up here for 20 minutes. Be sure to cool down and take your pulse again as you recover.

You can improve the pumping action of the heart as you get more experience with aerobic exercise. When you work out like this, your muscles demand increased oxygen supplies, and they get this because you inhale more deeply, taking more air into your lungs, which delivers oxygen to the blood. After you've been aerobically challenged for three or four months, your heart will get used to its harder work and will recover more quickly when you stop and relax after exercising. You'll find that a real aerobic session not only pumps you up higher but also gives you a deeper level of relaxation when you're finished. For tense individuals who have trouble relaxing, this is one of the most important benefits.

Because you sweat a lot when you do aerobic exercise, you rid the body of many toxins, some of which may be responsible for your feeling depressed, anxious, compulsive, and so forth. You can walk, jog, bike, swim, hike, dance, climb stairs (or use a Stairmaster), take a low- or high-impact aerobics class, do racquet sports, or join a martial-arts class in order to get a good aerobic workout. And the best plan is to cross-train, alternating types of exercise.

Strength Training, or Anaerobic Exercise: It will help your body to withstand increasing amounts of stress. If you can take on physical stress, with weight training or using a Nautilus system, you can shoulder any burden emotionally. This type of exercise is particularly beneficial to women who traditionally lack upper body strength and gain a lot of confidence by being able to lift free weights effectively. This static, or isometric, type of exercise increases blood pressure temporarily; however, it drops to normal quite quickly when you're done with your workout. The better you get at lifting, the faster your system will get back in balance.

Endurance Exercise: It will help you increase your abilities in all other types of exercise. You don't need a quick burst of energy for this kind of movement; rather what you are striving for is a method that allows you to increase intensity and stamina over time. Tai chi and yoga are particularly excellent forms of endurance exercise that train the mind to go on when the body might want to give in and say "stop."

Keep Going at Your Own Pace

You will find that no matter what type of program you choose, you will reach a plateau before you can see any more progress. This is very disheartening to many diehard exercisers. Remember that you are trying to beat only your own record, and the sooner you look on this as a friendly competition, the sooner you will be able to use physical exercise to enhance your mind and emotional well-being.

One way to relax more into your practice is to visualize yourself doing the exercise when you're just sitting or lying around. Athletes who imagine themselves doing well in addition to practicing become more proficient than those who restrict themselves to physical movement and don't use their mind to expand their exercise potential. Think of yourself as graceful, powerful, strong, and untiring, and you will become so.

Exhaustion

see also Anxiety, page 43; Fatigue, page 158; Stress, page 407

Everything tuckers you out. You get up and feel so tired you want to drop back into bed; you drag yourself to the office and feel so weak you can barely pick up the phone. You aren't available to your family when you get home, because it's all too much for you.

▓ What Happens When You're Exhausted

Physical stress that is unbearable leaves us feeling tired, worn out, weak, and under pressure. We feel as if we've just been through a long illness and are recuperating very slowly. There's not enough energy to get the willpower working, and this can become a vicious cycle. When we're physically tired, we don't attempt much, and by lying back and letting the world pass us by, we tend to feel drained—more out of it and less motivated to get moving.

Exhaustion is a natural component of illness, so if you're tired all the time you should be checked out for chronic fatigue syndrome or mononucleosis. If you're recuperating from a flu, or pneumonia, it's understandable that you would feel weak and tired. But other forms of exhaustion aren't tied to disease.

In the workplace, exhaustion often appears as burnout. When nothing you do on the job makes any difference and you're fed up with the system, you feel impotent and take on a "what's the use?" attitude. At home, it can manifest itself as indifference to loved ones and a total unwillingness to do chores and make a household run smoothly. Unfortunately, many individuals cope with exhaustion with destructive behaviors such as overuse of caffeine or taking "uppers," such as methamphetamines and cocaine.

Instead of drugging your mind to the problem, confront it. Deal with the physical aspects and then start to work for some emotional uplift.

Eat Your Way to Strength

It's important to get your physical being in good shape. This means you should eat as though you were recuperating from an illness—plenty of protein (preferably chicken without skin, fish and seafood, and legumes), lots of whole grains, vegetables, and raw fruits. You should keep dairy consumption to a minimum and strictly avoid refined sugars. (Don't eat a candy bar in the middle of the afternoon as a pick-me-up. This will bump up your blood sugar for only an hour, after which time it will plummet, leaving you more tired than you were before you ate the sugar.)

No More Caffeine

Caffeine (coffee, cocoa, or caffeinated sodas or teas) is absorbed into the bloodstream and from there travels to the brain. This stimulant makes the heart pump more blood; however, it decreases blood flow to the brain by constricting local blood vessels. Once it does get to the brain, it stimulates the cerebral cortex, so we feel alert, ready to think hard and stay awake longer.

Caffeine also deactivates enzymes within each cell, which modifies their activity level, and that's why we feel so restless after three cups of coffee. The more you ingest, the smaller the effect; this means that you're tempted to take more of it.

As with any stimulant, the period of arousal is followed by a period of withdrawal. At this time, we may feel markedly depressed and exhausted.

The best advice is to get off and stay off caffeine. This will allow the brain and body to stay on an even keel all the time. What do you drink instead? The most revitalizing liquid, pure spring water. At least eight to ten cups a day will hydrate the body and make you feel more alert.

Take Your Supplements

It's important to supplement folic acid (400 mcg. daily), pantothenic acid (250 mg. daily), Vitamin B_6 (25 to 50 mg. daily), Vitamin B_{12} (500 to 1000 mcg. daily), Vitamin C (500 to 1000 mg. daily), iron (15 mg. daily if deficient only), zinc (30 mg. daily), and potassium (1000 mg. twice daily).

Get on an Exercise Kick

When you're really exhausted, your body is telling you that it's not working hard enough. This apparent contradiction is evident if you talk to former couch potatoes who are now positively addicted to daily activity. IT IS ESSENTIAL TO GET YOUR DOCTOR'S OKAY BEFORE YOU BEGIN AN EXERCISE PROGRAM TO COMBAT EXHAUSTION. When you've got the go-ahead for exercise, start slowly and build stamina in a daily walking program. Your first time out you may barely make it to the mailbox several yards from your house; by the end of a week, however, you'll probably be able to walk a mile in 15 to 20 minutes.

Don't push yourself. Select an activity you really like and you'll stick with it. Walking, actually, has been found just as effective in building overall fitness as jogging or racquet sports.

Develop Good Sleep Habits

If you're tired, you need more rest—this doesn't necessarily mean more hours in bed but a more regular schedule. Be sure you tuck yourself in by 10:30 P.M. every night (even weekends) and are up by 7 A.M. The body has natural highs and lows, and if you're fighting them with late bedtime and late awakenings, you're draining yourself unnecessarily. Although these hours may seem out of synch with your current way of living, going to bed earlier and getting up earlier can make a big difference in the amount of energy you have throughout the day.

Melatonin May Revive You

The neurotransmitter melatonin is one of the body's best regulators of our daily rhythms. Our pineal gland produces a lot of melatonin in the dark, when we're sleeping, and stops producing it when we wake up and it's light out. The dosage and timing of this supplement is crucial in order to restore the good balance of your daily time clock—too much too early in the evening will make you drowsy or more exhausted. You should take the lowest dose possible (1 mg. is enough) after it's dark out (right before you go to bed). Take the hormone only for a week or two until you've balanced your body clock and your own system takes over. You can also eat melatonin-rich foods before bed, such as tomatoes, sweet corn, bananas, oats, rice, or barley.

Homeopathic Help

The remedy for mental exhaustion is Phosphoricum acidum.

Perk up with an Herb

If you are suffering from a lack of vitality, you can take Siberian ginseng, 1/2 teaspoon tincture two to three times daily, or oats (avena sativa), 1/2 to 1 teaspoon tincture two to three times daily (this preparation should contain oat seed and straw).

Flower Power

The Bach flower remedy for exhaustion is Bottlebrush. Take 5 to 6 drops under the tongue or mixed in half a glass of water as needed.

Take a Yoga Posture

Yoga is a wonderful discipline for integrating the different levels of your mind and body. You stretch your muscles in a pose and get your parasympathetic nervous system to relax you, but you also activate the endocrine and immune systems to protect you from fatigue and illness.

Try the following exercise.

Spinal Rock/Head to Knee Pose: Lie on the floor and bring your knees into your chest. Wrap your arms around your knees and begin to rock forward and back. You will be stimulating the entire spinal cord from the base of the brain to the coccyx. Finally, rock into a seated position and stretch your legs out in front of you. Put the sole of your right foot as high along your left thigh as you can. Now slowly lower yourself over the outstretched leg, reaching for your shin or ankle. Don't bounce.

Breathe into the posture, letting each inhalation take you lower. You will find as you practice that you don't need to pull yourself down—your body will elongate as you use your breathing effectively.

Change legs and repeat the exercise, making each breath deep and full.

Now bring both legs together stretched out in front of you. Then fold them in front of you into a tailor-sit. Tuck your head and roll it down toward your lap and take three deep breaths. Come back up to sitting posture.

You should feel energized and relaxed.

*F*ALLING ASLEEP, DIFFICULTY

see also Insomnia, page 248; Sleep Disorders, page 404

Even those of us who sleep soundly through the night are often plagued by the inability to drop off at one time or another. The causes are many—lingering worries about something that's occurred or is about to occur, excitement about some greatly anticipated event, overstimulation from a big evening with lots to mull over afterward.

■ *What Happens When You Have Difficulty Falling Asleep*

You lie there, unable to keep your eyes closed. You check the clock. You feel your muscles uneasily draped on your body, tense and tight. Your skin itches, and the sheets feel rough. You can't find a position that feels right. You lie still and then find it's impossible, so you turn again. The more you don't fall asleep, the more you worry you'll *never* drop off, and your anxiety about the next day keeps you awake even longer. Eventually, exhausted, you drop off. But the next morning, you may feel achy and fatigued from lack of sufficient sleep.

In order to drop off to sleep, you have to learn to relax. There are a variety of helpful techniques to try:

Bedtime Cocktails

A mug of warm milk contains lots of the amino acid tryptophan, which is a tried-and-true favorite with insomniacs. Mash a banana (which also contains this amino acid) and whip it with the milk for a calming presleep cocktail.

155

Feel Your Breath

Regulating the breath will help to regulate the amount of oxygen to your brain. Lie on your back and concentrate on your inhalation and exhalation. Clear your mind and watch your belly rise and fall with the rhythmic motion of your breath. You will find that there is an almost hypnotic quality about the easy flow of your breathing. Never hold the breath, but rather, let it reach its peak fully before starting down. Now imagine the breath moving in your brain like a great wave, settling the thoughts and feelings. You will feel drowsy in a while even if you don't fall asleep right away, and this will relax you sufficiently to rest and restore your body and mind.

Pressing Palms

Using acupuncture points, do the following:

- Palms facing you, cross your wrists—the right wrist on the outside. Curl your thumb and fingers around your opposite thumb. Hold lightly for three to five minutes. Then proceed with each of your other fingers, holding them for the same amount of time. (If you have not fallen asleep by this time, you can switch hands and repeat on the other side.)
- Lie on your side and pull your knees toward your chest. Place your hands back to back in between your knees and rest the palm of the left hand on the inside of the right knee. Hold for three to five minutes.

Run Yourself Ragged

You may not be falling asleep because you're not tired enough. Make sure you have at least a half-hour period of aerobic exercise at some point during the day (but more than three hours before sleep so that you won't be too revved up).

Yoga Slows You Down

The wonderfully relaxing postures of yoga send calming energy through the spinal column to the brain. Try the following half an hour before bed:

NECK ROLLS: Roll your head easily from side to side, touching chin to chest. Then complete the circle. Reverse direction. Repeat five times on each side.

HALF MOON SERIES: Stand up and raise your arms over your head. Gently bend to your right from your waist, then to the left. With outstretched arms, make your body a hinge and bend forward with a flat back, then round the back and bend the knees slightly as you bring your hands close to the ground in front of you. Roll up your spine, one vertebra at a time, and then reverse the posture, placing your hands on your hips for support and leaning back so that you are looking at the ceiling. Return to standing.

THE WARRIOR: Stand with one leg thrust forward, raise your arms over your head, and bend your front knee so that your thigh is parallel with the ground. Hold for a count of ten, then repeat on the other side.

THE SPHINX: Lie on your stomach, elbows bent, hands in front of your shoulders. Lift up your head and chest, resting the weight of your body on your forearms.

CAT STRETCH: On your hands and knees, round your back and lift your spine to the ceiling. Then reverse, arch your back, and lift up your head. Repeat five times.

CORPSE POSE: Lie on your back, arms and legs relaxed at your sides, and breathe into your limbs and back. You may wish to cover yourself with a light blanket as you become completely comfortable and relaxed.

Nighttime Herbal Elixirs

The following herbs will help you drop off: Jamaica dogwood, lime blossom, passionflower, valerian, wild lettuce, hops. You may take these as tea or tincture an hour before bed ($^1/_2$ to 1 teaspoon infused in a cup of water or $^1/_2$ teaspoon of tincture). Hops and lime blossom also can be sewn into small flat bags to place under your pillow.

Melatonin in Moderation

A very small dosage of melatonin supplements (1 mg. a day for a week or two) taken just before bed will help your own body clock get back on track.

Dump Your Sleeping Pills

If you have been taking tranquilizers or sleeping pills to help you drop off, you must get off them and should do so gradually, tapering yourself every other day and then every three days. Sleeping pills are addictive and usually lose their effectiveness after a few weeks, which means that you must keep increasing the dosage in order to continue falling asleep. They have a half-life that can result in daytime drowsiness and difficulty with concentration and coordination.

A Sense of Place

Use your bedroom only for sleep and sex—that way you'll always associate it with the activities that promote rest and relaxation. Try a hot bath before getting ready for bed.

FATIGUE

see also Anxiety, page 43; Blues, page 72; Exhaustion, page 149; Lack of Self-esteem, page 380; Sexual Dysfunction, page 387; Stress, page 407

It is natural and normal to have slumps during the day and even to go through weeks when you feel particularly tired. There are also certain times of life—pregnancy, menopause, advanced old age—when we are more prone to fatigue because we are using all the resources at our disposal to accomplish certain important stage transitions.

Fatigue differs from exhaustion in that it isn't triggered by physical stress. It is more a lack of vitality or a dimming of spirit than simply being tired. Fatigue is often a symptom of depression and seems to go with mood swings and headaches. Sometimes actually described as "the blahs," fatigue is harder to fight than exhaustion, which often vanishes with a good diet-and-exercise program.

■ *What Happens When You're Fatigued*

If you are under a lot of stress for a long time, you never have a chance to recover and recoup your mental and emotional resources. You feel drained, unable to motivate yourself to do anything, and it's virtually impossible to maintain a routine. After only a few weeks of being ruled by fatigue, your attention span gets weaker, and your problem-solving abilities lessen. It's as though mind, body, and spirit had given up.

There are several different causes of fatigue, and commonly, several of them co-exist, making you feel even worse:

- lack of energy-giving nutrients
- accumulation of waste products in body
- chemical imbalance from overexertion
- lack of communication between endocrine and nervous systems

When off your schedule, you will be more likely to be fatigued than not because your natural circadian rhythms are out of balance. (Think about how difficult it is adjusting to vacations and you'll realize how much we are creatures of the clock.) It's not just lacking the oomph to get through a day that's the problem. It's the fact that fatigue is a vicious cycle—we're too tired to do anything, so we can't motivate ourselves to get out of our slump. Once deeper in the slump, we feel more fatigued.

Most individuals suffer from long-term fatigue that starts small and grows to unmanageable proportions. (The incidence of chronic fatigue syndrome, where fatigue hits suddenly, has no apparent cause, and is not helped by rest, is very small.) The type of fatigue best known to us has either physical, psychological, or lifestyle triggers. Physical causes include illness and low-grade infections as well as imbalances in the adrenal glands (which control the stress reaction of the body). Psychological causes include poor self-esteem and lack of motivation. The way we live our lives can also cause fatigue, particularly when you consider that most people are engaged in the perennial rat-race of balancing job and home responsibilities.

Chronic fatigue is the most frequent complaint in doctors' offices today, and most physicians have no clue as to how to approach it. They will probably tell the patient to "take it easy," to enjoy themselves more and worry less, but these suggestions are all terribly amorphous.

There are, however, some good natural therapies that will help:

Get in Shape

If you haven't done so yet, quit smoking for good. Nicotine can rob your brain of necessary oxygen that will give you enough energy to carry on. If you're carrying a lot of extra pounds, get on a healthful nutrition and exercise program that will allow you to lose half a pound a week (losing any faster than that will make you weak and tired).

Get Off the Boob Tube

Television seems to be what we want when we're too tired to do anything else—actually it lulls us into a state of lethargy. When you have some free time and don't particularly feel like doing anything that requires physical oomph, read a book or magazine or sit and meditate.

Dump Your Stress

If you're the type of person everyone comes to with his or her problems, start saying no. You cannot possibly shoulder the burdens of the world and still have enough energy for yourself. Prioritize and learn what you can and what you can't do.

Pamper Yourself

An evening of complete luxury may revitalize your spirits. Turn off the phone, soak in a bubble bath, listen to quiet music, have a glass of wine or a cup of herbal tea. Asking your partner for a massage is a good idea, too.

Delicious Thinking

By eating right, you can boost the stress-managing effect of your adrenal glands. A high-potassium diet (3 to 5 grams daily) will ensure that your adrenals are functioning well and will keep your energy level on an even keel. Foods high in potassium are sunflower seeds, yams, Swiss chard, soybeans, and potatoes with skin.

Fat is a real problem for someone who's fatigued. Oxygen, carried by the red blood cells, can't get through if blocked by fat. A high-fat diet increases the incidence of atherosclerosis, which clogs the arteries and makes the heart work harder—which, of course, is very tiring to your system. Obesity (which comes with a high-fat diet) makes you tired, since it's harder to carry all that weight around.

Make sure you avoid caffeine and white sugar, both of which will provide an energy jolt, followed by an energy slump. Both increase blood sugar rapidly and oversensitize insulin response.

Stop Dragging, Start Exercising

If you're really tired, you should get out and exercise. Although it sounds contradictory, the best remedy for fatigue is improving your physical fitness, thereby boosting your energy level. Exercise also increases your metabolism, which helps you burn more calories and feel more vital and lively. If you start slowly and do some aerobic activity every day, you will find your fatigue lessening week by week. The other extraordinary benefit of regular exercise is that it increases endorphin production, which lightens your mood and makes you feel more awake and aware.

- *Walking:* A brisk two-mile walk, which should take you about 25 to 30 minutes, is the best and easiest method of improving your fitness level.

- *Racquet sports:* A partnered exercise program is excellent because it's social, and you depend on each other to be there and always keep the date.

- *Dancing:* The music itself is a mood elevator, but most people respond happily to getting out there on the floor and moving, whether with a partner or singly, in a dance class. You will find your fatigue melting away with each whirl around the floor.

Remedies to Perk up

The homeopathic remedies for fatigue are: Pulsatilla (if weary and worn out), Kali phosphoricum (after mental and nervous exertion); or Spongia tosta (after the slightest exertion).

Herbal Energizers

To reduce fatigue, try 5 to 10 drops with each meal for three weeks of any one of the following: ginseng, black cohosh, yellow dock, or dandelion. If you feel you need stimulation, make a tea with $1/2$ to 1 teaspoon of cayenne, ginger, or cinnamon powder.

Press a Point

Press the following acupressure points if you suffer from fatigue: (see pp 10-11 for acupressure charts)

St.36 : on the outside of the leg, with the leg slightly bent, between the lower edge of the kneecap and an inch and a half from the edge of the shinbone.

Ki.7: on the inside of the leg above the ankle, at the hollow between the muscle and the Achilles tendon.

Bach Flower Remedy

Use Olive to combat fatigue. Take 5 to 6 drops under the tongue or mix with a half-glass of water.

Tell Yourself You're Worth It

If you don't feel good about yourself—your relationships, accomplishments, goals—it's difficult to find the energy to get up and go. When you doubt that everything you do and say has worth, you begin to feel like nothing, like no one. This is a very exhausting perspective to take on your life.

Self-esteem building can be done in a psychotherapeutic setting, but you can help yourself to realize your potential in a variety of ways:

• Make a list of everything you've done (other than routine activities like eating, sleeping, getting dressed, and so forth) in the last two weeks. Look at the list as though someone else wrote it and star those items that seem unusual, creative, or full of fun.

- Make yourself a party. Go shopping for ingredients for a healthful meal with a friend, then come home, set the table with your best china and candles, blow up some balloons, and put on some music. Consume the meal slowly, enjoying each others' company.

- Set yourself a task that is a challenge for you and work at it until it's completed. Stand back and admire what you've done.

Get Rid of the OTCs and Prescriptions

You may not realize that the over-the-counter and/or prescription drugs you're taking are causing you problems. If you are under a doctor's care, you must speak with her or him about whether in fact your medications could be making you feel groggy or exhausted. If these are possible side effects, you'll want to taper off your dosages under a professional's care.

If you are self-medicating, slowly wean yourself off these drugs as you begin to use the natural therapies listed here.

FATIGUE ON AWAKENING

see also Sleep Disorders, page 404

If you are tired when your alarm rings in the morning, you aren't sleeping soundly. This means that you have not been able to get down to the deepest (Stage III and Stage IV) levels of sleep, which restore and replenish the body.

Any of the treatments for fatigue will be useful, in addition to the following:

Reset Your Clock

To readjust your sleep cycle, try going to bed half an hour earlier and setting your alarm half an hour earlier. Try not to drink any fluids after 6 P.M.—particularly not alcohol—so as to avoid the urge to get up to go to the bathroom in the middle of the night.

Remember Your Dreams

Keep a pad and pen by your bedside and when you wake at any time, write down your first impressions. When you begin these exercises, you do not remember much, but as you require yourself to record your dreams, you'll start to pick up details. Dreaming, during the stage known as REM sleep, is essential to waking refreshed because it allows for a normal, cyclic pattern of biochemical change over the course of the night and permits a discharge of biochemical accumulation.

*F*EAR

see also Anxiety, page 43; Palpitations, page 342; Panic Disorders, page 344; Trembling, page 428

A fear is a terror of something real, such as an abusive spouse or a sick parent who might die. (See Anxiety, page 43, for fears that have no immediate basis in reality.) Fear is our most primitive reaction to danger, and it's a healthy one. We should turn and look if we hear footsteps behind us on a dark city street; we should protect ourselves from a rabid dog. We can, however, exacerbate the fears we have unrealistically—if we are afraid of *all* animals, for example.

When we're afraid, we put out the "fight or flight" hormones that get our nervous systems racing and that produce the characteristic symptoms such as pounding heart, darting eyes, clammy hands, knot in the stomach. The more fear we fear, and the more often we feel it, the worse our physical and psychological condition. If we're in a constant state of agitation, our psychic "tone" is always on high, which can lead to problems such as headaches, stomach aches, allergies, and over the long run, chronic illnesses such as heart disease, stroke, and various cancers.

| CASE HISTORY |

Patricia was 37 when she had her first seizure and couldn't have been more relieved when a CT scan indicated a large amount of scar tissue in her brain from a bad knock on the head she'd had a year earlier. But two years after the surgery, when she started getting dizzy and seeing double, she had a sense of foreboding that whatever had been wrong had never been fixed.

Follow-up treatment revealed another mass in her head, and this time they called it cancer and gave her radiation. "It clicked into place—they had opened up my head for something that could never be cured. I was thankful not to have chemo, which burns your insides out, but I really couldn't believe the radiation was going to heal me. I didn't have a good attitude—I wish I'd been more in charge of my fear.

"I started meditating, sometimes to music and sometimes silently. My sister made me a tape with Tibetan bells that I used, but I found that I really wanted natural sounds—birds and bugs in the summer, water from a stream or river when I was near one. Water was good because it was a continuum—like my life. Everything in nature became so important—seeing the first buds on my tomatoes let me know that summer was coming; or the first frost, knowing I had to get stuff done in the garden.

"I got comfortable being alone, because after all, you can't take anyone with you on this trip. When I really listened to what was going on inside me, I understood that having cancer isn't necessarily more scary than walking to the mailbox—it's the *fear* that keeps you from dealing with it that's crippling."

Talk to Yourself—and Your Monster

When we were children, we often comforted ourselves by confronting a particularly scary thought by making it palpable. If you have a conversation with the monster inside you, it becomes less threatening. You will undoubtedly feel silly when you first try this exercise, but it can be a very liberating feeling to look the fear in the eye and tell it off. Make sure you write down your complaints and anxieties before you stage your conversation. Pretend you're going in to argue with your boss—you must have your points lined up before the actual confrontation.

Change Your Mind

Use cognitive techniques to relabel your fears. For example, instead of saying to yourself, *"I'm scared—I can't,"* switch the emphasis and say, *"I'm having one of those anxiety attacks again, but this time I'm going to deal with it."* If you feel frightened most of the time and don't have a specific cause, tell yourself that there may be no cause. Instead, it could simply be a reluctance on your part to avoid trying new things or meeting new people. You can overcome this worrying by thinking less and doing more. Distract yourself from the fear by participating in activities that give you pleasure and give yourself a reward every time you block the fear with a positive thought or action.

Turn on the Radio

Listening to music or the voice of a broadcaster is a proven way to deal with fear. The energy and rhythm of music distracts us from unsettling thoughts; the sound of friendly voices makes us feel that we're not alone.

Take a Big Breath

When we are frightened, one of the first things we do is allow the breath to rise to the chest and mouth instead of keeping it rooted in the belly. To feel strong and secure, try the yoga three-level breath.

Lie on the floor and place your hand over your belly. Now inhale and expand your belly. Keep your chest and throat uninvolved. Puff up your belly as big and hard as you can with the breath. When you cannot take in any more, slowly release and let the belly deflate.

On the next breath, inhale and expand the belly. When you cannot get it any bigger, let the breath move upward and expand the chest. When you have reached your capacity, let go, deflating first the chest and then the belly.

Finally, inhale and expand the belly. When it is full, let the breath move up and expand the chest. Then let it move up even further and open the throat.

When you begin to practice the three-level breathing, do only four complete rounds and then rest, so as not to become lightheaded. Each day, as you do a little more, you'll feel bigger and braver, and you'll increase your capacity for oxygen and energy.

As you get better at the breathing, you can practice it standing and seated as well as lying down.

Meditate Away the Fear

One of the best methods for gaining a calm, steady mind is to practice meditation. When we sit, not trying to go anywhere or do anything, we give ourselves room to explore the deeper ramifications of our feelings. We are also able to develop a sense of groundedness and stability. There is nothing to fear once we are at one and at peace with ourselves.

Sit comfortably, either cross-legged or in a straight-backed chair, and close your eyes. Let your thoughts enter and pass by, as though they were scenery and you were the passenger in a car. Begin to watch your breath, making each inhalation and exhalation as even and rhythmic as possible. Ask your mind whether it is all right to go to the depths of your fear, or whether, for now, you should stay near the surface, with your head above water.

Probably, at the beginning, you won't be able to tackle the big issues, and that's as it should be. Meditation teaches us not to reach for any goals, but rather, just to accept ourselves in the present. The more you sit, the more you will feel competent to look at problems you were too terrified to face.

Rely on the Wisdom of China

Traditional Chinese medicine looks at fear as a malfunction of the kidney organ network and would recommend acupuncture treatments specially designed for your personality and problem. The nature of fear is cold, so a helpful hint would be to place a hot water bottle on your lower back and keep the bottom of your feet warm.

Homeopathic Strength

Try the following homeopathic remedies for fear: Aconite, Belladonna, Causticum, Ignatia, Silica, Lycopodium, Phosphorus, Pulsatilla.

Let the Aroma Make You Brave

Aromatherapy offers a variety of herbs to combat fear: Orange flower absolute for shock and fear; Sandalwood to ease anxiety and nervous tension; Ylang-ylang to bring about a sense of well-being and alleviate anxiety.

*F*EAR OF ANIMALS

see also Phobias, page 346

Some of us have an irrational fear of wild beasts coming into the house; for some of us, it's the neighbor's dog or cat. An animal may be an ancient symbol for our own wild urges, which we suppress in everyday life but which could conceivably get loose and run amok.

▓ *What Happens When You Fear Animals*

You feel that you have no control, that the creature is out to get you and you are trapped. The phobia of being mauled or eaten by an animal actually reverses the traditional state of affairs where the animal is caged and the person is loose. What happens when we can't control the fear is that we feel trapped.

Animal phobias generally start before the age of seven and occasionally begin because of a particular event such as being scratched by a cat or bitten by a dog. Especially if the parents overreact to this event, the child may internalize the fear and it can perpetuate itself into adulthood.

When we're terrified, our levels of adrenaline and noradrenaline skyrocket. But when we are in control, the levels of these chemicals decline. In a study done at Stanford University Medical Center, women who were phobic about spiders were taught to cope with their panicky feelings and thus control their neurotransmitter levels. When they were finally able to handle the spiders and reduce adrenaline and noradrenaline, they also reported fewer frightening dreams and thoughts.

Behavioral therapy and desensitization are the most common treatments for all panic disorders and phobias. See also the therapies suggested below for some specifics if you fear animals.

Behave Differently Around Animals

First you must give your phobic situations grades, from the least to most fearful (seeing a pet would be at the bottom; having a pet leap on you and lick you would be at the top). Then you will begin to visualize situations at the bottom of your hierarchy and combine this imagery with a progressive relaxation.

As you lie on the floor, tense the muscles of your feet and think about seeing the animal at a distance. Now relax completely. As you work your way up the body, tensing and relaxing every part, allow the pet to get closer to you in your mind. When you can do this exercise without feeling anxious, you are ready to move up to another imaginary scene that is higher up on your list of fears.

Control the Critter with Your Mind

Self-hypnosis and densitization will allow you to calm your mind and make concrete changes in your behavior. To tackle this problem, you will need a friend with the type of pet you are currently repelled by. Before your friend brings the pet over, go into a trance state. Roll your eyes upward, close your eyes, and hold your breath. Then allow yourself to breath easily as you imagine yourself floating. Begin your trance state with the suggestion that your natural feeling of compassion and nurturing will help to overcome your fear of animals.

Then arrange to meet your friend. At first you will not be able to approach the animal, which will be leashed and kept at a distance. Keep repeating the suggestion you used in trance as you get closer. Over a period of days, you may be able to stay in the same room with the animal; finally, you may be able to pet his back as your friend holds him on a leash. After your sessions, reinforce the hypnotic suggestion.

During the next weeks, you can work your way toward petting the head of the pet, embracing the pet, being licked by the pet. You will find that the suggestion becomes stronger the more time you spend with the formerly dreaded animal.

Homeopathics Against Animal Terrors

Try the following homeopathic remedies when you are combating your fear of animals:

Fear of animals: Belladonna, China, Tuberculinum, Calcarea, Carcinosin, Causticum, Hyoscyamus, Lycopodium

Fear of birds: Natrum mur, Ignatia

Fear of cats: Tuberculinum, Calcarea, China, Medorrhinum

Fear of dogs: Belladonna, China, Causticum, Hyoscyamus, Pulsatilla, Stramonium

Fear of snakes: Lachesis, Belladonna, Carcinosin, Natrum mur, Pulsatilla

Fear of spiders: Calcarea, Carcinosin, Natrum mur, Stramonium

Breathe Away the Fear

When we are terrified, our breathing becomes shallow and we don't take in sufficient oxygen or get rid of sufficient carbon dioxide. Practice deep belly breathing for ten minutes twice daily, either lying down or sitting in a straight-backed chair. Place your hand on your belly to make sure you're expanding and contracting it with each inhalation and exhalation.

When you confront an animal, immediately use the trigger of putting your hand on your belly to start breathing deeply and fully. You will find that it's easier to relax mind and body as you concentrate on your breath.

Hang up a Baby Picture

Generally, kittens and puppies are less threatening than grown animals, and luckily, the purveyors of decorative arts have dozens of Hallmark-type photos ready for hanging. By keeping one of these pictures in sight, perhaps in your den or family room, you can desensitize yourself each time you pass it.

FEAR OF FAILURE

see also Depression, page 112; Phobias, page 346; Victim Mentality, page 433; Vulnerability, page 445

Most of us lack confidence once in a while, but if you constantly worry that you're going to fail, you are erecting your own impediment to doing well. It's difficult to muster the strength to motivate yourself when you assume you'll do poorly. Fear of failure is closely tied to fear of success—it's as though the accolades that others give us when we do well don't mean anything. We have no way to take the first step of the journey because we can't see ourselves completing it.

This fear is not technically a phobia, which is a terror of a specific object or activity. But like a phobia, this fear seems unreasonable to others and perfectly logical to you.

What Happens When You Constantly Fear You'll Fail

You have no will to tackle the simplest challenge because you think you'll mess it up so badly. You always defer to others, saying they have more ability than you, even when you know rationally that that's not true.

If you are disabled by the fear of failure, you will never try for a higher degree, never apply for a more challenging job, never ask a potentially interesting partner on a date. You probably won't decide to take up the cello or build your own log cabin, because the thought of ruining the project is worse than the excitement of starting something fresh.

Fear of failure is often a side effect of depression. If everything in life seems hopeless and you can't raise yourself out of the misery that surrounds you, trying an interesting activity will be too difficult. Most depressed people live lives of "quiet desperation," as Henry David Thoreau phased it, and don't permit themselves innovation or exploration.

Work on Your Self-esteem

It's useful to go through the various stages of your life and make an effort to record your successes. If you or your parents happen to be pack rats, you may even discover old papers from school with good marks that got put into a "must-save envelope." If you ever won a trophy for ice skating or bowling, that goes into your list of past greatest achievements.

Moving on to the present, make yourself a weekly chart of Great Deeds Done and go out and buy some gold stars. Give yourself a daily goal to do something you can be proud of—helping a friend through a crisis, volunteering at a local hospital, baking cookies for a church event. When you've completed your self-assigned task, put a gold star on your chart. You'll be amazed to see how many times you not only didn't fail, but you actually went over and above your desired achievement.

Take a Test

Whether it's the motor-vehicle test, a quick course to prepare you for the SATs, or a Red Cross certification in first aid or cardiopulmonary resuscitation, just do it. Dare yourself to complete the work and then take the written and/or practical test—and do well. Tell yourself over and over that you have the ability and knowledge to pass. And remember that you are not trying for A+. Any passing grade is a success.

Look at Your Dreams

Your dreams will be particularly telling, once you start recording them. Keep a pad and pen by your bedside and write down the feeling of the dream as soon as you awaken. Do you feel crushed or impotent because of something that occurred? Write down the important elements of the dream as you recall them and see if you can ask the images or characters why you aren't doing well. The answer may be that you just don't want to, that it's less work to keep muddling along at your accustomed pace. Determine to go back the next night and correct the failure.

Eat Hearty

When you have the right nutrients in your body, you feel stronger and more powerful. Start the day with a substantial breakfast high in complex carbohydrates—perhaps a baked apple and some oatmeal with soy milk. Your lunch can be a light meal, perhaps soup and salad, and dinner should be low-protein, low-fat, and high in calcium as well as vitamins and minerals. (You don't need dairy for calcium—green leafy vegetables, turnips, and fish with bones like salmon in the can are great dietary sources of this mineral.)

Get rid of caffeine and refined sugar in order to keep your brain chemistry balanced and your blood glucose level on an even keel.

Drink a Flower

The Bach flower remedy for fear of failure is Larch. Take 5 or 6 drops under the tongue or mixed in water.

Set an Exercise Goal

When you feel you'll fail, it's scary to think about trying something like a ten-mile mini-marathon, or swimming a two-mile lake. But this is one of the best ways to develop confidence and assurance that your body will not fail. The incredible rush of training for a competitive event will spur you on to do your best. If you finish—no matter how long it takes—you can't fail.

FEAR OF FLYING

see also Panic Disorders, page 344; Phobias, page 346

The very idea of going up in the air in a vehicle heavier than a herd of elephants is awesome, but to some people, it's sheer suicidal madness. The terror of sitting, strapped into a seat and listening to the engines rev, then tooling down the runway going faster and faster until finally the wheels lift off, is heartstopping for those who suffer from fear of flying. And staying up in the air for hours is tantamount to an eternal stint in Dante's Inferno.

■ What Happens When You Fear Flying

Your heart starts pumping as soon as you walk in the door of the terminal, you find your throat drying up as you hand the ticket over to the attendant at the gate. Your mind is numb, because you realize you are going to your doom and so are all the other people around you, and there's nothing you can do about it. As you sit in the aisle seat (the window is worse because you can see the ground rushing away from you), you feel your stomach drop out as the plane begins to move. The takeoff itself, which causes panic attacks in many, is not the end of the torment, because you know that as soon as you are in the air and the plane appears stable, this is the moment when it could just as easily fall to earth in a fiery blaze.

Fear of flying is accompanied by a fear of heights for most people, which is actually a fear of falling or a fear that you will not be supported if you begin to fall. Another part of this fear is the claustrophobic feeling of being imprisoned in a tight space for several hours.

Behavioral therapy and desensitization are the most common treatments for all panic disorders and phobias. See also some of the following therapies for more specifics if you fear flying.

Join a Desensitization Class

Several of the major airlines have cooperated with psychologists and social workers to stage a mock flight for those who suffer from this phobia. Several sessions are devoted to learning about flight, sitting in an airline seat, moving around the plane, and finally, going down the runway, taking off, and spending a few minutes circling the airport before descending. As in any process of desensitization, you are allowed to get a little closer to the frightening experience each time, so you can build resistance to the problem gradually.

Let Your Mind Control the Plane

Using self-hypnosis, you can take charge of this phobia. Sit quietly and calm your breath. Roll your eyes up, then close your eyes and hold your breath. Allow your breath to come easily now, as you tell your arm to levitate upward. Give yourself the suggestion that the plane is simply an extension of you, that it is controlled by your mind and muscles. Imagine yourself floating over the plane, which is attached by strings to your hand like a marionnette. You have ultimate charge over how high the plane flies, how fast it goes, and how it lands. When you are ready, take another breath and return to earth. After you have been able to put yourself into a trance state successfully for several weeks, the suggestion will come back to you whenever you have to get on a plane.

Breathe Yourself Into the Air

Many studies on directed breathing show that you can lower blood pressure and heart rate and calm the nervous system. You must practice your breathing when you are not in a terrifying situation, so that when the moment of flight arrives, you'll have your technique down pat.

Close your eyes and imagine yourself completely alone, comfortably seated on the floor or in a straight-backed chair. Inhale slowly, filling yourself with strength and initiative. You should feel like a balloon, lighter than air, able to float and, yet, covered with a resilient skin that will not pop, no matter how high the balloon goes. As you exhale, keep a core of this air inside you, but rid yourself of carbon dioxide and toxins that would bind you to the earth. Keep the breathing up, each time taking in a little more air, which will cushion you throughout any experience you happen to try.

FEAR OF GOING CRAZY

see also Confusion, mental, page 100; Panic Disorders, page 344; Phobias, page 346

Even the most sane among us may sometimes fear that we are abnormal. There are times when we think we're so different from the rest of humanity we can't stand it. As we might have as children, we paint ourselves into a box and surround it with everything bad. It seems as though real life has stopped and we are suspended in a frightening void when we can't tell reality from fantasy. Is it real? Is it stress overload? How do we know?

▓ What Happens When You Fear You're Going Crazy

You imagine that you're being followed down the street, you hear voices, you see the toaster move out of the corner of your eye. If the situation persists for several days, you feel worn down by the constant mental exercise of warding off the scary monsters of your mind. It's terribly stressful to think that you've snapped, and you may find that you're unable to do your work, relate to your loved ones, or find any peace of mind in activities you generally enjoy.

Most people who suffer from a fear that they're going crazy really aren't. They are just bombarded with sensations and are hypersensitive to them. The amount of stress in everyday life is sometimes overwhelming, and when we can't deal with it, we shut down. The walls aren't really closing in, but they seem to be because we haven't gotten our mental and emotional resources together to push those looming bricks away.

Behavioral therapy and desensitization are the most common treatments for all panic disorders and phobias. See also the therapies suggested below for some specifics if you fear you're going crazy.

IF THE THERAPIES BELOW DO NOT ASSUAGE THE PANIC AT ALL, IT IS POSSIBLE THAT YOU ARE HEADED FOR A PSYCHOTIC BREAK AND SHOULD BE IN A DOCTOR'S CARE. MAKE SURE YOU TELL A FRIEND OR RELATIVE WHO WILL BE ABLE TO HELP YOU GET HELP.

Meditate Every Day

You can't go crazy if you have a strong grounding in reality, and this is the gift that meditation brings. As you sit each day for 20 minutes, your mind is the basis for your feelings—whatever they are. In this haven, you are fully in control of your senses.

Begin by sitting cross-legged on the floor or in a straight-backed chair. Concentrate on your breath. See the purity of each inhalation and exhalation—feel that they are cleansing your system. When you have established a good rhythm, begin to focus on the parts of your mind that you wish to contact. You can take your breath to the cerebral cortex and use it to clear your rational thinking processes. You can bring it to the frontal lobe and strengthen your decision-making and problem-solving abilities. You can take it into the limbic system and soothe your emotions. Remind yourself that there is nothing to fear in your mind. Slowly come out of the meditation by becoming aware of the world around you.

Get Nutritional Help

It is possible that your diet is affecting the way you feel. Various toxins such as lead, mercury, cadmium, arsenic, and aluminum can cause mental distortions (excessively high amounts of aluminum have been found in the brains of Alzheimer's patients). You may also have certain specific food sensitivities, such as allergies to wheat or dairy products, or you may have reactions to preservatives in food that make you feel distraught and crazy. See a nutritionist for a comprehensive look at your diet and have your physician do a blood or hair test to check for heavy-metal toxicity.

Play a Game with a Child

Nothing brings us back to what's real as much as a child who is intensely involved with everything and anything, greedily learning about what's real by participating in it.

You might go to a playground and let the child lead you in and around the equipment. Make sand castles together in the sandbox, go on the swings or the slide and see what makes you laugh and enjoy yourself the most.

Relax Progressively

In order to calm down and get control over your "fight or flight" reaction, progressive relaxation or autogenic training will be helpful. In progressive relaxation, you'll lie down and work your way from toes to head, alternately tensing and then relaxing each body part. When you've completed your body inventory, stay relaxed and breathe yourself deeper into the floor with a suggestion that you are well and safe.

Autogenic training is another system for relaxing parts of the body. Lie down or sit in a comfortable chair. Begin with your right arm and say to yourself, "My arm is heavy and warm. It is totally relaxed." Give this suggestion to each body part and say the words aloud. By the time you have completed your tour of the body and head, you should feel rooted, like a huge tree growing out of the ground.

Try a Flower

Cherry Plum is the Bach flower remedy for a fear of mental collapse. Place 5 or 6 drops in a half-glass of water, or directly under your tongue.

Homeopathic Help

Try the following homeopathic remedies for a fear that you may be going crazy:

> For a fear of insanity: Calcarea, Anacardium, Cannabis indica, Pulsatilla, Natrum mur, Nux vomica, Phosphorus, Sepia, Staphisagria, Stramonium.

> For a fear that something terrible will happen: Ignatia, Sepia.

*F*EAR OF *P*UBLIC *B*ATHROOMS

see also Obsessive Compulsive Disorders, page 329; Panic Disorders; page 344; Phobias, page 346

A fear of having to deal with our bodily functions in a public setting usually harks back to childhood and an overly insistent parent attempting early toilet training. Mothers who constantly nag their children about getting dirty or soiling themselves or letting strangers see their private parts may be breeding a phobia in their child about urinating and defecating in public.

The element of losing control figures prominently in this phobia. If you are terrified of letting go (loosening your sphincter), it may be because you need to keep a tight rein on yourself. Of course, there is no way to regulate our bodily functions completely, which makes us feel powerless and impotent in the face of instinct.

▣ What Happens When You Have a Fear of Public Bathrooms

You hold it until the very last minute, feeling your muscles contract and your sphincters tightened to the limit. You feel disgusted even before you enter the room and may hold your breath, anticipating a bad odor. You may not wish to look into the toilet, anticipating a view of what should not be seen. Most individuals who have a dirt phobia will cover the toilet seat with toilet paper and will stand or crouch over the toilet rather than sit down on it. This can produce muscular aches and pains that you always associate with going to the bathroom. Many men, anxious about the extremely open view at a urinal, will attempt to find an available cubicle with a door rather than stand next to anyone who might catch a glimpse of their genitals.

The more uncomfortable the experience, the more avoidance. The more avoidance, the more discomfort from trying to hold yourself back from natural release.

Behavioral therapy and desensitization are the most common treatments for all panic disorders and phobias. See also the suggestions below for therapies relating specifically to a fear of public bathrooms.

Clean the Space with Your Mind

You will use self-hypnosis to assist in your progress with this obsessive-compulsive disorder. Roll your eyes up and close your eyes, holding your breath. Feel that you are floating, that your left arm cannot remain in your lap but must float upward. When you are in trance, tell yourself that you emit a powerful disinfectant that will immediately wipe out any germs in your vicinity. You are also folded into an invisible protective shield that will keep you safe from any foreign or dangerous elements. As you enter a public bathroom, understand that you have the ability to keep yourself intact, because you respect and care for your body.

Get Flooded

Just do it. Although many behavioral therapists take a gradual approach, working your way slowly as you become desensitized to your fears, some experts feel that phobia is best abolished by using ungraded exposure. That means you must be at a maximum state of panic until at last the panic drops. (This approach is not advisable if you have a heart condition.)

FEAR OF PUBLIC SPEAKING

see also Anxiety, page 43; Nervousness, page 304; Panic Disorders, page 344; Phobias, page 346; Stage Fright, page 407

Half the population has nightmares about being onstage in front of thousands of people and not knowing what they're supposed to do. The extreme embarrassment of having everyone stare at you—everyone judging you—is the ultimate in terror for many individuals.

A little stage fright is good—it gives actors and speakers the edge they need to put on a terrific show. When your adrenaline is pumping, you are experiencing eu-stress, or the good stress that challenges us to work harder and do better. But for some, the feeling of panic is overwhelming.

What Happens When You Fear Public Speaking

Your throat closes up, your heart seems ready to jump out of your chest, and you can barely catch your breath. This means that you are in the midst of distress, a crippling condition that can be remedied by appropriate use of the following therapies:

Keep the Beat

Although speaking in front of a group can present many problems, often singing does not. Using self-hypnosis, you will give yourself a suggestion that if you keep the beat and stick with it—like a metronome—you can't go wrong. The rhythm of your speech will carry you through the fear. Roll your eyes up and close your eyes as you hold your breath. Now in a trance state, you can imagine yourself floating above the crowd. You are in complete charge, orchestrating the event as though you were a great composer and conductor. The words will flow out of you like music, rhythmically taking care of their own meter, pattern, and volume.

Practice Makes Perfect

The more you do it, the less anxiety-provoking it will be. Take any opportunity to get up in front of people and speak:

a party, a classroom setting, a PTO meeting at your child's school. Ask a group of friends over and play a game where everyone has to stand up and tell one interesting thing that happened to him or her that day.

Have a Relaxing Drink

A glass of wine (just one) often loosens your tongue and makes you feel a little more relaxed. You can also have a glass of warm milk—the amino acid tryptophan makes you slightly sleepy and less jittery.

Bach Flowers to the Rescue

Try 5 or 6 drops of Rescue Remedy under the tongue just before you go onstage.

Homeopathic Help

Try the following homeopathic remedies for stage fright; doses can be taken every half hour if fear is acute:

> Fear of public performance: Lycopodium
>
> If you feel weak in the knees: Gelsemium
>
> If you are a musician with a knotted stomach: Anacardium
>
> If you are so terrified of performing that you have diarrhea: Argentum nitrate

FELDENKRAIS THERAPY

Moshe Feldenkrais, a physicist and engineer who also held a black belt in judo, lived in Israel and Europe in the early days of this century. He discovered that many athletes he worked with had chronic pain that did not respond to massage or rest. Experimenting on his own, he developed a method of movement that combines awareness, attention, and imagination. It eliminates the need or desire to work for any goal, but rather, teaches each individual to discover what makes him or her comfortable. There is no right or wrong in Feldenkrais movement—only a better accommodation to your own body and mind.

This therapy is an educational process rather than an attempt to cure or fix what's wrong. Each person attends to his or her own feelings and thus discovers slowly and subtly how he or she holds tension in the body and how only he or she can relieve it. The therapist is there to suggest, but never to create a specific pattern or form for you to follow.

There are two types of Feldenkrais work—Awareness Through Movement, which consists of or group classes, and Functional Integration, which are private sessions with a therapist. In both cases, the principles are the same.

In a class setting, the theme of the day might be freeing up the range of the arm. You'd be asked to lie on your side on a mat on the floor and circle your arm above your head. As you play with this movement, you'll be able to see whether you can make a whole circle or are restricted to an oval; whether you have pain at any segment, whether you can touch the floor when your hand comes around, whether you can move your arm at the same speed at all points on the circle, and so forth. Since we are all accustomed to moving our arms in particular ways for effect, for example, to lift or push or pull, the experience of using abstract movement can be liberating.

In the individual sessions, which are usually for those who feel they want more intensive work or have a specific problem, the therapist will have you lie on the table and remain passive as he or she moves your body for you. It will be apparent where you are holding tension only after many tries to let it go, but the revelation of Feldenkrais is that one moment when you suddenly feel free or comfortable.

Because each student discovers this secret for himself or herself, the process conveys a great deal of self-esteem, self-confidence, and self-respect. Often, depressed people who always walked around with shoulders slumped and chest caved in will suddenly discover how wonderful it feels to straighten up. Breathing is easier, alignment of the bones and muscles is liberating, and years of being cramped inside your body can fall away in an instant.

The development of self-awareness is a wonderful tool for delving deeper inside. Feldenkrais therapy is useful for people who are into their bodies, such as dancers and athletes, but it may be most beneficial for people who live in their minds and are afraid to acknowledge the input of their bodies. Very often, individuals who were physically or sexually abused as children can find a path out by discovering what feels good. People whose physical tension is a remnant of a childhood command to "sit tight and don't squirm" can suddenly open up and move the way they want to.

Any mental or emotional problem that involves letting go can be helped by Feldenkrais, as can disorders that involve the body directly, such as Anorexia, page 34, Bingeing, page 59, and Bulimia, page 84, or Distorted Body Image, page 118.

You can take a quick course in Feldenkrais (most are six, eight, or ten weeks long), or you can make it a lifelong pursuit like yoga or tai chi. Very often, therapists will suggest that their clients combine meditation with Feldenkrais.

*F*INANCIAL EXTRAVAGANCE

see also Bipolar Disorder, page 67; Gambling, page 187; Impulse Control, page 246

Spending wildly is often done to impress others, and it can be a way to bolster a deficient ego. If you don't think much of yourself, but you have *things*, this proves to the outside world that you're substantial—you're "made of money."

▓ *What Happens When You're Financially Extravagant*

You purchase things without a thought to their cost, or to whether you'll have any need for them after the whim to buy has past. You don't tally your checkbook or record your credit card purchase, because to do so would be to acknowledge that you're in the red. You are very ostentatious about your purchases and want others to know what everything cost.

Financial extravagance is sometimes a symptom of bipolar disorder. When you are in a manic, euphoric state, everything seems wonderful; anything is possible. This means that you don't count pennies (or dollars), but simply spend for the sake of spending. This is not always a selfish pursuit; many people with bipolar disorder buy incredible gifts for friends and never think twice about the consequences. Even the appearance of bills at the end of the month doesn't quash the excitement of coming home laden with boxes and bags.

If you spend more than you have, your checkbook doesn't balance. If you max out your credit cards, you lose the ability to purchase more. Overspending can lead to a host of other problems—not leaving enough to buy necessities such as groceries or to pay the rent. The difficulties in getting out of long-term debt are massive and should be avoided at all cost.

Make a Budget

Sit down and add up exactly what you need to live on each month—no more and no less. You should factor in living expenses, food, gas, upkeep of your car if you have one, medical and pharmaceutical expenses, and personal upkeep such as haircuts and clothing for work. Then figure out what you need in your pocket per week for incidentals such as newspapers, snacks, or a necessary purchase from a drugstore.

At the beginning, you'll be astounded as to how fast the money goes, and it may take you several weeks to adjust your daily expenditures. Keep at it! This is the best way to make the theory of money into something real and concrete.

Don't Carry Any More Cash Than You Need

Once you have your budget set, understand that you can take this much and no more from an ATM machine at the beginning of the week. (You should, of course, keep an extra allowance available for emergencies, but you should define in advance what a financial emergency is.) Take only the amount you'll need for the day with you. You cannot borrow from subsequent days, although if you have money left on any particular day, you can use it the next day.

Cut up Your Credit Cards

Unless you have a debit card (where money is deducted directly from your checking account when you use it), you shouldn't have access to plastic. If you are concerned about getting and keeping a credit rating, get an American Express card, which must be paid monthly.

Write Down Everything You Purchase

Whether it's a newspaper or a silk blouse, write it down. Keep a daily tally of everything you spend and how you pay for it and check it each night. You will be amazed to see what actually goes out, and this in itself can restrict your spending the following day.

Get Support

Tell your friends and relatives what you're doing and request their participation in getting on a sensible spending program. You may also be able to find a support group in your community—either Gamblers Anonymous or Overspenders Anonymous—where you can attend meetings and have a buddy or mentor you can call when you feel an urge to open your wallet too wide.

Say an Affirmation Daily

Remind yourself that you're on a positive track and you can stick to it. Each morning, look yourself in the mirror and say,

I'm important without my possessions,
The riches of personal experience are worth millions,
I don't have to buy presents in order to be loved.

Though you may feel fake when you first begin to repeat these maxims, they will take on meaning as your program for spending less money becomes more familiar to you.

GAMBLING

see also Impulse Control, page 246

Once in a while, we all take a chance and bet on a long shot. But when the compulsion to wager makes you center your life around getting the money to gamble, it's an illness. Approximately six million Americans (between 1 and 3 percent of the population) have serious gambling problems and debt brought on by the problem that often ruins family life and career.

■ What Happens When You Have a Compulsion to Gamble

You cannot pass up a lottery ticket or a card game. You will go out of your way to place bets on sporting events, and the only vacations that give you pleasure are those where casinos are the major entertainment. You casually bet a friend that something will or will not occur, and you make sure the stakes are high and that your colleague is able to pay up if you win. You gamble because the excitement of not knowing where the chips will fall gives you a high; you gamble to relieve stress in your otherwise humdrum life; and you gamble to "chase" your losses—in other words, to pay off your debts.

Problem gamblers are usually highly competitive men in their thirties who work in an environment of high risk, such as investment, business, or law. They are gregarious, energetic individuals, concerned with the approval of their peers. They overflow with generosity—if they have a big win, they'll buy extravagant presents for family and strangers. When they cut back on their gambling, they become restless and irritable. A typical remark on hearing the lottery numbers read on the news is, "I almost played that number!"

Gambling is closely associated with crime. When you borrow from loan sharks and can't pay up, you and your family may be in serious danger. The mental anguish of never knowing when your number is up can't possibly be as bad as the threat of real physical harm coming to those you love.

Get Away from the Temptation

Just as recovering alcoholics cannot visit bars, recovering gamblers must stay out of casinos, betting parlors, and even 7/11s selling lottery tickets.

Reward Yourself in Other Ways

As you pass up an opportunity to place a bet, put that money aside to pay your debts. But keep a special envelope for a "reward" fund and place a dollar in it each time you resist temptation. At the end of the month, buy yourself or someone you love a gift.

Let Gravity Ground You

Because gambling typically causes a "high," you will feel agitated and nervous not gambling. A north-pole oriented, 800- to 1000-gauss magnetic field under your head as you lie on a massage table can help to relax the anxiety.

Don't Carry Cash . . . or Credit Cards

In order to revamp your spending, you will have to make most of your payments by check. Especially if you have had bad debts in the past, it's a good idea to explain to your creditors that you are in a recovery program and must account for every penny. By writing a check (even for bread and milk at the convenience store), you'll see exactly where your money is going.

Let Your Body Release

Bioenergetic therapy (and other bodywork) may get you in touch with some deeply buried feelings that drive you to risk everything you've got for the unknown. The breathing stool is an excellent medium for allowing the rage and pain to get out. Under the direction of a therapist, you will bend backward over the stool and breathe deeply. You may find that your thighs begin to shake, or that you feel like crying or yelling. Anything is permissible. Over a period of months, as you learn to release the stored tension in your body, your urge to gamble may dissipate as you develop real feelings of excitement for life.

Get Rid of Stimulants and Sedatives

If you're taking any type of medication to stay awake (so that you can gamble longer at a casino), or if you're a coffee addict, this is the time to stop. If you drink heavily so that you won't remember what you did the previous night, this is the time to stop. You will find, when you don't stimulate or sedate yourself, that clear-eyed reasoning is easier for you. You will also like yourself better when you're not on uppers or downers.

GASTROINTESTINAL DISORDERS

see also Anxiety, page 43; Stress, page 407

That rumbling in your stomach when you have to go into your boss's office—those butterflies banging around your intestines before an important event—that crippling diarrhea every time you think about your impending wedding!

Everyone has had stomach aches and gastrointestinal disorders that apparently have no organic cause. In fact, stress can cause the body to behave as though you had a virus or had eaten bad food. It's just as uncomfortable and just as real.

What Happens When Your Stomach is Upset

You may have cramps, pain, gas, diarrhea or constipation (or both), an empty or hollow feeling in your gut, a lot of noise and rumbling, as well as a jumpy "butterfly-in-the-stomach" feeling.

One reason that feeling upset can upset your stomach is that you actually have a secondary nervous system in your gut. The enteric nervous system lines the esophagus, stomach, small intestine, and colon. It is a network of neurons, neurotransmitters, and proteins, and it works independently of the brain to produce a variety of feelings. Interestingly enough, it puts out the same secretions as the brain does; serotonin, dopamine, nitric oxide, and even chemicals called benzodiazepines that relieve anxiety. Colitis and irritable bowel syndrome come from problems in this secondary brain, which has more neurons in it than the spinal cord.

When you feel distress or anxiety, the brain in your head releases stress hormones that prepare you for action. At this point, the gut's "brain" is stimulated by those hormones as well. If you're really terrified, you may experience a bout of diarrhea; if you're standing onstage and can't think of your lines, you may find that you can't even swallow because the neurons in your esophagus are overly stimulated.

The question is, can we control our enteric brain as we do our other brain? If we consider it a mirror of the brain in the head, then perhaps we can achieve calmer gastrointestinal states once we've mastered relaxing the primary brain.

So the calmer you can be, the better off you are. This means that rather than dealing with the stomachache, you must first ascertain the cause of the distress and deal with that.

CASE HISTORY

Barbara said she'd had stomach aches since she was 16. She had repeated GI series over the years, but no doctor could find anything wrong with her. They all told her it was stress and that she should learn to relax. After the birth of her second child, she was in such enormous distress that a friend recommended a nutritionist. Although Barbara knew nothing about alternative therapies, she decided to give it a try.

"I got to this man's office late at night and he opened the door himself. As he ushered us in, he asked if I'd like to sit down because I had a stomach ache. How did he know? I was really thrown for a loop.

"He examined me and the stool sample I'd brought along at his request. Then he told me to avoid all meat and dairy products, to take the list of vitamins he was going to prescribe, and to dance for two minutes every hour I was awake. I must say I didn't stick to my dancing, but I did everything else, and within six months I was completely fine. He kept fine-tuning the vitamins and minerals over the years as my body and mind changed. My nervous stomach quickly became a memory, and in the last 20 years, I haven't had any problem with gastrointestinal upsets."

Barbara currently takes a multivitamin powder with lots of E and lecithin in it daily, B_6 (500 mg.), Vitamin C (1000 mg.), CoQ10 (60 mg.), magnesium taurate (125 mg.), and pantothenic acid (1,000 mg.).

Breathe Into Your Stomach

The traditional Chinese method of healing breath and exercise, known as *qi gong* or "breath work," uses a point three inches below the belly button and about three fingers in as the center of the body. This point, known as the *tan tien,* or "field of elixir," is thought in Chinese medicine to be the source of energy and sustenance in the body. When you breathe in, you inhale oxygen along with energy—in a sense, filling up your bank account with a healthy deposit.

Inhale through your nose, contracting your stomach muscles and pulling everything into your center. Exhale and push the tan tien out, making a tight seal. As you repeat this exercise ten times, keep your hand on your belly, giving it resistance as you inhale and exhale. The more work you get from this part of the body, the more your internal organs will be able to counteract whatever nervousness and anxiety you may feel.

Let the Machine Guide Your Gut

Biofeedback has been shown to be effective in dealing with chronic gastrointestinal distress. Your "involuntary" muscles in your stomach and intestines contract and release as they send the food you've eaten along their journey down the alimentary canal to the excretory organs. While this is happening, you are also secreting various enzymes, to break down the food and make it easier to digest. Stomach acid, of course, is acid and can cause a lot of discomfort to the intestines.

Biofeedback techniques involve placing electrodes on your skin around the stomach area. By watching the screen and listening to auditory signals, patients learned to increase and decrease the frequency of stomach contractions by imagining the pattern the muscles are making and consciously watching that pattern slowing down. Another method of doing this is placing a stethoscope on your stomach so that you can listen to the intestinal digestive sounds and think about controlling them. As you relax more, the muscle movement does, too.

Be Kind to Your Stomach

Stay away from greasy, fatty foods and also from highly spiced foods. Never eat beyond your satiety level—if you're not hungry any more, stop eating. It's much better to have six small meals than three large ones daily. Pay attention to the temperature of the food as well—what you eat shouldn't be too hot or too cold. Make sure you're ingesting plenty of fiber so that your digestive system can get on track and function efficiently.

Drink to Your Stomach's Content

You should consume eight to ten glasses of liquid daily, preferably fresh spring water, herbal teas, and fruit juices. Don't drink carbonated beverages, which add gas to the digestive tract. Keeping your kidneys clear of waste is vital, and drinking a lot will help you avoid constipation.

Eat Slowly and Mindfully

Don't ever eat standing up or sitting in front of the TV. Each meal or snack should be a pleasurable experience, prepared and consumed lovingly and with attention to detail. Savor each bite, roll it around in your mouth, and chew thoroughly before swallowing. Be grateful for the nourishment that keeps you energetic and alive.

Inhale the Odor of Calm

The aromatherapy oils, Geranium and Neroli, are both sedative and uplifting. Put a little honey or brown sugar into an ounce of hot water and add two or three drops of either oil. Inhale this mixture once an hour for a few hours prior to a stressful event.

Go to the Bathroom When You Need To

If your gastrointestinal upset is caused by nervous tension, you may be eliminating more than usual. Don't worry about that—if you get your diet under control and start exercising, you'll get back on schedule. But remember that it's better to get waste and toxins out of your body. This means you shouldn't delay when you think you have to go.

Herbal Relief

Chamomile, fennel, peppermint, ginger, hops, and wild yam all ease spasm and inflammation in the digestive tract. Use $1/2$ to 1 teaspoon of dried herb in a cup of water three times daily or as needed.

Jog Your System

Exercise helps in the process of digestion and elimination. Make sure that whatever you do—jogging, swimming, racquet sports, dance, or martial arts—you do on an empty stomach. Aerobic activity will also temper your appetite, so that you'll eat lightly when you come in from an exercise session.

Practice Yoga

There are several yoga postures that are particularly beneficial for gastrointestinal disorders:

STOMACH LIFT: Stand with your feet apart, hands on your knees, like an umpire. Exhale completely and swallow, keeping your throat in the swallow pose. Then contract the front muscles of the abdomen and draw your stomach back toward your spine. Right before you need to inhale, release the abdomen.

STOMACH ROLL (NAULI): As you become more accomplished and can hold the stomach lift longer, you may move the stomach right to left, left to right, and around in a circle.

YOGA MUDRA: Sit cross-legged on the floor and circle your right wrist with the thumb and third finger of the left hand. Exhale and bend over as far as you can go, then breathe into the posture. As you feel more comfortable, try to touch the floor with your forehead, then your chin, then your chest.

GRIEF

see also Aging, page 17; Broken Heart, page 78; Depression, page 112; Death, thoughts of, page 109; Tearfulness, page 421

To grieve over a loss is a natural, emotional release of feelings. After a death, a divorce, the loss of a job—or in fact, any serious loss—we have to settle with ourselves. Grieving is a ritualistic way of making peace with whatever has been taken away from us.

■ What Happens When You Grieve

There is nothing in you but pain. You can't possibly stop the
tears or the anguish because they are part of your state of
mind. You are more than sad, more than angry, completely
involved in the experience of losing something you can
never again have back. Other people's comfort usually means
nothing, and you cannot imagine a time in the future when
you will once again be interested in life, work, sex, friends, or
a movie.

There is nothing wrong with grieving—as a matter of
fact, in some non-Western groups it is considered a highly
valuable state, one in which we lose touch with ordinary reality and submit ourselves to pure feeling. We become like the
frenzied, raging maenads who followed Bacchus, the god of
wine, and tore their hair and rent their clothes. The ritualistic tribal keening that follows the death of a relative sounds
inhuman, like the mourning wind, and yet it is an integral
part of the death practices of cultures around the world.

Grief does interfere with everyday life, and perhaps it
should. If we passed off our losses as though they meant
nothing, then our lives would be very shallow indeed. If a
person grieves too long or too wildly, it tends to be embarrassing for those around him or her, which is the reason family members beg their physicians for Valium and other soul-
deadening medications right after a traumatic loss.

The best thing to do with grief is to let it have its days.
There is nothing wrong with periodic bouts of tears, even if
they go on for months. If, however, you feel that the grip of
your grief is too strong to handle, you may wish to try some
of the following natural therapies.

Draw on the Right Side of Your Brain

Many of us tend to try to analyze our problems; we grasp at
whatever intellectual straws will help us to make sense of
tragedy. But often, it's more useful to allow the right brain
free access. This imaginative, emotional hemisphere can tell
us a lot about our grief.

You may use any artistic medium you choose—a crayon,
pen and ink, clay, or perhaps, if you're not artistically
inclined, a collage made of clipped-out photos. You do not

have to draw a picture of what happened or the person you lost, but rather, you should put together a visual impression of your feelings. Try not to think about what you're putting out—allow your hand to move the writing utensil or grip the soft clay in a way that feels right to you. A particularly useful tool designed by psychologists is a sand table. A heap of sand is laid out in front of you, and you can move it, dig it, swirl it, or place small dollhouse-type figures in it to represent what's going on in your emotional life.

Let Yourself Go

Dancing is a traditional means of expressing strong emotion. Many cultures use dance at funerals to allow the mourners full range of movement. What does it feel like when you throw your head back, when you spin wildly in a circle, when you jump in the air, or crouch on the balls of your feet? Put on some music and experiment with your limbs and torso. You may find that the unrestrained movement frees your stuck emotions; you may begin to laugh, cry, or make sounds that are aren't familiar to you. Don't be self-conscious—just let yourself release everything.

Homeopathic Help

Try the following remedies for grief: Aurum, Causticum, Ignatia, Lachesis, Natrum mur, Phosphoric acid, Phosphorus, Sepia, Staphisagria.

> For grief, if you cannot cry: Ignatia, Natrum mur, Nux vomica, Pulsatilla
>
> For love, with silent grief: Ignatia, Natrum mur, Phosphoric acid
>
> For anger, with silent grief: Aconite, Ignatia, Lycopodium, Staphisagria, China, Natrum mur, Phosphoric acid

Dream a Little Dream

This is a wonderful opportunity to communicate with your unconscious mind. Although you may feel as though your thoughts are all centered on the tragic event that causes you such grief, it is sometimes interesting to see what other elements appear to us in our dreams.

Keep a pad and pencil beside your bed. Tell yourself before sleep that you intend to remember your dreams. As soon as you wake, write down the pervasive mood—are you actually sad, or mad, or feeling as if you want to run away? Then begin to piece out elements and characters in the dream. Figure out first how you would like the dream to improve and then discuss it with the imaginary characters. See if you can make changes in the way your mind handles the grief and surrounding emotions. Maybe you can make peace with whatever has occurred in your unconscious life, and that will assist you in repairing the damage done in your waking life.

Get on Your Knees

When we are transported beyond ourselves in prayer, we realize that we're not alone and that sheltering forces are looking out for us. Whether or not you believe in a higher power, or whether your faith has been shattered by this terrible event, prayer can be a healing remedy. It is worthwhile to examine your feelings in the light of something bigger than yourself and your tragedy.

Use Chinese Wisdom for Your Sorrow

Traditional Chinese medicine sees grief as a malfunction of the Lung organ network, and deep breathing is recommended to open up the blockages here. You can also massage clockwise the two points on either side of the chest in the hollows made by the collarbone and the top of the ribs.

Plant a Garden

The change of seasons is a balm to tortured hearts. Even in the death of winter we can begin to see snowdrops growing under the snow. If you have access to soil and some seeds, plant a garden. You may find that growing new life is the best symbol for rebirth of the spirit you have.

GUILT

see also Anxiety, page 43

Guilt is the fear that you've done something wrong. Even if you aren't quite sure what it is, it eats at you, often taking away from your enjoyment in every other part of life. You may feel guilty that you spend so much time at work away from your kids, or guilty that when you're with your kids you're apparently not as interesting to them as their friends are. You may feel guilty about spending too much on a new car, or feel guilty that you bought an inexpensive used one which may not be in good shape and might get you and your family into accidents.

It is said that certain ethnic groups have cornered the guilt market—Catholics start with original sin and feel guilty for an act none of them (or even their ancestors) were alive to commit, and Jews are quite expert at instilling guilt in their children for not doing enough, amounting to enough, or even feeling guilty enough.

Although we make fun of our guilty feelings, they do symbolize an underlying fear that we have erred along the pathway of life, and some day someone is going to call us on it. In early life children can hit each other or kick the dog and go on about their merry way, but as they pass the age of six or seven, they realize that they are responsible and must take the blame. A child whose superego becomes terribly strong will take the burdens of others on her shoulders.

What Happens When You Feel Guilty

A sense of dread or looming terror is always with you. The sinking feeling in the pit of your stomach gets worse when you try to make light of your questionable behavior. You look over your shoulder, sure that someone else is about to point the finger and realize that you're the one placing the blame.

As good as we may be at our *mea culpas,* we are often helped along by spouses, parents, children, and friends who let us know they know how awful we are. If we are dependent on the opinions of others as to what constitutes appropriate behavior, we relinquish our power to make decisions and stand by them.

Of course, all of us occasionally do make mistakes that we'd prefer no one else find out about—the guilt we feel for covering up an extramarital affair or not reporting a big check to the IRS is reasonable punishment for moral lapses. But sometimes, making one real error can start us mulling over all our behavior—good and bad. It's when we start feeling guilty for anything and everything that it becomes a full-time, unrealistic job.

Take a Flower to Heart

The Bach flower remedies for guilt are Pine and Hyssop. Take 5 or 6 drops under the tongue or in half a glass of water.

Look at It Logically

Cognitive awareness will teach us to put different labels on our behavior so that we can see it clearly. Let us assume that you have a lot of guilt about your mother, who lives alone several states away from you. You think that you should invite her to live with you, yet you realize that this would alienate your husband and children. Besides, you don't want to have her around all the time.

But when you have her on your mind, it's as good as if she's there with you. Think about the irrationality of the following statements:

> *The only time my mother isn't miserable is when she talks to me on the phone.*
>
> *I haven't called her in four days.*
>
> *I've made my mother miserable.*

Look at the sequence of thought and see how you have put yourself at the center of your mother's world. If you don't call her and she's miserable, that's her fault. She ought to be calling others (or you, if she needs you) or getting out and doing something that would brighten up her day.

By identifying the false elements in your thinking, you can alleviate your guilt—at least some of the time.

Trash the Guilt

Write down on a piece of paper whatever you feel guilty about, whether it's a real or imagined offense. Crumple the piece of paper or tear it in shreds and drop it in the trash can. This completes your obligation; now you can think about something else.

Affirm Your Rights

You can come up with statements that will boost your self-esteem and record them on a tape recorder so you can play them back when you're in the midst of a guilty fantasy. Try some of the following affirmations:

> *I have a lot to offer to others.*
>
> *I live by a strong moral code and do unto others as I would have them do unto me.*
>
> *Other people's opinions don't count unless I really respect them.*
>
> *Whatever I've done is over with; it's time to move on.*

Alternate Your Nostrils

A particular type of yogic breathing, known as "alternate nostril breathing," not only relaxes you but also allies the two hemispheres of the brain. By concentrating on your inhalation and exhalation, you can stop the self-punishing thoughts as you allow cleansing breath to permeate your mind and soul.

Place your right thumb over your right nostril and inhale through your left nostril. Exhale through your left nostril and then close it off with the pinky and fourth finger of your right hand, releasing your thumb as you do so. Inhale through the right, exhale through the right, close the right with your thumb as you release your pinky and fourth finger. Repeat for ten minutes once a day.

*H*ALLUCINATIONS

see also Fear of Going Crazy, page 175; Panic Disorders, page 344

When you see, hear, or feel things that are not actually there, this is classified as a hallucination. Technically, what's happened in the brain is that acute fear and panic has stimulated the sensory cortex without any stimulus receptors being present.

■ *What Happens When You Have Hallucinations*

For a moment, you are certain that something terrifying has brushed your hand or called out to you. Out of the corner of your eye, you know you saw a bizarre figure. And then, a second later, you realize there is nothing, and you feel as if you're going out of your mind.

Hallucinations aren't common, but they can occur during a panic attack when the stress hormones are pouring out and you feel your heart pounding, your breath coming in gasps, and your head spinning. Your higher brain isn't functioning at peak to discard the stimuli that have invaded your mind. Usually, these visions or feelings pass quickly as the panic subsides.

Some individuals who are grieving over the death of a beloved spouse or relative may have hallucinations of that person coming back and talking with them. This experience can be comforting, and may actually help ease the transition over the loss.

Visual, auditory, or sensory hallucinations are also a component of drug or alcohol abuse and of schizophrenia.

Get Rid of Substances

If you have a drug or alcohol problem, or even if you're overusing caffeine or nicotine, this should be warning enough that it's time to stop. Understand that if you curtail the abuse cold turkey, you may suffer serious withdrawal symptoms. IF YOU HAVE BEEN HAVING HALLUCINATIONS, YOU SHOULD HAVE PROFESSIONAL SUPERVISION TO COME OFF AN ADDICTIVE SUBSTANCE. YOU MAY HAVE TO BE HOSPITALIZED OR KEPT UNDER OBSERVATION UNTIL YOUR SYMPTOMS DISSIPATE.

Breathe Yourself Whole Again

Breathing without visualization can be helpful to relax the spirit. You shouldn't try to think of anything or even to conjure up pleasant images. Your sensory apparatus has been oversensitized, so what you must do now is calm it down.

Sit in a quiet, comfortable place. If it makes you feel safer, you may wish to surround yourself with pillows or bolsters. Close your eyes and begin to feel your accelerated breathing getting slower and slower. Don't consciously try to alter the pace; simply let the natural rhythm in your body guide your inhalation and exhalation.

Tell yourself that there is nothing in the world right now except for this quieting breath. Feel it expand your belly, your lungs, your kidneys, your cardiovascular system. Open your heart to the warmth of your breath. Understand that you have nothing to fear and no time constraints. You may stay here and breathe as long as you like, and the longer you do it, the more benefit you'll derive from it.

When you're ready to finish, let your eyes open just enough to plant your gaze on the floor about two feet in front of you. When you're able to take in this much of the outside world, begin to listen to the sounds of life around you—doors opening and closing, footsteps, traffic, and so forth. If you allow your breath to lighten your spirit, you will be able to determine which of these sights and sounds are real.

Try a Flower Remedy

Cherry Plum is the Bach flower remedy if you fear mental collapse and loss of control. Rescue Remedy is also a good idea when you're in a panicky state. Take 5 or 6 drops under the tongue.

Go for a Blow

A sharp rap on the cheek or both hands is a strong—and real—sensory stimulus that can bring you back to reality. If you can tell a friend to smack you lightly, do so—otherwise you'll have to do it to yourself.

HANDWASHING BEHAVIOR

see also Obsessive-Compulsive Behavior, page 329

Repeated handwashing behavior is a type of obsessive-compulsive disorder, which is defined as a chronic or recurring pattern of ritualized behavior (compulsiveness) to accommodate a phobia (the obsession). About 1 percent of the population is afflicted with this condition, although many more people may at times exhibit behavior over which they feel they have no control.

What Happens When You Are Compelled to Wash Your Hands Repeatedly

You are desperately afraid of contamination from dirt or germs. Therefore, you have an aversion to touching people or objects and avoid household and other tasks that involve use of your hands. If you have to perform them, you may wear several pair of gloves. If you're unable to complete the rituals you have established to comfort yourself, you may be overcome with panic attacks, palpitations, trembling, and other symptoms of extreme stress reaction.

Desensitization

This behavioral approach is considered the gold standard of treatment for obsessive-compulsive disorder. Early diagnosis is the key.

Desensitization involves getting over your terror and revulsion by throwing yourself into the midst of it. In order to stop handwashing, you have to accept germs, dirt, and contamination by others.

The program consists of behavioral learning therapy; that is, you must learn new, healthy behavior by practicing it over and over. Exposure begins slowly, and you are not expected to escalate to the more difficult steps until you can do the early ones without anxiety. Relaxation and visualization are an integral part of the process.

- You will look at a picture of a dirty shoe and try to breathe deeply, relaxing your muscles as you see the picture. When you are able to do this without great anxiety, you can move on to the next stage. If you begin to feel panicked, you can go back to the stage before.

- You will look at a dirty shoe while a therapist holds it and talks to you calmly about the positive qualities of the shoe.

- You will stand beside the dirty shoe until you are able to look at it without anxiety.

- You will hold the shoe with one hand by the laces. You may not wash afterwards.

- You will hold the shoe on the sides with both hands.

- You will touch the bottom of the shoe and rub the dirt on your hands. You may not wash afterwards.

Therapy can be initiated in a psychologist's office (even in a hospital if symptoms are severe), but must be practiced at home with the cooperation of your friends and family.

Change Your Behavior

In order to change behavior, we must first have the motivation to do so. It's best to start by making a list of positive forces that would help to change the behavior and opposing forces that perpetuate the behavior.

On the side moving toward change and healing, you can say that handwashing doesn't eliminate all germs, that it takes a great deal of time and energy and roughens your skin. Your obsession keeps you distant (physically and otherwise) from those you love. On the other hand, the forces that keep you from changing are your fear, your desire for control over situations, and the fact that you've had this habit so long you do it without really thinking about it.

The next step is to find certain interventions that will keep you on track. For handwashing we would use proscriptive lists (when you may not wash), activities such as "contaminating" a towel by letting another use it and then using it yourself. We'd also employ positive self-talk with diary and tape recordings. The following is a typical program:

Tell Yourself You're Okay

Start the day by looking into the mirror and repeating positive phrases such as,

> *I am doing well, I feel great.*
>
> *Nothing can harm me.*
>
> *The world is a sparkling place, full of interesting people and things for me to explore when I feel ready.*

Play Back Some Good News

Tape record the above message, and others you may read from sources that give you inspiration, such as the works of F. Scott Peck or Louis Buscaglia or Marianne Williams. Play them back to yourself when you feel a need for a supportive boost. Just hearing your own voice saying these positive things is a spur to healing your behavior.

Write Yourself a Contract

You will create a contract for yourself and sign it in the presence of witnesses. Make your own list of promises to yourself and be as imaginative as you can, adding elements you really find difficult (remember to escalate to the harder ones slowly and to move back to the easier ones if you are having too much anxiety).

Contract with Myself

I promise from here on to follow the pattern I have designated:

- I will allow myself only two handwashes a day and one bath or shower a day.

- I may keep a bar of soap in my office or bedroom, but it must remain wrapped and dry.

- I will practice preparing a snack or cup of coffee for my family or friends—I will use utensils and cups and saucers they have already touched ("contaminated").

- I will take a cup or glass from a friend or family member who has already sipped from it and take a sip myself.

- I will accept pencils or pens that others have used or carried around and write with them.

- I will use towels that have already been touched by other family members. I may not carry a towel or "wet wipes" with me when I go out.

- I will put on gloves or other clothing that has already been worn by a friend or family member.

- I will practice going to restaurants and using napkins and utensils that have been previously touched by the waiter.

- I will touch toilet seats in my own house, take out the garbage, and pick up my family's dirty laundry and put it in the hamper.

I agree to stick with this program because I know it will work for me!

Signed _____.

Join a Group

You don't need an already established group to make use of this valuable therapy—friends and family can serve as your team. Set up meetings to discuss your progress and to ask for advice about new projects you might tackle. Be sure you are getting positive as well as critical feedback. Because there is a real value to being able to help others as well as receiving help yourself, you might want to start a general group in your area and invite people who are phobic or obsessive or have other types of psychological problems. Many ongoing groups are already in place at hospitals around the country; check with the public relations department of your local medical center to see if there is one appropriate to your needs.

Get Touched

Throw yourself into an activity where you have to be "contaminated" as part of your desensitization training. Partnered dancing is a great option, and you may want to choose the type according to the music you like best: folk dance, square dancing, line dancing, or ballroom dancing. This therapy is excellent for obsessive-compulsives because the patterns of touching and being touched are set in advance—there are no surprises. The choreography of the dance will give you advance notice about when and where you'll make contact with your partner.

Try a Little Tai Chi

Although most people think of tai chi as a solo form, you can also work with a partner. "Push hands" tests your own balance and your partner's—the goal is not to push someone over but in fact to discover where you are vulnerable and where you are centered and rooted. This is particularly beneficial for compulsive handwashers who have a dread of losing control of the "germ" situation.

Partners stand facing each other, right feet forward and parallel, left feet slightly back and angled 45 degrees out. Right wrists are touching, and the left hand is supporting the partner's left elbow. Together you are making a circle with your arms. Partner A initiates movement and shifts his or her weight to the front foot, pushing toward B's chest. B yields to his or her own back foot. So as not to be pushed over, B shifts his or her hips to the left away from A and continues the circle, now pushing toward A's chest. The circle continues ad infinitum— you can challenge your partner as you get more experienced by angling your hands and hips differently. Remember to keep your head up and the alignment of your spine perfectly straight. And let yourself be pushed as often as you have to be. The idea is not to resist but to go with the flow.

Breathe as You Touch

In the push hands exercise above, inhale as you yield to your partner and exhale as you push forward. Think of taking in oxygen through your belly and allowing it to travel throughout your body, expanding each tissue and organ it touches. As you inhale, keep your mouth and teeth closed and contract the abdomen; as you exhale, let air out through your nostrils and just a small stream of air out through your slightly parted lips.

No matter how unbalanced you may feel when your partner is pushing, never let all the air out but keep a core of it at your center in order to strengthen your actions. You will find, as you concentrate on the breath, that you don't have to think so much about pushing and yielding and that your fears of being touched and touching will be reduced.

Get a Gentle Rubdown

A person who has trouble touching because of a fear of contamination may also feel afraid when he or she is being touched. A licensed massage therapist who is used to dealing with very sensitive clients is a must; you can also ask a friend, partner, or family member to do gentle massage on you.

As in any desensitization process, you must work from a more to a less anxious feeling. You may direct the masseur to touch or to remove touch from you at any time.

Ask the masseur to start on a part of the body you are most comfortable with—it will probably be your back and shoulders, and you will probably wish to be clothed. For the first few massage sessions, only light touch should be used on these areas. After a while, the masseur can proceed to your head, neck, legs, and arms, and finally to your hands. Remember that if you are feeling anxious, you can go back to any earlier stage and work your way up again.

Full-body massage with just a sheet as a covering will undoubtedly bring up a great deal of emotion, and you may find yourself crying, shaking, or even laughing. This is perfectly normal and is part of the therapeutic process of letting go of your obsession.

Remedy the Situation

Try the following homeopathic remedies:

> For emotional upsets: Phosphorus (This remedy has long-lasting effect, so don't repeat it often.)
>
> If you feel fearful, anxious, and dizzy: Aconitum napellus
>
> If you are irritable, impatient, hypersensitive to touch, noise, light, odors: Nux vomica

Imagine Yourself Healthy

Sit in a comfortable, quiet, dimly lit spot and begin by closing your eyes. Support your back with a cushion if you need to and keep your hands on your knees, palms turned upward.

Breathing lightly from your abdomen, start to think about the feeling of air on your body. It lightens all your cells, swirling from outside to inside. The energy from this air is able to infuse all your tissues and organs with power and vibrant health. Now see this air as a loving hand, stroking you and calming your spirit. The hand moves from your spine up to the top of your head, one vertebra at a time, and finally coasts over your scalp and inches down your chest, coming to rest on your own hands. You will have a sense of nothing touching you and yet being enveloped in a protective warm cloak. Feel this gracious hand taking yours, as though you were a child and it were your mother. Enjoy the sensation of your hands being held by this capable, life-affirming spirit.

Take three more healing breaths and slowly allow your eyes to relax open.

*H*EADACHES/*M*IGRAINES

see also Anxiety, page 43; Stress, page 407

When your head pounds, it's hard to think and even more difficult to feel good about life. If you suffer from frequent headaches, it may seem as if you're encased in a vise of steel and can't escape. This terrible agony may leave you constantly stressed, unable to deal with others or with your daily activities.

■ *What Happens When You Suffer from Headaches*

There are two general categories of headache: tension headaches and vascular headaches (of which migraines and cluster headaches are the most common varieties). Headaches stemming from physical causes such as eyestrain, hangover, or sinus conditions will have many of the same symptoms and will respond to the same treatments.

TENSION HEADACHES result from sustained contraction of skeletal muscles around the face, back of the neck, and forehead. When the muscles contract, they don't get enough oxygen, and there may also be an accumulation of toxins that cause pain. When you're upset or anxious, the dull, nonthrobbing pain of a tension headache is a logical result. This type of headache is generally on both sides of the head and responds better to heat (to open blood vessels and relax muscles) than to cold.

MIGRAINE HEADACHES are more common in women and have certain distinguishing characteristics. The pain is generally one-sided, can last anywhere from 4 to 72 hours, has a pulsing or throbbing quality, makes the sufferer nauseated and sensitive to light and noise. Additional symptoms may sometimes include an awareness of flashing lights and shimmering zig-zag lines or blank areas in the visual field. The vascular-type headache responds better to cold (to contract the blood vessels) than to heat.

A migraine is a type of nervous system overexcitability that creates neuron imbalances and changes in the regulation of blood flow throughout the head and body. The various migraine triggers set off a rush of chemical messengers, including serotonin, dopamine, histamine, and norepinephrine. At the same time, they depress the ability of the brain to produce endorphins, the natural pain killers that might stop a headache in its tracks. The overabundant supply of neurotransmitters in turn sets off reactions in the blood vessels. This combination of nerve sensitivity, muscle spasm, dilated blood vessels, and low endorphins create what we think of as a migraine.

These headaches can wreak havoc with your life; if you're getting them frequently, you may be out of commission and out of social contact for a day or two during the headache and then for a couple of days' recovery afterward.

Some migraines ("classic" migraine) give notice before they arrive—the person has an aura or a sense that something is about to happen. The "common" migraine doesn't offer this protection. But if you suffer from the first variety, you can do something effective while you're still *compos mentis*.

CLUSTER HEADACHES Are almost always found in men and are cyclical. They occur in groups of four to eight a day, daily or every other day for one to three months, after which you may have a respite of several months or years before they reappear. They have been described as "a red-hot poker going through my eye to my brain," and in fact have driven some sufferers to suicide. Although they are also vascular headaches like migraines, there is an element of hormonal imbalance as well.

Some of the following treatments work for both types of headaches; if they are designed only for vascular headaches, this will be specified below.

Learn a Relaxation Technique

Meditation, progressive relaxation, autonomic suggestion, self-hypnosis, and guided imagery are all successful methods of dealing with tension and vascular headaches.

If your main symptom of stress is that pounding or vise-like grip, you have to do some personal work on your tendencies to be ambitious, conscientious, a perfectionist, and a workaholic.

Set yourself a half hour a day to sit by yourself with no goals and no challenges. You may breathe quietly, listen to music, or imagine a succession of fluffy white clouds passing through your head.

Do this as a preventive exercise even if you aren't having headaches.

Put Your Head in Someone Else's Hands

A visit to a chiropractor or osteopath for manipulation may be the key to success for you. Myofacial and craniosacral therapies, (see page 104) are even more specific treatments for headache that some migraine sufferers swear by.

Chiropractic theory is based on a belief that the slightest misalignment of the spine can create pressure on nerves that may impinge on many different parts of the body. Subluxations (alterations of the normal placement of vertebrae) can occur at any part of the spine, increasing or decreasing the flow of nerve energy to the organs or tissues connected with this nerve.

A headache, therefore, may evolve from a subluxation of the cervical vertebrae, which can affect blood supply to the head and cause headache, nausea, dizziness, and ringing in the ears.

Your chiropractor or other professional who is trained in manipulation won't work only on your upper spine. The entire body is involved in a headache and must be adjusted to reestablish normal blood and nerve function.

Let the Machine Train Your Mind

Biofeedback has been used successfully in the treatment of migraines since it was discovered that hand temperature rose dramatically (about ten degrees) at the onset of a headache. The patient's hands are hooked up to a machine that provides feedback (either a visual picture on a screen or a blinking light) when the correct response is given. The patient uses imagery and autogenic suggestion ("My hands are heavy, my hands are warm") as well as the prompting from the machine in order to learn to control temperature. After it's evident that the patient can alter temperature with thought process, the machine isn't needed anymore. In this way, at the onset of a headache, the patient is in control of skin temperature and can literally *think* it back to normal.

A second method uses an electrode attached to an artery in the scalp, and the patient is taught to control blood flow. In a classic migraine, there is a period of time when the blood vessels in the head constrict, but prior to that, if you can think about opening the vessels you may be able to ward off the headache.

Biofeedback is also used for tension headaches. The headache sufferer is connected to the machine via electrodes that measure the muscle activity at rest and when an upsetting thought or feeling is experienced. If the muscles are tight, a high-pitched tone pierces the air; when the patient learns to relax these muscles, the tone lowers. The idea is to lower the tone as you relax progressively, and this will take care of your tension headache.

Press Your Points

Acupressure is a wonderful way to release tension, since pain is often caused by blocked nerve impulses at particular sites throughout the body. Press the following points for 20 seconds, release for 10 seconds. Repeat the process four times at each point:

- the web of skin between the thumb and forefinger
- the top of your foot between your big and middle toes
- outside your shinbone, just below the knee
- both temples together
- the back of your neck at the base of your skull on either side of the spinal column (at earlobe level)

Try a Chinese Herbal Elixir

This is a common mixture for headaches that are accompanied by cold hands and feet, loss of appetite, nausea, tension in neck and shoulders, and/or migraine: *wu ju yu tang* (Euodia decoction), made from euodia, ginseng, Chinese jujube, and fresh ginger. If your headache or migraine is accompanied by pain, nausea, congestion in the chest or solar plexus, and profuse perspiration, you might try *gui jir ren sheng tang* (cinnamon and ginseng decoction): cinnamon, licorice, atractylis ovata, ginseng, dried ginger.

Take one of these decoctions morning and evening over three to six months on an empty stomach. (These should give short-term as well as long-term relief.)

Get a Breath of Sea Air

Ions are positively and negatively charged particles—in a natural setting such as the mountains or seashore, the ratio of positive to negative ions is five to one. Indoors or in polluted environments, however, we don't get enough negative ions.

A study at Columbia University directed its headache participants to take a walk by the sea and take advantage of the negative ions released into the air by the crashing ocean waves. More than half the participants felt relief of their symptoms within half an hour.

Watch the Weather

Stay out of the sun, or at least wear a hat and sunglasses if you absolutely must be in it. Hours spent under those beating rays can dehydrate you and dry up fluids responsible for cushion-

ing the spinal cord and brain. As blood vessels rub on surrounding tissues, you can develop a whopper of a headache.
An environmental trigger of migraines is any rapid change in
humidity, altitude, or barometric pressure. If you are going
on a trip where you may hit serious weather, stay out of the
thick of the storm. If you love mountain climbing, do it slowly, making sure you adjust to each increase in altitude gradually.

Get Sexual

The classic excuse for not having sex is having a headache.
However, there is a growing body of evidence that sexual
stimulation can actually ward off a headache in progress, and
there are anecdotal reports that enough good sex can stop
migraines for good.

When we are sexually aroused, there is a flow of neurotransmitter production that makes us feel good. These natural opiates actually turn off the pain center in the brain when
the pleasure center is activated. At the same time, we are able
to direct blood flow from the head down to the genitals,
which become engorged as they prepare for orgasm. By
diverting capillary and vessel activity in the head to the lower
part of the body, we are depriving the migraine of the "food"
it needs to flourish.

No Happy Hours

Alcohol is one of the most common triggers for migraines or
clusters. If you often have these headaches, don't ever have
more than two drinks; and if you haven't eaten or if you're
particularly stressed out, don't have any. A tension headache
might initially respond well to one drink because alcohol
relaxes muscles; however, you may well replace the tension
headache with a vascular one if you overindulge.

Slow Down, Cool Off

The feeling of being rushed and overheated often starts a
migraine. So give yourself plenty of time to do whatever you
have to and wear layers of clothing, so that you can take off
the top layers if necessary.

Don't Disco

The nervous stimulation of loud noises and flashing lights can often trigger a migraine. Make sure you avoid situations where you might encounter these phenomena.

Watch What You Eat

Approximately 20 percent of migraine sufferers have some food sensitivities. Some triggers for migraines include all caffeinated products, MSG (often found in Chinese restaurants) and certain spices such as garlic and onion powder or meat tenderizers, certain legumes (fava, soy, and lima beans, lentils, onions, peas), nuts and seeds, pickles, and many fruits (citrus fruits, bananas, figs, raisins, papaya, raspberries, pineapples). The additive tyramine (similar to the amino acid, tyrosine), is a real culprit; it is found in anything made with yeast, in aged cheese, processed deli meats, soy sauce, eggplant, and sour cream.

Also, never skip meals. When you do so, your blood sugar level plummets, which may trigger a migraine.

Supplements for Your Head

Large doses of calcium can stop headaches in their tracks. Take 500 to 1000 mg. up to four times daily.

Inhale Some Relief

Massage one drop Peppermint oil into each temple when you have a headache or migraine.

Homeopathic Help

Try the following remedies for headaches:

For throbbing, swelling and pressure: Apis

For right-sided headaches, throbbing, fullness in the forehead, pain coming and going quickly: Belladonna

For bursting frontal headache: Bryonia, Lycopodium

For a band around the head, blurred vision: Gelsemium

For a thousand hammers knocking, pain in the eyes: Natrum mur

Hold the Hormones

It has been found that excess estrogen not only triggers migraines but makes them more severe. If you are a woman currently taking hormone replacement therapy (HRT), you may wish to talk to your doctor about discontinuing this medication.

IF NONE OF THE ABOVE NATURAL TREATMENTS HEALS YOUR HEADACHES, YOU SHOULD SEE A DOCTOR AND POSSIBLY HAVE A CT SCAN OR MRI OF YOUR BRAIN TO BE CERTAIN THE PAIN IS NOT CAUSED BY A TUMOR. THIS RARE TYPE OF HEADACHE IS CHARACTERIZED BY VISUAL, SPEECH, OR PERSONALITY CHANGES, PROBLEMS WITH EQUILIBRIUM OR GAIT, SEIZURES, AND PAIN THAT BECOMES INCREASINGLY WORSE.

*H*ERBALISM

see also Aromatherapy, page 46

Herbs are natural drugs, probably the oldest pharmaceutical medicines that exist. The versatility of plants is what makes them so desirable in terms of their healing powers: you can use the root, the rhizome, the flower, the leaves, the bark, and the seeds to produce a tea, an infusion, a tincture, or a powder to be put in a capsule; you can turn it into a cream for topical application or capture its essence in aromatherapy by inhaling it or rubbing it on the body.

The active compounds in plants either promote certain reactions or inhibit certain cell processes. But although many herbal compounds are used to create drugs, there is a major difference: Herbs work on the whole person with a battery of ingredients, whereas drugs filter out just one chemical element from a plant and target the disease with that one active ingredient. When you drink a tea or take a tincture, you are getting a combination of vitamins, minerals, enzymes, and hormonal precursors. Each herb has one main action, but also possesses many supportive factors that benefit your entire system.

■ *Tonics and Nervines Soothe Mind and Body*

When we think of using herbs to take care of a mental or emotional condition, we think first of tonics, and then, of nervines.

A tonic strengthens the whole system; it will treat an acute problem and a chronic condition simultaneously. A tonic works directly on the target organ or system that needs help, but at the same time, it works slowly on the body as a whole over a period of months. Dandelion, for example, is a wonderful general herb that helps strengthen the heart but contributes to the well-being of both body and mind as well; it also supports the liver, which means that it helps to process toxins that might otherwise diminish your good health.

A nervine works specifically on the nervous system. Most tend to relax you, acting something like a tranquilizer, and others stimulate you; however, all these plants strengthen the system at the same time. The holistic effect of taking a nervine is that you feel more awake and aware, but also calmer and revitalized.

The best known nervines are:

oats	damiana
scullcap	vervain
wood betony	black cohosh
black haw	lemon balm
California poppy	motherwort
chamomile	pasque flower
cramp bark	passionflower
hops	rosemary
St. John's wort	hyssop
Jamaica dogwood	lady's slipper
lavender	

If your condition involves a sense of fatigue and weakness or despondency about life in general, you may not want an herb that will calm you. Rather, you would do better with a nervine stimulant. These herbs give a boost to the nervous system without the side-effects of "uppers." Something such as ginseng or peppermint is useful in this case, as are wormwood and mugwort—two bitter herbs that stimulate the whole metabolism.

The whole plant concept is essential to herbal therapy. The one active ingredient that alleviates your depression or calms your fear is not sufficient to heal. However, the body can best utilize this ingredient by taking it in while it is balanced by the various other constituents of the plant. Not only can we reap the benefits of the particular nervine factor, we can gain a stronger system in general by ingesting all the other parts of the plant that heal and nourish.

Herbs work in a synergistic way, that is, all the properties of the plant enhance each separate property. If you are taking several herbs at once, the effects of some will be highlighted more than if you took just that herb alone.

■ *How to Buy and Prepare Herbs*

Most busy individuals don't have time to pick their herbs, dry them, and keep them fresh for months. Because the timing of herb gathering is an art unto itself (certain herbs lose their maximum potency if picked at the wrong time of day or the wrong season), it's better to purchase what you need in a health-food store or through a mail-order catalogue (see Resource Section, page 475). It's best to buy organic, domestic herbs that have not been sprayed with chemicals; don't experiment with varieties that have not been tested in this country. After six months, loose herbs are practically worthless, so buy small quantities—just what you need for a month or two.

Herbs can be taken as teas, infusions, tablets or capsules, tinctures, and as essential oils for aromatherapy.

TEA: One heaping teaspoon dried herb in tea ball, in one cup water. Generally, teas are too weak to offer real medicinal benefit, but are good as a general tonic and can be calming and comforting throughout the day. (Herbal teas contain no caffeine, which would stimulate rather than relax you.)

INFUSION: One ounce of cut-up leaves or flowers in a pint jar, cover with boiling water and steep (leaves for four hours, flowers for two). Drink two cups of infusion a day if you weigh from 125 to 150 pounds; three cups daily if you weigh from 150 to 200 pounds; four cups if you are over 200 pounds. If you find the mix too bitter, you can sweeten with a little juice.

DECOCTIONS: Use one ounce cut-up hard root, bark, or seeds in a pint jar, covered with boiling water and steeped. A decoction can be stored in the refrigerator for months. Use the same dosage as for infusions, above.

CAPSULE: These are freeze-dried extracts of the plant, packed into gelatin capsules. Depending on the herb and the size of the capsule, take two to three capsules, twice or three times daily.

TINCTURE: This is prepared by soaking the fresh or dried herb in an alcohol or vinegar-based solution. Depending on the herb and the concentration, take 1/2 to 1 teaspoon two to three times daily in a quarter cup of water. Shake the bottle well before filling the dropper.

AROMATHERAPY OILS: Mix 2 drops of the specified oil in a carrier oil (sweet almond, wheatgerm, or grapeseed oils are typically used) and use in a vaporizer or bath or for massage.

Dosages

Most experts suggest different dosages for different purposes, and dosages for children should be half the amount required for an adult.

FOR INCREASED ENERGY: Take one dose daily on an empty stomach; either 2–4 capsules/tablets or 10–18 drops tincture or 1 cup tea (made from 1 ounce fresh or dried herb).

FOR VITALITY/NUTRITION: Take two divided doses, one with breakfast and one with dinner daily; either 4–6 capsules daily or 10–15 drops tincture daily or 2 cups tea (made from 2 ounces fresh or dried herb).

FOR RELIEF OF SYMPTOMS: Take several doses throughout the day between meals (every 4 to 6 hours): either 2 capsules/tablets every four hours or 15 drops tincture under the tongue or mixed with a glass of water every 4 hours or 1 cup tea every 4 hours.

Safety of Botanical Medicine

Although we think of botanical medicines as being safer than drugstore pharmaceuticals, with far fewer side effects, they are powerful compounds and must be carefully dosed. Herbs can be harmful—even lethal—if used improperly, and the effect of taking several herbs in combination can be totally different from taking one at a time. Be sure you start with the *lowest dosage* and gradually increase if you need it.

Certain stimulant herbs are contraindicated if you have chronic hypertension, and others are prohibited during pregnancy because they may start uterine contractions. Do not use the following herbs if you are pregnant (those starred are recommended throughout the book as useful for mental and emotional problems):

sweet flag	pleurisy root
barberry	beth root
Oregon grape root	yarrow
*ginseng	*feverfew
ma huang	arnica
tansy	shepherd's purse
juniper	pennyroyal
camphor	licorice
flax	mistletoe
blood root	devil's claw
*passion flower	thuja
lavender	greater celandine
opium poppy	pokeroot
wild cherry	red and yellow cinchona
rue	chilis
lovage	*vervain

The following should be used with caution during pregnancy, only with your health-care provider's approval:

*burdock	*mugwort
marigold	*German chamomile
watercress	fenugreek
*motherwort	catnip
*lemon balm	angelica
wood sorrel	*gotu kola
Queen Anne's lace	

The laxative herbs (cascara, senna, rhubarb, and aloe) are also restricted in pregnancy, as are coltsfoot and comfrey because of their particular alkaloids.

The following herbs are strongly hypoglycemic and should never be used by anyone with chronically low blood sugar:

cayenne pepper   garlic (Kyolic garlic is okay)
goldenseal   onion
pau d'arco

A small dose of one herb may do nothing to affect the way you feel, but an overly large dose could aggravate or even worsen your condition.

You will notice that you rarely get an immediate effect; the healing that comes with herbal treatments is cumulative and works slowly, changing your system over a period of months. It is always best to consult a professional herbalist as well as your regular health-care practitioner before using any herbal preparation.

HOMEOPATHY

The root *homeo* means "similar"; the suffix *pathein* means illness. In the holistic practice of homeopathy, *like cures like.* When Dr. Samuel Hahnemann came up with this concept in the eighteenth century it was because he believed that there was more to illness and wellness than a set of symptoms. He felt that personality and circumstance often dictated what went well and badly in the body and mind.

The homeopathic system (as opposed to the conventional allopathic system that supplies a drug to act in opposition to the disease) offers the patient a small dose of something that in large dosages would be toxic or upsetting. The remedy may be so diluted that there will not be any of the original substance left; however, the energy of that substance directs the body and mind toward its own healing course.

Although there are homeopathic remedies for anything that might ail you, they are particularly effective for emotional and traumatic conditions. The first diagnosis by any homeopathic physician deals not only with symptoms but with ways in which you react to life in general. So a broad-spectrum description of what a remedy does might include sensitivity to cold, sensitivity to what people say about you, and the fact that distant music causes you sadness. In order to select a remedy that's right for you, you must know something about your inner self, not just your outer symptoms. Any aches, pains, or mental or emotional problems you have represent disharmony and imbalance in the whole person.

The premise of this type of medicine is that any symptoms you have represent your own personal way of fighting illness. By taking a remedy that is similar to your reactions, you are pushed a little further toward reorganizing yourself around a higher state of health.

The Hierarchy of Symptoms

It's important to chart all the various feelings you have, and according to the homeopathic system, *unusual or peculiar* symptoms (such as if your bones feel like shattered glass or it feels as if an animal is trying to escape from your stomach) come first. These strange manifestations of the disease state would give a homeopath a clear picture of the particular remedy necessary.

If no such symptoms occur, the next place to look is at mental and emotional problems. They rank second highest in the hierarchy of symptoms because they are greatly indicative of personality disturbances. A very aggressive person who is angry and has heart palpitations would need a different remedy from a very shy person who is upset and has heart palpitations.

The next level of inquiry is general problems and includes all relevant symptoms that relate to appetite, sleep, body temperature, and function of the reproductive organs.

Finally, particular symptoms show obvious signs of illness, such as fever, sore throat, rash, intestinal upset, and so forth. These are the least important symptoms in the hierarchy because they are simply the outward manifestation of the lack of internal harmony.

In treatment, the "law of cure" states that the first problems to vanish are those that came last. Usually, the vital organs such as the lungs and heart will heal before the less crucial ones, such as the skin or throat. Symptoms move from inside the body outward, dispelling toxins through the bowels, urine, vomit, and so forth. And the symptoms usually move from top to bottom—a rash might move from the leg to the foot before disappearing altogether.

How the Remedies Work in Body and Mind

The homeopathic system is based on restoring and conserving energy in the body and mind. This means that you do not need a potent drug that acts on a target organ to heal; rather, you simply need a trigger that will boost the energy inherent in a dynamic system such as the body.

Homeopathic remedies are derived from plants, flowers, animals, and minerals, some benign, some—such as bee-sting and snake venom—deadly if used on their own. But no remedy is used as it is found in nature. Rather, it goes through a process of diluting and shaking so that eventually only the "phantom" or remnant of the original substance is left.

A remedy is first diluted by being ground up and mixed with water or alcohol—one part substance to nine parts inert substance. This is called the "mother tincture," and the dilution process is called *potentiating*. The result is then taken through a process of shaking, or *succussion,* before being potentiated again and diluted even more. The smaller the amount of original substance, the more powerful the remedy. At a level of 1 to 30,000, there is nothing left of the mineral, flower, poison, or whatever you started with, but the vibrational energy remains.

The potency of each remedy is designated by an X, a C, or an M (diluted by 10, by 100, or by 1,000). Most homeopaths counsel you to take lower dosages such as 6X or 12X once or twice an hour and higher dosages such as 30C once or twice a day. Though in this potency there is no longer any active substance left, the energy vibration of the remedy is very potent indeed, and this can resonate with your own energies, stimulating your natural healing force.

Common Remedies for Mental and Emotional Problems

In order to choose a remedy that's right for your condition, you will have to examine yourself closely. You can't just think about your particular mental or emotional problem when choosing a remedy; you must also consider your basic personality, your likes and dislikes, and any physical symptoms you might have.

The remedy should be taken until it removes the first level of your problem (perhaps heart palpitations or a chronic upset stomach). As one layer of dysfunction disappears, you will probably have to choose a new remedy for the next level. Certain remedies cannot follow one another because they have opposing actions. The individual listings under symptom headings will specify if there are any remedies you should not be taking.

Follow these directions when choosing your remedy:

- Start with the remedy that most closely matches your symptom picture.

- Begin with two doses in the correct time period, following the instructions on the tube or bottle. For problems involving the nervous system, it's best to stay in the medium range of dosages (30X to 30C). Take 3 tablets or 10 pellets daily.

If you are having an acute problem, consult a homeopath for more specific recommendations.

- Do not touch the pellet with your fingers, since the skin carries its own energetic force. Use the top of the tube as a dispenser and place the pellet or drops directly on your tongue.

- Avoid ingesting anything else—foods, liquids, caffeine, medicines—for 15 minutes before and after taking any remedy.

- Stop taking a remedy if you feel much better or if your symptoms persist unchanged, in which case you need another remedy. Check the symptom picture again and select the next remedy on your list of possibles.

- If your condition improves, continue until the symptom vanishes.

If you cannot seem to find a remedy that helps you, it's a good idea to consult a homeopathic practitioner for a diagnosis.

Some homeopathic remedies typically associated with mental and emotional problems are:

Phobias	**Anger**	**Sadness**
Aconite	Nux vomica	Natrum mur
Arnica	Lycopodium	Ignatia
Arsenicum	Aconite	Aconite
Sulphur	Ignatia	

Anxiety	**Bulemia**	**Sleep problems**
Lycopodium	Natrum mur	Coffea
Arsenicum	Calcarea	Nux vomica
Ignatia	Ferrum phosphate	Pulsatilla
Phosphorus	Pulsatilla	Aconite
Calcarea		Chamomilla

Safety of Homeopathic Treatments

One of the most exciting things about homeopathy is that there are virtually no side effects to the remedies. They can be taken alongside conventional medication, and you will see effects even if you haven't yet really gotten on track with a healthy nutrition, exercise, and stress-management program.

If you stay with a remedy longer than you should, you may note new symptoms cropping up. These are just a manifestation of the fact that you don't need this remedy anymore. Having already passed one stage of your illness, if you continue to take the same remedy you can inadvertently turn your healing path back in the opposite direction.

Understand that you aren't taking the remedies just to remove a symptom, although that will happen. Rather, you are aiming for a global difference in the way you feel and act. As homeopathy begins to work for you, you may get up in the morning feeling that you've slept very well and have more energy. Your appetite will improve, and you'll desire better foods. If you were drawn to high-fat, high-sugar foods in the past, you may now notice a craving for whole foods—fresh fruits and vegetables, whole grains and legumes. You may discover that you are motivated to get up and jog two miles with your dog or bike along the river. With the correct remedy in place, you should feel generally better within a couple of days.

And this in itself may give you the impetus to wean yourself off antidepressants or serotonin reuptake inhibitors. One of the biggest problems of being on medication that makes you feel better is that you may be worried that your comfort and confidence is all chemically based. Starting a course of homeopathy can be an incentive to speak with your doctor about reducing your medications and eventually tapering off them altogether.

The first principle of homeopathy is that our natural state is a healthy one and that we all have the ability to return to it even if we get off the track for a while. Even if you have been chronically depressed, anxious, angry, despondent, or stressed out, this healing course can make a difference in your mental and emotional state.

HOPELESSNESS

see also Alienation, page 28; Depression, page 112; Death, thoughts of, page 109

Most of us have days or even months where everything goes wrong. But if we feel that change is not only possible but inevitable, we can deal with the bad times while they're happening, expecting that a new day will bring some ray of light.

Without hope, however, there isn't much purpose in going on. It's like being stuck in a tunnel, where you can't even tell which way to go to get out; like being buried alive when no one even knows you're missing. There's simply no exit, or if there is, you don't care to try and find it.

▩ *What Happens When You Are Hopeless*

If you have no hope, there is no reason to believe that anything will ever improve. You will always feel miserable and overwhelmed; people will always take advantage of you, and the days will pass one after another with inexorable tedium.

Many people at the depths of a depression lose all hope and feel that death is the only solution. Hopelessness is in a way more difficult to deal with, however, since even moving toward death requires some effort on the part of the sufferer. If you have no hope, you can't see yourself escaping.

Let There Be Light

Light therapy has been found effective in relieving the debilitating lack of energy and constant level of sadness in many individuals. One hour daily in front of a 10,000-lux white-light box can make a huge difference.

Walk By the Ocean

The rhythm of the tide's ebb and flow, the salt air and the negative ions released by the crashing waves, the feeling of sand between your toes, even the mournful cry of seagulls, can fill you with a sense of wonder at the fact that the universe goes on despite you. If you have no access to an ocean, try listening to an audio tape of waves, but make sure you listen outside in the fresh air.

Spend Some Time With Others

If you can do something for someone who needs you, you will realize there is a purpose to your being here. Volunteer at a hospital or learn emergency medical training and ride an ambulance. Help illiterate people learn to read, or make yourself available at your local church or synagogue for jobs that need doing. It's amazing, when you receive the gratitude of others, how you suddenly see the world—and your place in it—differently.

Learn the Value of What You Have Inside

Daily meditation will take your mind off the anguish you've been feeling and allow you simply to be. Because there is no goal or desire in the act of meditating, you are free to explore the various feelings that you may have denied were there.

Sit quietly and concentrate on your breathing. Allow whatever thoughts that pass through your mind to flow like water, leaving you washed clean. Keep returning to your breath and see it as a glowing light you can move around inside you. First you may wish to light up your center as you breathe into your belly. Then as you feel more comfortable, move the breath upward to your mind. The light will infuse every corner, warming and protecting you. Expand the energy within and allow it to break up blockages and permeate the cold numbness inside. When you sense a peacefulness within, you can let your eyes relax open.

Flowers in the Soul

The Bach flower remedy for extreme hopelessness is Gorse. Take 5 or 6 drops under the tongue or in a half glass of water at least four times daily on an empty stomach, or as needed. It's best to take the remedy out in the sun and feel the healing energy permeate your mind and body.

Homeopathic Help

The remedies Symphytum and Aurum metallicum are excellent during a depression when hopelessness is a major factor.

*H*UMILIATION

see also Aging, page 17; Guilt, page 197; Sexual Dysfunctions, page 387; Shame, page 393; Victim Mentality, page 433; Vulnerability, page 445

Humiliation is a state of dishonor and disgrace that causes a painful loss of dignity. This terrible loss of self-respect generally comes from the outside: Your reputation is tarnished, and you have no way to defend your good name. You don't necessarily have to do anything to be humiliated by another person, but usually your inner policeman takes over and casts shame as well as humiliation on the offense. (See Shame, page 393). There are individuals who feel they are always being judged and will always get the toughest sentence, despite the fact that they aren't guilty.

What Happens When You Are Humiliated

You are in deep disgrace. The entire community knows you have done something so terrible, it's too embarrassing to admit. The problem is that your private infraction has become public knowledge.

It is also possible that you have really done nothing, but someone else has wronged you. Many women who are raped or abused by their partners feel humiliated; they take the punishment because deep down, they feel that they caused the attack, that they merit every bad thing that happens to them. The same may be true of a person who discovers that his or her spouse has been having an affair—the feeling is one of being used and ridiculed, particularly if he or she was the last to find out.

Challenge Your Self-Esteem

You know whatever it is you've done that's bad; but do you really know what you do on a daily basis that's good? Make a list of everything—from organizing the files at your local community center to helping your elderly mother pack for a trip. Tabulate your good deeds as weighing twice as heavily as the bad deeds (because good deeds have rebound effects and make others happy as well as you). You may be pleasantly surprised to realize that you are worth quite a lot in the big scheme of things.

Get Out of Town

Suppose you've done something worthy of censure: You had an affair with your boss's wife, or you cheated on your taxes and were found out, or you got terribly drunk and ran naked through the streets of town one night.

All right. It's done. The cat's out of the bag and others do blame you for your flagrant behavior.

If you cannot live with the shame, it may be because others around you remind you of what you did. To preserve your self-respect, you may have to make a drastic move and actually transplant yourself. Even if you don't get out of town, you may find it healing to abandon all your old haunts and start fresh with a new circle of acquaintances. This is not running away from the problem, but simply removing one of the major obstacles to healing, which is others' opinions of you.

Change Your Behavior

The behavior that got you in trouble is just an action. It is not your personality or temperament and therefore can be altered. Using the model for behavior change (see Behavioral Therapy, page 55), you are going to make yourself a list of driving forces and restraining forces that keep this behavior in place. Then figure out interventions you will use to help to change the behavior. If you're guilty of mismanaging funds, for example, you will now become scrupulous to the penny. You will account for your expenditures and attempt to save money for the company whenever you can.

The ability to change shows you how strong and self-reliant you really are. You can be proud of yourself and your commitment to living differently.

Join a Group

Sometimes, being alone sets us back into old patterns and beliefs. But when we spend time with others who don't know us that well, we get to see ourselves in a new light. If you can join a support group—perhaps one for depressed people or those going through a crisis—you may be astounded to learn that others hold you in high regard. Be honest about whatever it is you've done (or what you believe you've done) and then really listen to the reactions you get. You are undoubtedly your worst critic, and if you can learn something about yourself that's really good, you may be able to temper your harsh judgment.

Say an Affirmation Daily

Even if you've done something terrible, it can't be that terrible (or you'd have been thrown in jail or an institution, or your misdeeds would be all over the newspapers). Just repeat the following positive statements daily:

I'm not all bad. I can hold my head up.

I have a lot to offer the world.

It's more important for me to trust in myself than to expect others to trust in me.

Try a Remedy

Homeopathic remedies that may be of some assistance are

For self-blame: Aconite, Arsenicum album, Aurum, Hyoscyamus, Ignatia, Natrum mur, Pulsatilla

For feelings of disgust: Kali carbonicum, Mercury, Stramonium, Pulsatilla, Sulphur

For feelings of rejection or desertion: Aurum, Pulsatilla, Stramonium, Argentum nitrate, Lachesis, Mercury, Platinus

*H*YPERVENTILATION

see also Anxiety, page 43; Palpitations, page 342 Shortness of Breath, page 397; Stress, page 407

If you become very anxious and your breath becomes shallow and quick, you soon discover that you can't get enough air. In a desperate attempt at a deep breath, you begin gasping like a fish out of water. You may feel lightheaded and dizzy, or panicky and terrified that you're dying.

What Happens When You Hyperventilate

You take inhalations more rapidly, closer together, and end up expelling too much carbon dioxide without taking in enough oxygen. The lower the level of carbon dioxide in the blood, the slower your respiration. As your air hunger becomes greater, you may experience palpitations and panic attacks. This, in turn, makes your breathing even faster and shallower. If you can't calm yourself down, you will pass out, and this is actually a good thing, since it allows the body to relax. Without the interference of your anxious mind, your respiration returns to normal.

Hyperventilation is a frightening event because you feel as though your body has taken over and is out to get you. In fact, it's your mind that has deregulated the process of inhaling and exhaling. If you can snap the chain of panic, you can regain your ability to breathe.

Discover the Real Value of Breathing

When you learn to do it right, you have a useful tool for any emergency. Practice breathing each day as you sit calmly in a straight-backed chair or on the floor with your legs crossed tailor style. Begin to watch the breath as though it didn't really belong to you. Think about standing outside yourself, allowing the breath to come in naturally and leave naturally without an effort.

You may watch the breath at various locations. First, concentrate on the nostrils. You might want to put up your hand to feel the warm air coming out as you exhale. Then you can watch the expansion and contraction of your chest and know that the lungs are processing oxygen and carbon dioxide efficiently. Finally, you can lie on the floor and watch your belly raise and lower as you inhale and exhale. Understand that this miraculous process, which happens whether you try to make it happen or not, is what keeps you alive and well.

Put a Bag on Your Head

Breathing into a paper bag traps the carbon dioxide and allows you to inhale it again. This is a long-proven strategy for preventing blackouts in individuals who faint a lot. If you're prone to hyperventilating, keep a grocery bag folded up in your jacket pocket or purse.

The Water Cure

A quick splash of cold water in your face and throat will slow your heart rate and give you a moment's pause during which you can get your breath back to normal.

Laugh It Up

Laughter changes your breathing patterns. When you're feeling panicky, quickly think of a funny joke, or if you can't do that, simply make mechanical laughing sounds. When you're calm, rent a Marx Brothers or Three Stooges movie and teach yourself what it feels like to let go and relax. (The next time you're panicky, you'll be able to recall one of those side-splitting scenes and it will be easier to let go of your anxiety and laugh out loud.)

Feedback Some Information

Biofeedback can be helpful if you're not aware of your breathing. In a laboratory setting, hooked up to a machine, you will be asked to breathe and watch the monitor as you inhale and exhale gently. Now you will be asked to think of a stressful situation. When your breathing starts getting irregular, you will trigger lights and sounds from the machine, indicating that you are starting to hyperventilate. By using conscious relaxation techniques (see Autogenic Training, page 48; Progressive Relaxation, page 361; Visualization, page

442), you will be able to stop the sounds and lights and return the machine output to normal.

Get Into Bodywork

Learning to use the powerful tools of Alexander, Feldenkrais, or Bioenergetic bodywork can train both body and mind to cooperate differently in a difficult situation. Working with a therapist, you will learn how to use your head, limbs, back, and legs differently when you are in unusual physical positions. As you become aware of the angle of the head when you're angry or depressed, or the way you hunch your shoulders under stress, you will develop an arsenal of positive corrections to use when you begin to hyperventilate.

Press a Point

The acupuncture point Pe. 6 on the inside of the arm, about an inch and a half up from the crease of the wrist, between the two tendons, will help you calm down. You can also press the two points known as *ding chuan,* about an inch and a half out from the spine on either side right below the first vertebra in the cervical spine (the bone that projects out farthest when you bend your head down.)

Yoga for You

Each yoga posture becomes easier as you breathe into it. Here are two that will help you out when you feel panicky.

THE PLOUGH: Lie on the floor and bring your knees into your chest, then lift your buttocks off the floor and slowly begin to straighten your legs. Let them act as a counterweight as you support your back with your hands. Allow the legs to rest on the floor behind your head. Be sure to tuck your chin into your chest to take strain off the back of your neck. Breathe into this posture and feel the legs sink into the floor behind you. After a few minutes, reverse the posture, bringing your legs down in front of you. Lie flat on the floor and breathe easily.

THE UPSIDE-DOWN DOG: Get on your hands and knees and tuck your head between your shoulders. Stretch your arms out in front of you, leaning on your elbows; allow your legs to straighten. Keep your toes on the floor. As you breathe into the posture, try to get your heels to touch down. Breathe deeply and easily. After holding the posture for a few minutes, bring your knees to the floor and your arms back in to your shoulders. Breathe comfortably here for a few more minutes.

Remedy to the Rescue

The Bach flower remedy for panic is Rescue Remedy. If you're prone to hyperventilation, carry it with you and put 5 or 6 drops under your tongue if you have an attack.

Powerful Spirits

Spirits of ammonia are an old-fashioned but still valid method of shocking the system. The ampules are available in most pharmacies—you crack one open and wave it under your nose when you're hyperventilating or feel you're about to faint. The strong odor passes from the nostrils to the brain and stimulates various brain centers, including the reticular activating system in the brain stem, which regulates metabolism and breathing.

*I*MPATIENCE

see also Anger, page 31; Anxiety, page 43; Impulse Control, page 246; Jitteriness, page 260; Nervousness, page 304; Stress, page 407

If you can't wait for the toast to brown in the toaster and it's difficult for you not to finish your friend's sentence for her, you need to learn patience. This is an almost unheard-of concept today in our busy world where we are rewarded for hurrying and for doing twelve things at once. The cursory attention you give to your job, your love life, your home, and your relationships is hardly missed when everyone around you is impatient, too.

But the feeling of impatience actually destroys the fabric of life; you can't drive well if you're always trying to beat the guy in the next lane, you can't listen to your children if they have trouble explaining their problems, and you can't pay attention to the book you're reading because you're never in the present moment but always looking ahead to the future.

▓ *What Happens When You're Impatient*

You tap your foot, watch the clock, and feel your gut churning when others hold you up or slow you down. Nothing moves briskly enough for you, and other people's interests bore you. You have ants in your pants, and no amount of jumping around will relieve the itch. You live with the remote control—changing channels, switching cuts on your CDs, opening the garage door before anyone is ready to get out of the house.

235

Impatience is a symptom of anger and implies an underlying dissatisfaction with life and everything in it. The great
Chinese philosopher Lao Tsu expressed his disdain for people
who rush into and out of everything when he asked, "Can
you be patient? Can you wait for the mud to settle and the
water to clear and the right action to arise by itself?" He wisely stated that battles are lost by rushing in precipitously. But
by remaining alert and aware of what's around you, you gain
an edge on your enemy.

If you calm your body and mind, if you stay in the
moment, you have all the time in the world. Patience is a
virtue, as the old saying goes, and the beneficial impact it can
have on the rest of your life will make it worth the wait.

Mind What You're Doing

If you concentrate on one thing at a time and you have nothing else in mind, you will find you're less impatient.

Pick one activity that you do routinely, such as washing
your face. You are going to explore every facet of this behavior mindfully, in minute detail, so as to block out any other
thoughts that might occur. First, look at your face in the mirror, and examine its planes and angles. Touch your face with
your hand and feel the texture of the skin, how it changes
when you get to your lips, what your eyebrows feel like. Then
turn on the water, feeling the cold and hot liquid splash on
your hands. When you have regulated the temperature so that
it is comfortable, enjoy the sensation of splashing it on your
face. How is your face different wet from the way it was dry?

Now pick up the soap. How does the bar or gel feel in
your hand? Explore the slippery feeling, passing it from hand
to hand, watching the bubbles foam on your skin. Smell the
soap and take the scent into your lungs fully, deeply. Now
bring your hands to your face and shut out the rest of the
room. Imagine the tiny world you have created as you close
your eyes and bring your soapy fingers up toward your nose
and cheeks. There is nothing else around you—simply water,
soap, skin, and air. Now slowly begin to use your hands to
massage your face, taking each area of skin separately. First
the forehead, then the eyebrows, the delicate eyelids, the
cheeks, the nose, the upper lip, the chin, the neck. How is
each area significant to you? Are some more sensitive than

others? Do you like some better than others? See where the bumps, pimples, or scratches are and how they react to the soap and water.

Now splash warm water all over your face and rinse it off. Or use a washcloth and carefully pat or rub the various parts. At last, turn off the water and listen to the silence in the room. Then see the drips as you hold your head over the basin. Grasp a towel with your hands and sense the fabric; put it to your face and smell the detergent as you burrow into it.

Now look at your face again, clean and shining. Enjoy the sight of yourself and the long process it took to get to this state.

If you are paying close attention to each element along the way, you will relish your patience as you move slowly from step to step.

Focus Your Mind

It's hard to be impatient when you meditate, since there's no goal and no desire to reach any conclusion. The Zen attitude of nondoing is the one you adopt as you sit and just exist. Cross your legs and place the backs of your wrists on your knees. Breathe slowly and gently, taking all the time you need to relax. Take air in, let air out—wait patiently for the inhale to complete itself before the exhale begins. Sitting for 20 minutes to half an hour a day will teach patience.

Homeopathics for Patience

Try the following remedies:

> For impatience: Chamomilla, Ignatia, Nux vomica, Sepia, Silica, Sulphur

> If you are always in a great hurry: Arsenicum album, Belladonna, Ignatia, Mercury, Natrum mur, Nux vomica, Silica, Sulphur, Tarantula hispania, Aconite, Arnica, Nitric acid, Pulsatilla

Take up a Game

If you dedicate yourself as seriously to playing as a child does, you'll find you develop an abundance of patience. Chess is great therapy for someone who is never satisfied with what's going on in the moment, as is backgammon. You might also try a knitting or beading project that will require close attention and a commitment to finishing what you started.

Drink a Flower

The Bach flower remedy for impatience and irritability is Impatiens. Take 5 to 6 drops under the tongue or mixed in half a glass of water, four times daily.

Practice Tai Chi

Once you have learned one of the choreographed patterns of tai chi, you repeat them over and over. Mastery is an accolade that is awarded to very few (usually after 20 or 30 years of practice), which means that a veteran tai chi player may be doing exactly the same postures as a beginner. The difference, of course, is in the subtlety of detail, the combination of inner and outer energy, and the coordination of mind, body, and spirit.

Try the following exercise and repeat it several times daily:

Stand with your feet shoulder-width apart, your right foot pointed straight ahead, your left at a 45-degree angle, and about two feet behind the right. The legs should feel springy and released, with a slight bend in the knees. Bring your left hand up from your side and press it into your right wrist as you put your weight on your right leg and straighten the left. Now withdraw both hands back toward your chest as you sink onto the back leg and bend both knees. Finally, bring your hands forward in a pushing motion and once again, straighten the back leg as you bring your weight onto the front.

This "press, withdraw, push," is one of the most common combinations of the Yang-style tai chi form. The more you practice it patiently, the more variation you will find within the one theme.

Impending Doom, feelings of

see also Anxiety, page 43; Death, Thoughts of, page 109; Depression, page 112; Panic Disorder, page 344; Stress, page 407

"The sky is falling," said Chicken Little when an acorn fell on his head. He had no reason to fear the worst, and yet his anticipatory anxiety was so great that he blew everything out of proportion. If we sense that something is wrong, we can either downplay our intuition or use it as a catapult into the terrors of the unknown.

What Happens When You Have a Feeling of Impending Doom

You have no rational or reasonable excuse for the sensation of dread that overwhelms you. The sky seems to darken, and the sinking feeling in the pit of your stomach is real. Even the ring of the telephone can be a portent of something evil.

Sometimes we feel as though the world is due to end because of some unusual event—a letter about the death of a distant relative or your boss looking at you funny. But most often, this sensation arrives for no reason. Women more than men tend to say that they've had an aura or an intimation that something is about to happen. Their intuition gives them a direct line to the future, and they are sure they're not imagining it.

In the past, seers were considered wiser than the rest of us because they were in touch with the nether world. Today, shamans are also reputed to be able to communicate with the dead and with those spirits who influence our current and future lives. Because we really have no way of proving that ours is the only ongoing universe or time, it's possible that intuition is simply another type of intelligence and that we should pay attention to it.

However, it's also likely that feelings of impending doom can be present in a very anxious individual who always sees the glass as half empty. If you anticipate terrible things happening to you, you may bring them about simply by your negative attitude and lack of initiative to change the unpleasant situation. It is for this reason that you should not throw up your hands and say that it's out of your control, but instead, should apply yourself to several of the following natural therapies:

Eat for a Better Future

You will feel better within days if you strictly avoid caffeine, nicotine, refined sugar, and alcohol. Since many anxious individuals stave off their frightened feelings by having a drink or cigarette or consuming a lot of coffee and sweets, getting free of these substances will make a big difference in your blood sugar and energy levels.

You might also consider giving up red meat and restricting your consumption of chicken and fish as well. As your system adjusts to a diet of legumes, complex carbohydrates, whole grains, and fresh vegetables and fruits, you will find that you no longer have the logy feeling that has hung around you for years. Be sure to eat lots of green leafy vegetables and low-fat dairy products to increase your calcium, which has been found to curb extreme anxiety.

Supplement Your Attitude

You should be supplementing all the B-vitamins (50–100 mg. daily) as well as pantothenic acid (500 mg. twice a day) and folic acid (400 mcg. daily) to reduce stress. You should also supplement calcium and magnesium (1,200 mg. and 600 mg. respectively), Vitamin C (1000 mg.) and Vitamin E (400 IU). Zinc (30 to 50 mg.) daily is helpful for your depressed state, as is the amino acid tryptophan (100 mg. available as part of many herbal stress formulas).

Get Out of the Dark and Into the Light

It is more typical to fear that something awful is going to happen in the winter, when it's dark and cold outside. For those who suffer from SAD (see Seasonal Affective Disorder, page 373), just 30 minutes a day of light therapy can make a difference. The light boxes can be purchased for home use (see Resource Guide, page 475), or you may wish to visit a therapeutic center near you. Therapy consists of sitting one to three feet away from a 10,000-lux fluorescent light each day during the winter months. This therapy can lighten your load and assure you that life will go on as you wish it to.

Look at Your Dreams

The symbolic content of your dreams may offer a key to your real fears. If you have been having nightmares or dreams that incorporate a feeling of doom, you may be carrying the feeling into your waking life. When you wake up from the dream, quickly write down the feeling you have. Are you panicked? Expectant? Resigned? Do you feel vulnerable and unable to stand up for yourself?

Next, practice visualizing different endings for the dream and replay the new scenario until it feels real to you. You may wish to include a character (you or someone you admire) who comes to your rescue or lightens the load you are carrying in your dream. When you go back to sleep, you may do so with a sense of comfort that you've put the pieces in place already. By redreaming your attitude toward potential danger, you may be able to change your anticipatory anxiety when you wake up.

Say an Affirmation Daily

The more you tell yourself that things are good, the less time and energy you have to spend on your awareness of doom. Say to yourself:

> *I am fine!*
> *I am allowed to enjoy myself.*
> *Things are going well in my life.*
> *Being alive is being happy.*

Flowers to the Rescue

The Bach flower remedy for persistent unwanted thoughts or preoccupation with a worry or event is White Chestnut. You might also take Aspen for apprehension, foreboding, and fears of unknown origin. Take 5 or 6 drops under the tongue or mixed in half a glass of water, four times daily.

IMPOTENCE

see also Sexual Dysfunctions, page 387

The word "impotent" implies failure, and for this reason, the medical establishment has changed the name of this sexual problem to "erectile dysfunction." Although this phrase is still pretty much of a downer, at least it describes the problem objectively.

The old joke about the difference between fear and panic tells it all. Fear is the first time you can't get it up twice; Panic is the second time you can't get it up once.

■ What Does It Mean to Have an Erectile Dysfunction?

A man is classified as having an erectile dysfunction if he is unable to achieve and maintain an erection hard enough for penetration and ejaculation three out of four times.

Most men fear the lack of potency more than anything else. They say that they are unmanned, emasculated. The problem, which may be physical, psychogenic, or both, tends to affect men more as they get older. Although impotence is not necessarily a function of aging, about 55 percent of all men over 75 have experienced erectile dysfunction at some time.

The reasons are many and varied, and usually overlap.

PHYSICAL PROBLEMS: Over 75 percent of all cases are physical in nature, resulting from inadequate blood flow to the penis (insufficient vascularization, sometimes caused by athero-sclerosis), diabetes, endocrine problems (low testosterone), a thyroid condition, muscular dystrophy, spinal cord injury, epilepsy, chronic pain, chronic obstructive pulmonary disease, alcoholism and drug abuse, and use of antihypertensive medicines.

A chemical imbalance may also affect erection. A defect in the nitric oxide system of the penis may prevent the smooth muscles of the penis from relaxing. This, in turn, keeps the blood vessels in the penis from opening and allowing the cavernous bodies to fill with blood, which is what produces an erection.

PSYCHOLOGICAL PROBLEMS: Lack of or inhibited desire, sexual repression (disgust at vaginal penetration), anger at your partner, having a new partner, boredom with an old partner, financial worries, legal problems, anxiety, depression, bereavement, stress may all weigh too heavily on the penis to let it stand up.

Trying too hard is one of the major reasons for erectile dysfunction. The feeling of urgency is often connected with anxiety—the more you can't do it, the more you feel you're disappointing your partner and you *have* to do it. So you furiously apply yourself and still can't function. It's a vicious cycle. But most cases with a psychogenic basis can be improved if not cured completely. And even individuals with chronic disease can be greatly helped.

Any man who can physically achieve an erection does so several times a night during sleep when he experiences NPT (nocturnal penile tumescence). In order to rule out physical problems, you can take a test with a monitor that slips around the penis and tightens during an erection. However, the treatment of psychological difficulties can be far more difficult because it involves a major change in your attitude about lovemaking and your irrational need to take charge and be "manly" all the time. (Most women, by the way, are nowhere near as interested in a hard penis as they are in playful affection.)

Here are a variety of natural treatments to try for erectile dysfunction. BE SURE TO CHECK WITH YOUR PHYSICIAN IF YOU HAVE A HEART CONDITION OR CHRONIC RESPIRATORY DISORDER.

Focus on the Rest of You

Sensate focus, an exercise recommended by sex therapists, is an opportunity to explore your sexuality without having to have an erection, although men are very often so stimulated they have one anyway. Explain to your partner that you are going to take turns stimulating each other—for the first 20 minutes, you will touch, kiss, caress, lick, and thoroughly pleasure her. However, you will not make contact with her genitals. She is simply to lie back and passively receive your ministrations; although she can express her pleasure, she should not ask you to change anything you're doing. Then, for the next 20 minutes, she will do the same to you.

You will do this exercise at least three times a week, without attempting to have intercourse or ejaculate. (She can come to an orgasm if she wants to.) By the end of the second week, you will find that your desire and awareness of your own pleasure have both increased exponentially and that your fantasy life is much richer.

At this point, you can allow your partner to stimulate your penis to erection. Still, you are not permitted to come. If you feel close to ejaculation, tell her to stop stimulation until the feeling subsides (your erection probably will, as well). Practice getting excited and stopping yourself for another week. At this point, if you are having an erection regularly, you may proceed to orgasm.

The Aphrodisiac of Choice

Although many foods and herbs have been suggested as increasing sexual interest and potency, the only one that seems to have an actual effect is derived from the bark of an African tree and is called yohimbine. Three commercial varieties—Yocon, Yohimex, and Aphrodyne—are currently prescribed by sex therapists to increase sexual desire and appear to have no detrimental side effects. In studies, about a third of the men suffering from psychogenic erection problems improved after ten weeks of herbal therapy.

Do It by Yourself

If your problem is psychogenic, your partner may be your biggest concern. Many men are able to masturbate to ejaculation with no trouble at all, using fantasy, a vibrator, lubricant, erotic magazines, or erotic films. Try it for yourself, allotting enough privacy and time. You may find that the lack of pressure and performance anxiety make a big difference in your ability to have and to keep an erection.

Use a Vacuum Pump

If your problem is physical, you may wish to try an erection aid. (These are commercially available for about $400. You must see a urologist who specializes in erection problems in order to get one.) A plastic cylinder is placed over the penis and you use a pump to draw air out, creating a vacuum. This draws blood into the penis and causes it to become erect. A velcro band is then placed at the base of the penis and the vacuum removed. This aid creates a floppy erection, but one that works well.

Let the Band Play

A constriction band (otherwise known as a "cock ring" or "performance ring") may be leather, metal, or plastic. These are useful for men who can achieve an erection on their own but can't sustain it through ejaculation. The band is placed around the base of the penis and kept on throughout intercourse.

Change Your Medications

Tranquilizers, diuretics, antidepressants, barbiturates, and drugs for stomach ulcers can all create erectile problems. Prozac actually curbs the desire for sex, so you never even get to the erection stage.

Certain beta blockers (antihypertensive drugs) have been shown to cause erectile dysfunction. These drugs lower the heart's demand for oxygen under stress, blocking the effect of the sympathetic nervous system on the heart muscle and taking the stress off the arteries. The drugs Inderal, Blocadren, Levatol, and Corgard are particularly problematic for someone with an active sex life.

Taking multiple antihypertensive drugs usually enhances the effect of each one. If you have a heart condition and are currently taking one of these drugs, you may wish to discuss lowering your dosages or changing your type of medications entirely.

The Herbs of the East

Chinese medicine is prolific on the subject of impotence, since the male essence of life *(jing)* is supposedly contained in the ejaculate. By strengthening this factor, the belief is that a man will live longer and stronger. However, many Chinese physicians feel that treating the symptom (inability to get an erection) is a wrongheaded approach. If, for example, the problem is a combination of vascular difficulties and depression, taking an herb to increase potency could overly stimulate the heart and be exceptionally dangerous.

Most Chinese physicians diagnose this problem as deficient Kidney *yang* (Fire) energy, and they attribute it to a combination of physical and psychological factors. There are several formulas used for impotence, and many contain different amounts of many of the following ingredients. One of the most popular mixtures is called *dzan yu dan* (assist nature elixir), which contains rehmannia, atractylodes, angelica, Chinese wolfberry, eucommia, curculigo, morinda root, dogwood tree, horny goat weed, broomrape, cnidium, allium seeds, cinnamon, ginseng, aconitum, and deer horn. IF YOU ARE TAKING ANTIHYPERTENSIVE MEDICINE, YOU SHOULD NOT TAKE A CHINESE HERBAL TO INCREASE POTENCY.

Homeopathic Help

Try the following remedies twice a day for up to five days:

> If your erection isn't firm enough for penetration: Agnus castus.
>
> If you have a surge of desire but anticipate failure: Lycopodium
>
> If you lack desire or feel an aversion toward sex: Graphites
>
> If your erection doesn't last: Conium
>
> If your erection occurs when you're half asleep but disappears when you awaken: Caladium
>
> If you have difficulties caused by grief or disappointment about a previous relationship: Ignatia

*I*MPULSE *C*ONTROL

see also ADD and ADHD, page 13; Compulsive Sexual Activity; page 97; Financial Extravagance, page 183; Gambling, page 187; Jealousy, page 257; Kleptomania, page 261; Risk Taking, page 367; Violence/Aggressive Behavior, page 437

In Freudian terms, the ego is the guardian of our consciousness and memory and mediates between the primitive id, which is ruled by instinct, and the strict superego, which develops after the age of six or seven and acts as the policeman for the id. When a tempting opportunity comes along, it's the job of the ego to monitor its appropriateness and allow either the id or the superego to permit or prohibit certain activities and behaviors.

Most of us grow out of the childhood tendencies to do whatever we want whenever we want. But what happens if the superego falls down on the job and the id goes wild?

When you cannot control your impulses, you have no limitations or barriers. You act in the moment because that's what you feel like—it's only afterward when the consequences look dire that you feel guilty for what you've done.

Impulse-control problems range from monetary extravagance (shopping and gambling) to theft (kleptomania) to personal violence (trichotillomania or hair pulling) to violence and aggressive behavior against things or people (pyromania and running "amok," which amounts to going on a wild rampage). It may also be relevant when looking at behaviors that are normal in moderation (sexual activity and exercise) but problematic when out of control.

Impulse control is not linked to biological causes in the brain; however, the repeated activity—whatever it is—causes a sudden release of endorphins, the natural opiates that alleviate pain and fill us with a sense of well-being. When off on a spree (whether gambling, having sex with strangers, setting fires, or getting into fights), the person suffering from lack of control is on a high. The behavior is so exciting it's impossible to stop.

The cyclical nature of this problem makes it difficult to treat—the compulsive shopper generally has very low self-esteem (and low levels of serotonin), and her behavior makes her feel better emotionally. So if she's depressed, she may go out and buy herself a new wardrobe. But when the bills come in a month later, she is once again depressed and has to go shopping to cheer herself up.

A person suffering with stress, anxiety, or depression generally hurts only himself. However, the problems associated with lack of control usually hurt others as well as the individual with the dysfunction. A compulsive gambler or shopper may incur a great deal of family debt and may actually put his family in personal danger if he borrows money from a criminal source; a pyromaniac may destroy property and lives; a violent individual takes out his or her anger in physically abusive ways.

Is there a kind of moral "stupidity" at work here, or is the person flagrantly violating society's norms just to see if he or she can get away with it? Usually, with impulse control, the person is not delusional and does have an awareness that his or her behavior is out of line, but the person simply can't stop doing it.

Because it is so difficult to resist the types of lures that hook the person with a lack of control, outside pressures to stop behavior are usually more successful than inner-motivated ones. Group therapy and support groups are the gold standard of treatment as well as practical restrictions. The shopper must not have access to credit cards and checks; the pyromaniac must never get hold of matches or a lighter; the hair puller must wear a hat or wear hair up rather than loose; the violent individual must be kept away from guns and knives. Since some people suffer from impulse control only periodically and are quite temperate the rest of the time, it's important for the individual to understand when a cycle of asocial activity is beginning so that it can be stopped quickly and effectively.

Treatments to try: Acupuncture/Acupressure, page 7; Behavioral Therapy, page 55; Body/Mind Therapies, page 74; Breathing, page 76; Cognitive Awareness, page 94; Homeopathy, page 221; Meditation, page 292; Mindfulness, page 296; Magnetic Healing, page 285; Self-esteem, page 380; Support Groups, page 414.

*I*NSOMNIA

see also Sleep Disorders, page 404

One of the most infuriating and frustrating problems is the inability to fall asleep when you want to. Although you can tolerate a night of this torture every so often, insomnia that stems from depression or anxiety tends to repeat itself. The more you can't sleep, the more you fear you won't fall asleep, and sure enough, it becomes a self-fulfilling prophecy. The next night, there you are awake again and the more debilitated you feel the following day.

■ *What Happens When You Have Insomnia*

You toss and turn; your mattress feels like a bed of nails. You try every position, and they're all impossible. The thoughts racing through your mind are enough to drive you crazy. And after a few nights of this misery, your body begins to tell the tale: You rise from bed disoriented, irritable, unable to concentrate or relate to others. Insomnia is surely worthy of a place in one of the circles of hell.

Forty percent of all Americans over 60 battle this problem; ten million individuals a year consult a physician about their difficulty, and half of those get a prescription for sleeping pills. Unfortunately, medication often exacerbates the problem because you need increasingly more of it over time to cause drowsiness.

Say No to Caffeine

If you do nothing else, get yourself off this stimulant. It should take about a week to wean yourself from coffee, tea, soda, and cocoa, but you will find the difference astounding. You can substitute herbal teas (some sleep-inducing) and roasted grain beverages such as Pero and Roma Kaffree.

Make a Sleep Cocktail

Take a cup of warm milk and place it in a blender with a banana. Whir into liquid and drink before bed. Both ingredients contain tryptophan, the amino acid that relaxes muscles and promotes good sleep. Although the supplement L-tryptophan was taken off the market several years ago because of adverse side effects and some deaths from contaminated sources, you can still purchase combination sleep remedies in the health-food store that contain less than 100 mg. of tryptophan.

Make Sure You're Tired

It's difficult to rest properly if you're tossing and turning, your body in knots or ready to spring into action. If you aren't physically tired, your wired system is saying, why fall asleep? In order to get proper rest, you must have proper exercise. Get up early and run two miles, mow the lawn, vacuum the house, do some gardening, paint the deck. Any activities that really get you moving will use all those muscles that have to be restored during a night of peaceful sleep.

Don't Nap

If you're exhausted during the day, you may be tempted to lie down for a few brief winks. But because naps are typically short (in the daytime, the body doesn't produce enough melatonin to knock you out for eight hours), you don't get down to those deep layers of Stage III and Stage IV sleep that restore the body and mind. Fight off the inclination to sleep during the day by doing some deep breathing, meditation, yoga, or tai chi. Then you'll be ready to conk out at night.

Prince Valerian to the Rescue

Valerian is a traditional herbal sleep remedy and works for nearly everyone. Take 1/2 to 1 teaspoon of the tincture half an hour before bed. In some individuals, it causes headaches, however, and if this proves true for you, you may wish to try other sedative herbs such as hops, Jamaica dogwood, passionflower, or wild lettuce.

Homeopathic Sleep Aids

Try the following remedies to help you sleep:

> If you are sleepless and restless, with anxious dreams: Aconite
>
> If you are wide awake in the evening, have restless sleep, and wake unrefreshed: Pulsatilla
>
> If you talk and twitch in your sleep and awake frequently: Sulphur

Press Your Points

Acupressure can be useful when you're trying to drop off. (Consult the acupuncture charts, page 10, for the exact location of these points.)

> Press the inner side of your forearm: Pe. 6
>
> Press the inside of your wrist crease in line with your pinky: Ht. 7

Imagine Yourself Sleeping

The following visualization can be helpful to calm your mind and let you drop off. Lie down in a darkened room and cover yourself with a light blanket in case you should fall asleep in the middle of this treatment.

Breathe slowly and gently, feeling the rhythm of your breath encompassing your mind and body. As you inhale and exhale, picture yourself in a place where you've always been secure and happy—a mountaintop at dusk or a sunny day by a lake, or sitting by a fireplace looking out at a snowy night. See yourself blending into this natural landscape, feeling at peace. You have nowhere to go, nothing to do.

Now concentrate on your limbs and feel how heavy and relaxed they are. First your right leg—it is warm, heavy, and free of tension. Then your right arm, so heavy you could not lift it even if you wanted to. Now turn your attention to the left side of your body. Your left leg is heavy and relaxed, sinking deep into the bed. Your left arm is totally comfortable, weighted and stable, right where it is.

Let the thoughts that come to you drift by like leaves across a pond. Let yourself sink and drift away. You are drowsy, ready for sleep. You are completely relaxed.

*I*NTERRUPTED *S*LEEP

see also Sleep Disorders, page 404

Is it worse not to be able to get to sleep and stay asleep, or to be awakened from a sound sleep, unable to get back? Those who wake continually during the night may be having physical or psychological components of the problem, or both.

What Happens When You Have Interrupted Sleep

You doze, then start awake and stare at the clock. You never seem to get down to the deeper levels (Stage III and Stage IV) of sleep that restore and refresh the body, so you get up in the morning feeling groggy, as though you hadn't slept at all.

Women during menopause often suffer from night sweats because of hypothalamic disturbances that cause quick and immediate releases of heat in the upper body. Men and women both occasionally suffer from sleep apnea, when they stop breathing for a short period of time and hold their breath. When the sleeper runs out of air, he or she compensates with a violent snort that often wakes him up. And having to get up and urinate—common in pregnant and menopausal women—also contributes to sleep awakening. Poor sleep hygiene (napping during the day or maintaining an irregular sleep schedule) may also contribute to the problem.

Make the Bedroom the Sleep Room

Make sure that everything is conducive to sleep (right temperature, right number of covers, no light, no noise, window open a crack) and designate this room your sleep room *Only.* Other than making love, there should be no other activities in this space.

Put a Nightshirt by Your Bed

If you are typically drenched from night sweats, you will experience far less waking if you quickly strip off the wet shirt you're wearing and put a dry one on at once.

Think Calm Thoughts Before Sleep

Progressive relaxation, (page 361) meditation (page 292), and visualization (page 442) before sleep can get your brain in the mood. Concentrate on your breath as you release every part of your body.

Don't Just Lie There

If you're not achieving sleep after half an hour, get up and do something. Read a magazine or a nontechnical book or listen to quiet music—do nothing that would stimulate the brain so much it would want to stay awake.

Forget The Hot Toddy

Many people still believe that an alcoholic beverage prior to bed will ensure sound sleep. It *does* make you sleepy enough to drop off, but because it disturbs brain patterns, it may cause briefer REM periods and may not allow you to get down to deeper layers of sleep. It's common to wake in the middle of the night after drinking too much alcohol, unable to drop off again.

Melatonin May Put You Out

By supplementing the body's own melatonin, we can achieve better sleep. It works best when taken an hour or two before bed: Start with 1 mg. daily, increasing your dosage gradually only if necessary. You cannot overdose on this supplement—high doses of 40 to 80 mg. have been used in studies and with older individuals; however, you may get very sleepy at doses over 5 mg. daily.

Take a Warm Bath

You may do this before bed or after you wake in the middle of the night.

Homeopathic Help

Try these remedies for interrupted sleep:

> If you can't sleep after 3 A.M. and get up feeling awful: Nux vomica
>
> If you are wakeful, sleep until 3 A.M. and then only doze and your mind is very busy: Coffea

Stay Away From OTC Drugs

Over-the-counter medications to induce sleep usually contain mild antihistamines that dry your mucous membranes and give your mouth a cotton-wool feeling. They also have a half-life that extends beyond your sleep period, which makes you wake up drowsy. You also need increasing amounts of these drugs as you become habituated to them. The best course is never to start taking them.

*I*RRITABILITY

see also Aging, page 17; Anger, page 31; Mood Swings, page 297; Stress, page 407, Violence/Aggressive Behavior, page 437

When you are irritable, you feel rubbed the wrong way by everything and everybody. Irritability is a form of suppressed anger—nothing is ever bad enough to cause an explosion, so you linger on the limits of your tolerance, ready to lash out at the next person who says or does anything stupid. You overreact to everything because you can't accept the disappointments and interruptions that keep your life from running smoothly. Chronic irritability is a true social problem; naturally, your friends and family will begin to stay away from you if they grow to expect a prickly person who is always critical and disgruntled.

What Happens When You Are Irritable

You are in a constant state of annoyance, and each little thing—the car not starting, a snippy comment from a co-worker, the fact that the supermarket is out of your favorite brand of ice cream—gets you going. You see the world as an adversarial place, and the chip on your shoulder gets bigger and heavier as more unpleasantries pile up.

Calm Down with Homeopathy

Try the following remedies for irritability: Nux vomica, Sepia, Lycopodium, Colocynth, Aconite, Nitric acid.

Take a Deep Breath and Hold It

Although slow, rhythmic, belly breathing is an excellent way to calm yourself down when you're angry, it may be more helpful to try the following exercise for irritability: Take a really deep inhalation and hold it. See how much more air you can take in at your peak—you want to feel close to explosion (which is the way you feel emotionally). When you can't keep it in anymore, let the air out with a yell. Repeat seven times, and then restore your breathing to a quiet, normal pace. You will find that the release of tension has calmed you inside and out.

Examine Your Annoyance with Logic

Use cognitive awareness to look deeper into your reasons for feeling so rotten. Think carefully each time something happens and relabel it.

For example, if the cleaner put too much starch in your shirts, your tax burden is higher than anticipated this year, and your partner forgets to kiss you on her way out the door in the morning, your reaction might be:

I feel physically uncomfortable with this stiff collar.

I feel poor and put upon—where will I get the money to pay?

I feel neglected and unloved.

The consequence is that you feel the world pressing in on you; you are sure there is a relation among the three annoyances.

But instead, you can put different shine on each one and separate them, making it possible for you to deal with each problem. Your new take on the day will be:

I'll stop in at the cleaner on the way home and get them to do the rest of the shirts over.

My accountant can file for late payment, and that way I'll be able to keep the money longer in my own account.

Maybe if I were a little more affectionate when my wife came home in the evenings, she'd reciprocate in the mornings.

These clear-thinking solutions can take the irritability out of your day.

Run Around the Block

There is nothing as beneficial as exercise to trigger the production of endorphins, the natural opiates in the brain that make us feel good. Make a date with yourself to start the day with a brisk two-mile walk, jog, or bike ride; or to take a lunch break to go swimming or play racquetball. You will be astounded when you see how the petty worries you've had melt away as you work out.

Greet the Sun

The yoga sun salute one of the most renewing patterns for both mind and body. Practice this exercise four times each day and work your way up to ten repetitions daily.

Stand with your feet together, your hands together at your chest as though you were praying.

Lift your hands over your head and stretch back.

Roll down your spine to touch your toes, swing your right leg back, but don't let your right knee touch the floor. Lift your head and breathe.

Swing your left leg back. (You are now in push-up position.)

Touch your knees, then your chest, then your chin to the floor. (Your rear end is now up in the air.)

Flatten your back, point your toes, bring your upper chest off the floor.

Put your weight on your hands and knees, then bring your rear end up in the air, making a bridge. Your weight is on your palms and toes.

Swing your right leg forward between your hands.

Swing your left leg forward, hang over with straight knees.

Slowly roll up your spine and place your hands in prayer posture in front of your chest.

Jealousy

see also Impulse Control, page 246; Worrying, page 452

The unreasonable gnawing in your gut is described as a "hostile rivalry" with another individual over someone or something you hold dear. The most common assumption of a jealous person is that his or her beloved is being unfaithful with someone else. Usually, you are jealous of both individuals—your primary love object and whoever or whatever is taking him or her away from you. The problem with jealousy is that the anger, turmoil, and confusion exist whether or not your suspicions are founded in fact. Jealousy is an insidious beast—as Shakespeare puts it, "a green-eyed monster."

What Happens When You're Jealous

You have a visceral reaction to seeing the two of them together, even imagining the two of them together. You monitor phone calls, address books, the credit-card bills, and question your mate unceasingly about his or her whereabouts, his or her feelings toward the other person, and the reasons you intuit for his or her lack of interest in you. You may begin to make demands on your partner's time or behave in an overly protective and smothering manner even when the other person is nowhere near.

By restricting your relationship, of course, you further alienate the person you love. This is possible whether you're jealous of a potential lover for your mate, a baby-sitter or grandparent for your child, your parent's new spouse, or a new colleague on the job who has gained the boss's favor.

Since jealousy breeds mistrust, you may find yourself questioning everything about your previously solid relationship.

Where does jealousy come from? Usually it's a type of insecurity about your participation in a relationship that seems shaky. You assume that others are better, more attractive, more clever than you, and you project your fantasies about being shunted off into a corner on any likely candidate that has caught your partner's interest.

If you arranged your life so that no one else intruded into your partner's world, you two could be hermetically sealed together. But you'd also be cutting off your mate from the type of social stimulation that makes him or her a well-rounded person. You'd also begin to resent the fact that you had to be all things to this person. If it's true that no man is an island, it's also true that no relationship exists in a vacuum. You need others around you in order to gain perspective on the special bond you have for each other.

Remedy Your Jealousy

Try the following homeopathic remedies for jealousy: Nux vomica, Pulsatilla, Hyoscyamus, Ignatia, Lachesis, Phosphorus, Staphisagria.

Wrestle Down the Problem

Sometimes we shy away from confrontation about jealous feelings because we don't know what to say. It can be liberating to use nonverbal communication with your partner, but you must gauge your own reactions and be certain not to let your anger turn this exercise into a pitched battle.

Tell your partner that you would like to have a wrestling match and that through the use of throws and holds, you will be able to work out some of the suspicious feelings you can't shake.

Pick a room with a nice soft carpet, clear the furniture out of the way, and begin by linking arms. You may grapple, shove, and constrict your partner; you may not punch, hit, head-butt, bite, or do any other potentially harmful actions.

The key issue here is trust; you are relying on each other not to get hurt. On the other hand, you want complete and full physical contact, so that you can feel each other's breath and touch each other all over. The point of the exercise is that neither of you should "win," but rather, you should both gain respect for each other's strength and energy.

Bolster Your Self-Esteem

If you constantly suspect your partner of carrying on with someone else, you must view yourself as pretty insignificant. For this reason, you need to appreciate all you are and what you offer others. Start by deciding what it is you think your partner has stopped liking in you, and you will actually discover what *you* have stopped liking.

Is it your looks? You may want to think about getting on a good nutrition and exercise program to improve your physical self-image. Is it your energy level, or your passion for life? How about taking an adult-school course in a subject that's always intrigued you? Is it your sexuality? Think about taking your partner away for a romantic weekend or surprising him or her with a seductive evening in your own home.

Get Some Sleep

Your preoccupation with something going on behind your back may be keeping you from getting the healing rest that will restore your spirit. Get to bed by 10:30 each night, even on weekends, and get up by 7 A.M. Be sure to restrict caffeine and alcohol—or cut them out entirely. If you have trouble falling asleep, see the suggestions for Insomnia, page 248. As you lie in bed, tell yourself that you are protected and comfortable and that nothing is out to get you. Breathe gently and easily as you fall into sleep.

Try a Flower

The Bach flower remedy for jealousy and suspicion is Holly. You may also try Chicory if you are overpossessive and demand attention. Take 5 to 6 drops under the tongue or mixed with half a glass of water, four times daily.

J*ITTERINESS*

see Agitation, page 21; Anxiety, page 43; Nervousness, page 304; Panic Disorders, page 344; Stress, page 407

*K*LEPTOMANIA

see also Impulse Control, page 246

We all know we're not supposed to take what doesn't belong to us. But to a person afflicted with kleptomania, the compulsion to steal is overwhelming. The desire to take things— usually small, insignificant items—is a symbol of a larger problem. The kleptomaniac enjoys the game of stealing and knows it's wrong. She or he might get caught. But a person who has a terrible need to be noticed feels that some attention is always better than none.

▓ *What Happens When You Have Kleptomania*

You don't really need whatever it is you're going to steal. You may be in a hardware store and feel you've got to pocket a box of nails; or in a jewelry store where the temptation to snatch a pair of earrings becomes too tempting to resist. You are not a shoplifter; it's not that you can't afford an item and feel you need it. Rather, you are someone who plays fast and loose with society's rules.

Kleptomaniacs are mostly women, and some are very affluent (celebrities—rock stars and movie stars—have been known to commit these acts). Some individuals do it once, get away with it, and never do it again. Others do it sporadically with long periods of remission, and still others are chronic kleptomaniacs, stealing with impunity on a daily basis.

Because they don't need the material goods they take (very often, they aren't even interested in the item, for example, the box of nails), they may be very generous, giving away their spoils to the next available person they meet. Others hoard their ill-gotten gains, keeping them as proof that they succeeded in their endeavor.

It is only when they are caught red-handed, by a store guard or a video monitor, that they become aware of their problem, and even then, they may regard their admonishment and punishment as part of the game.

The treatment of kleptomania requires you to examine the various reasons why you need negative feedback. Only when you have healthy outlets for your attention-getting can you stop the behavior.

Learn a New Behavior

Behavior change is probably the most urgent and most effective treatment. You are going to create a program for entering and leaving stores and other people's homes and offices that will prevent you from taking anything you haven't paid for.

For the first two weeks of the program, you should not be alone when you shop or enter a strange home or office. Make sure you get a friend or family member to accompany you.

Start by writing down the driving forces to steal and the restraining forces that keep you from stealing. You'll also need some interventions that you can put into practice immediately, such as snapping a rubber band on your wrist or turning your ring around on your finger when you have the urge to take something.

You'll need to keep a diary of places you enter and pinpoint objects that tempt you. As soon as you have the urge to take something, write it down. Indicate the time, place, occasion, and what was going on emotionally for you just before you wanted to steal.

If you find the urge is overwhelming, you must go up to the shopkeeper or owner of the item and tell them exactly what's going on. Explain that you are in recovery and wanted to express apologies even before you've done anything.

You will find that the combination of recording your feelings, interventions, and embarrassment at having to "tell" will subtly alter the high you get from stealing.

Join a Group

When you have others around you who understand your problem and are possibly having the same or similar impulses, it's easier to stick to your new behavior. A group such as Gamblers Anonymous or a support group for those with problems of impulse control may be already in place at a local hospital or community center. Most have weekly discussions and a buddy system, so that if you feel the urge to steal, you can immediately call your partner and work out the problem. No one who has ever had your problem will let you get away with excuses or self-pity; you'll find that surrounding yourself with those who have been on the other side and come back is the best way to stick to the straight and narrow.

Meditate on the Problem

Deep down, you know what you've been doing is wrong, but in the hurry and stress of daily life, it's hard to find the roots of your need for attention. Meditation will take you inside yourself so that you can explore the hurt and neglect that have led you to kleptomania.

Sit quietly, either on the floor with your legs crossed or in a straight-backed chair. Close your eyes and begin to breathe evenly and deeply. Tell yourself that you are in good hands—your own—and that you are about to take a journey that will offer keys to your future healing.

Imagine a white light outside your body that approaches slowly and steadily. It surrounds you with its warmth and seeps through your pores. It is a kindly presence that gives you all the support and love you need. Let this light come inside and touch your pain; allow it to circle your heart and give you peace. When it travels upward into your mind, understand that you now have a guide and mentor inside you who will stay your hand if it should ever feel a temptation too great to handle.

Take a final cleansing breath and allow your eyes to relax open.

Volunteer Your Services

Because impulse control involves a deregulation of tradition-al moral values, it's helpful to strengthen your ethical pur-pose. Volunteer in a soup kitchen, a hospital, an emergency squad, or donate your time to help underprivileged children. Spending a few hours a week with those who can't afford the things you steal will give you a better perspective on your behavior.

Give Away Your Goods

The Native American tribes of Oregon and Washington used to have a tradition called the "potlatch" where they hosted parties to give away their worldly goods. (The guests receiv-ing these riches were expected to host their own parties later on and return the favor.)

It may be helpful for you to do some housecleaning and get rid of unnecessary material possessions. Part of your prob-lem has been an inability to put a value on things—and on yourself. So distributing your wealth to others, especially giv-ing up a few items that really do mean something to you, can be a useful teaching tool. In this way you may discover the true worth of things that money can't buy.

Get Some Attention

Since kleptomania involves attracting negative attention, you need to find out what to do to attract positive attention. You might teach a course at your local community college, run for local office, or mount a talent show in which you get to perform. When you see that others can appreciate the good things you do, you won't need to misbehave to feel included in life.

LACK OF CONCENTRATION

see also Confusion, Mental, page 100; Distraction, page 121; Stress, page 407

All of us have occasional lapses in concentration when we're preoccupied with a problem and can't finish a newspaper article or when our mind is a jumble of thoughts and feelings that refuse to sort themselves out. But when you can *never* concentrate, you feel disjointed, lacking direction as well as focus. Unlike distraction, where you can be drawn away from your thought by a sound, a sight, or an event outside yourself, lack of concentration is a particularly difficult inner turmoil.

What Happens When You Can't Concentrate

You suffer from "monkey mind," the freewheeling, overwhelming mentality that jumps from subject to subject, lighting on one for a brief moment and then moving on to several more. Your thoughts and feelings run together; sometimes you feel elated as you juggle images of home, work, fantasy, and future goals; at other times, you sense a dragging, annoying clutter as you try to deal with too much going on at once in your mind.

Other people perceive you as ungrounded and rootless, and you may actually find that your eyes wander in the same fashion as your wayward ideas that come and go like ripples on the surface of a lake. If you can't concentrate, you can't complete your work (or do it well) in a timely fashion; you can't finish a book or a project; you may have trouble staying with the thread of a conversation; and it can be very tough to work out emotional difficulties in a relationship.

The real reason for lack of concentration is often stress. When you don't take care of each moment at a time, they all tend to escape. You can't pay attention to your lover because you're thinking about the bills; you can't pay attention to your child's play because you're thinking about your mother's recent accident. When you are overwhelmed with too much to do, you don't prioritize, and everything seems equally urgent. It can also be a convenient cop-out, because you can't handle all the things you think you're responsible for and end up doing nothing rather than everything.

In order to train your concentration, you have to focus on the moment and remove all excess thoughts.

Remedies for Rushing Thoughts

The homeopathic remedies for rushing thoughts are: Belladonna, Lachesis, Phosphorus, Arsenicum album, Calcarea, China, Ignatia, Kali carbonicum, Pulsatilla, Silica, and Sulphur.

Do One Job Well

Select a task that you haven't done in a while that will require a lot of attention. It can be something as basic as alphabetizing a pack of names or stringing beads for a necklace. Make sure that the room you're in is comfortable and quiet and that there are no outside distractions—don't play music or have the TV on or try to carry on a conversation.

As you work, devote yourself to the task, no matter how simple-minded you think it is. Look at the handwriting on your cards and focus on the loops and dots in the letters. Examine each bead and see the shape and color as distinct from the one next to it. By working attentively, you will begin to see how important each action and each moment is. You will find yourself more interested in what you're doing; and you will finally see what it feels like to concentrate completely and fully on the task at hand.

Write a Poem

Whether or not you consider yourself creative, you can find the rhymes for a limerick or brief verse. First make a list of easy words that might end a sentence: "you," "too," "flew," "grew"; or "best," "dressed," "test," "rest." Then select a topic and clap out a rhythm that will be the meter of your poem. It will take a lot of concentration to combine your topic and your pre-designated rhyming words and still manage to make each line scan in meter. Don't worry if it's not Shakespeare. The idea is to get your mind to combine several complex elements.

Tell a Story Without Words

Charades is a wonderful way to plant your mind on an objective and carry it through to completion. In this exercise you will go back to the type of gestures you did as a child, creating meaning from movement to explain what you're doing to others. You might act out a song or movie title or portray a character from history. You will discover, when you are restricted in your means of "telling," that you have to concentrate keenly on all your other faculties. You can make this a greater challenge by giving yourself a time limit to get your audience to understand what you're doing.

Prioritize Your Chores

Make a list of everything you have to do for the next week in order of importance and a second list of those things you'd like to do if you have time. You may not start one chore until you have finished the one before it—this means you will have to concentrate hard on each one in succession.

A Flower Will Heal You

Indian pink is the Bach flower remedy for lack of concentration. It will help you feel centered and focused even under stress. Take 5 or 6 drops under the tongue or mixed in half a glass of water, as needed.

Use a Mindful Meditation

Stand in front of a blank wall and focus your eyes on a spot of your choosing. Begin to watch your breath as you slowly inhale and exhale. Try to imagine the breath as connected to that spot on the wall, tied to it by a string. You can move the spot wherever you choose—in a circle, up and down, off the wall, and down onto the floor. Your whole focus is directed to keeping the spot the same size and color and to directing it precisely where you want it. The more deeply you allow yourself to get into this meditation, the better your concentration will be.

LACK OF SELF-CONFIDENCE

see also Fear of Failure, page 171; Loneliness, page 277; Self-Esteem, page 380;
Shyness, page 400; Victim Mentality, page 433; Vulnerability, page 445

Very few people feel confident all the time. Most of us question our choices or actions sometimes, and this isn't all bad—it's prudent to second-guess ourselves before making a big decision. If, however, you always lack confidence in yourself, if you have no pride at all in your own ideas or abilities, you effectively cut yourself off from trying new things and meeting new people. By hesitating, you can easily be lost.

■ What Happens When You Lack Self-confidence

You assume that you're wrong and others are right. You never take a challenge because you're sure you'd fail. You have no response when anyone asks what you think, because you never even bothered to form an opinion. If pressed, you'll speak out, but you feel miserable, certain that nobody really credits what you have to say, and they'll probably make fun of you if they're listening. Any new endeavor is a project, whether it's learning a new card game, going to a party, or being assigned to a new team at work.

Many people who lack self-confidence were taught at an early age that they were no good, stupid, or in the way. If your parents made you feel inferior when you were small (and when you naturally looked up to authority figures), you may have carried these feelings of worthlessness with you through the years. It will take a good amount of healing to repair the damage and to feel whole again.

Tape an Affirmation Daily

Tell yourself you're good! Sit down in front of a tape recorder and say the following:

I am a valuable member of society and this household.
Other people know they can count on me.
I try as hard as I can.
Even when I'm unsure of myself, I make an effort.

Play these affirmations (and others that relate to your specific qualities) each night before you go to bed. You might ask your partner, children, or friends to suggest a few for you if you have trouble coming up with statements that sound to you like boasting.

Give Yourself a Prize

You are going to examine everything you do at work and at home and reward yourself for your real successes. Buy yourself a box of gold stars and make yourself a chart. Did you bandage your child's cut knee? You have mastery as a parent. Did you finish your taxes on time? Give yourself a star for promptness. Did your family enjoy the Sunday outing to the beach? Congratulate yourself for being a great host or hostess. You will find, if you poke beneath the surface of the routine activities you do every day, the real worth of those chores. By caring enough about yourself and those around you, you intuit what has to happen and provide what's needed. These are qualities to be proud of.

Trust in a Trance

Using self-hypnosis, you will slowly plant suggestions that you are worthwhile and you deserve to feel proud of yourself. Take half an hour each day to sit in a quiet place in a straight-backed chair. Let your eyes roll upward, take a deep breath and hold it, then close your eyes. You will feel very relaxed, but alert, and ready to receive the following suggestion. While in trance, you will tell yourself that you have a light switch inside you. Whenever you are in a situation in your daily life when you feel unsure of yourself, as though you were in a dark tunnel, you will turn on the light switch. This will illuminate your intentions and make them clear to you and to others. Now you can sit and allow this light to become part of you and warm your entire body. When you are ready, you may slowly come out of the trance and open your eyes.

Relax Progressively

Sometimes we hold body tension like armor, waiting for some terrible event we feel unprepared to handle. The sooner we can let go of that, the more confident we'll feel about greeting the world.

Lie in a comfortable space on a blanket or mat. Feel your arms and legs fall away from your body; allow your body to sink into the floor. You are going to clench one group of muscles and then quickly let them go, starting with your toes. Put all of your attention first in your toes. Clench them hard, then release. Move onto your arches, the whole foot, then the ankle, the calf, the knees, the thighs, the hips and pelvis, the buttocks, the lower back, the waist, the solar plexus, the upper back, the shoulders, the neck, and the upper arms, elbows, forearms, wrists, and fingers. At last you will move up to the head to tighten and then release the chin and jaw, the mouth, the nose, the cheeks, the eyes and eyebrows, the forehead, and finally the scalp. When you have completed this body scan, tensing and relaxing each part, you will think of the whole as the sum of all your parts.

Tighten every muscle of your body. Feel in complete control as you work everything together. Now release every muscle of your body. Sink deep into the floor and feel as though you own it. By identifying and alleviating your own tension, you now can understand and respect the power of your physical being.

Flowers to the Rescue

Bach flower remedies can offer confidence. Take 5 or 6 drops under the tongue or mixed in half a glass of water, four times daily. The appropriate remedies are:

Mimulus, if you don't feel up to meeting challenges and feel paralyzed in difficult situations

Larch, for confidence, spontaneity, and creativity and for feelings of inferiority and a fear of failure

Homeopathic Help

Try the following homeopathic remedies to gain confidence:

If you are deeply insecure and need a lot of support: Arsenicum album

If you are tearful and shy with a tendency to yield and give way to others: Pulsatilla

LACK OF TRUST

see also Anger, page 31; Anorgasmia, page 38; Jealousy, page 257; Loneliness, page 277

As humans, we are fortunate in that we exist in a society of others like us, and part of the reason for our success as a species has been the way we trust enough to bond together to achieve goals. It is possible to trust too much; you can be misguided in your decision to lean on others. But when you feel you can't rely on anyone but yourself, you are a very lonely individual.

▪ What Happens When You Lack Trust

You can't delegate authority because you're the only one who can do the job right. When others promise you that they'll be there for you, you're convinced that they are just mouthing meaningless words. You are suspicious of offers of friendship; you are even wary of those closest to you and are always checking up on them to be sure they are toeing the mark.

It's one thing to mistrust strangers, but when you feel you can't rely on your partner or members of your family, you are even more likely to sour on life. The people closest to you should be the ones you come to as your port in any storm, but when you shut them out, you close the door to getting any help when you might really need it.

When you can't trust anyone, you burden yourself with the responsibility of being the only one who can do the job, who can make the relationship happen, or who can take care of a crisis. And the problem is that none of us alone can manage everything—we have to trust in others at some point to keep going. You can't control every element in your life, and once you realize that you'll be a great deal happier. Even if others can't perform the way you might like them to, if you decide you're going to trust them, you may be surprised by how much they'll accomplish.

Let a Group Support You

Joining a group of any kind—a chess club, a martial-arts school, a pickup softball team—will force you to rely on others. Since there is no way you can do these activities alone, you will be compelled to acknowledge that those around you are not quite as ineffectual or irresponsible as you thought.

Fall Back to Go Forward

Get a group of friends or acquaintances to help with this exercise. Stand with your back toward the group and ask everyone to form a half-circle around you. They are going to catch you when you fall backward. At first, you'll want your friends as close as possible, so that you have only a short distance to go; but as you gain trust in the fact that they are going to break your fall and not let you hurt yourself, you can ask them to move back a bit.

Physical trust is something we develop (or don't develop) in infancy. If you can recreate the feelings of being protected and cared for in this group situation, you will have gone a long way toward establishing your sense of emotional trust.

Have a Massage

When you let someone else lay hands on you in a gentle massage, you derive much more benefit from it by relaxing. The more you yield to this touch as though you were clay being molded by a sculptor, the more open you become. You may ask your partner or a friend, or you can book a professional massage. Be sure to tell the person who is working on you your goals for this therapy before you begin the session. You will probably want the therapist to start on some nonthreatening part of the body such as your back and shoulders. As you feel more comfortable, you can give the practitioner permission to work on other parts of you.

Pray Over It

If you feel that you have been wronged by someone or by life in general, it can be restorative to put your faith in something bigger than yourself and other human beings. Even if you're not an observant individual, you can lift your spirits by letting go of the control you feel you have to have over your life and trusting in a higher power.

Eat Right to Feel Right

Cutting out junk food may help you feel less heavy and suspicious. A body that exists on fat and sugar isn't getting the
nutrients that nourish the various organs, including the nervous system. Stick to a whole-foods diet—a well-balanced
combination of proteins, carbohydrates, and just a fifth of
your daily calories from fat. Make sure you eat lots of fresh
fruits and vegetables, legumes, and whole grains, and cut
down on meat, poultry, and fish. You'll feel lighter inside and
out.

*L*IGHT *T*HERAPY

see also Bipolar Disorder, page 67; Death, Thoughts of, page 109; Depression,
page 112; Hopelessness, page 226; Mood Swings, page 297; SAD, page 373;
Sadness/Despondency, page 375

Light therapy (or phototherapy) has been proven enormously
effective in those individuals who find their moods fluctuating
with the seasons. The changing pattern of daylight and darkness during the winter months often affects sleep cycles and
can wreak havoc with sensitive systems. The use of light to
treat depression and sadness has been around for centuries—
Hippocrates supposedly used sunlight to treat his patients.

Most individuals have a free-running clock, that is,
when shut away from natural light and a watch, most of us
would probably sleep longer and stay up longer than we do,
for a total of 25 or 26 hours a day. But many depressed individuals and those with bipolar disorder occasionally have
natural cycles that are less than 24 hours. When our biological clock is off its timing, when the cycle moves too fast, for
example, the peaks and valleys of our hormone production
are thrown off. Some people are highly sensitive to circadian
rhythms (the word means "around a day") and cannot seem
to function when they don't have an equal amount of light
and darkness throughout the day.

For some of us, the functioning of the pineal gland in
the center of the brain is crucial to our feelings of well-being.

When our eyes detect light, this gland produces serotonin (the neurotransmitter that gives us a sense of well-being) and just a little melatonin (the one that affects our circadian rhythms). But when it's dark, the pineal gland begins to convert serotonin into melatonin and pumps it directly into the bloodstream. During the night, we are infused with this hormone that makes us sleepy and allows us to rest. Like a bear in hibernation, when we have too much melatonin at high peak in our system on a regular basis, we begin to feel logy, listless, and exhausted. Melatonin levels in most people peak from midnight to about 2 A.M., but in people suffering from SAD (seasonal affective disorder), the levels peak later at night and remain high for four rather than just two hours.

SAD is caused by an imbalance in circadian rhythms and irregular melatonin peaks and valleys. So by artificially replacing the sunlight lost in the winter months, we can bring the circadian rhythms back into alignment. Therapy must be preventive, that is, you must start using a light box in November, *before* the darkest time of the year and the heaviest peaks of melatonin production have hit. Most experts agree that early-morning light is the most essential, so you should set your lamp on a timer that goes on about two hours before you're due to wake up.

Light therapy has been used with partial success in individuals who have other types of depression and mood swings, as opposed to significant success in those with SAD.

If you find that you feel down and logy all the time, if you lack energy and can't get yourself up in the morning, if you feel as if you've lost your creative edge, if you have a greater than normal need for sleep, and if you're eating a lot more than usual, you may benefit by the use of a light box.

This therapeutic tool—a 10,000-lux light box—contains a full-spectrum fluorescent or incandescent light (about 10 to 30 times as bright as ordinary indoor light). There are now many clinics around the country dealing with disturbances in circadian rhythms where you can be exposed to full-spectrum light. You can also perform this therapy at home by purchasing a unit and sitting in front of it for an hour a day during the dark months. A typical box is about the size of a VCR and costs from $200 to $600.

LISTLESSNESS

see also Alienation, page 28; Fatigue, page 158; Numbness, emotional, page 313;
SAD, page 373; Sadness/Despondency, page 375

Some people seem to fade into the woodwork, as though they were almost invisible and wished to remain that way. Listlessness is a combination of an imbalance in mind, body, and spirit: the sufferer feels physically weak, can't think clearly, and has no will to improve his or her situation.

What Happens When You Feel Listless

You are weaker than a kitten, with scarcely the energy to get up, prepare food, or go to work. Nothing grabs you, so you have no motivation to change your attitude. You aren't really tired, just disinterested in everything and everyone. There seems to be little purpose in doing or saying anything, and you have no strong opinions—one perspective is as good as another, and none is particularly appealing.

When trying to get to the root of your listlessness, it's important to find out what you're avoiding. The numb feeling will usually start to dissipate once you discover the elements that have either scared or frozen you into nonaction. The barriers you've set up to any emotional response to life will slowly dissolve as you use natural therapies to bring yourself out of your fog.

Chinese Herbs for Strong Qi

The diagnosis in Chinese medicine would be that your qi or life energy is weak and needs tonifying and nourishing. Any of the following herbs can be used: astragalus root, ginseng root, atractylodes rhizome, black dates, dioscorea rhizome, eleutherococcus, codonopsis root, licorice root, polygonatum rhizome, and pseudostellaria root. These can be taken as a tea or can be cooked and eaten. Because Chinese medicine is a complex system that does not target just one symptom, the person with depleted qi might also need additional support for depleted Blood and would require herbs that help with circulation. A Chinese physician might also prescribe herbs to warm the Spleen, which when out of balance might make a person lethargic and insecure.

Eat Hearty

Spice up your life with interesting food with strong aromas that will entice you to eat. Experiment with all types of chilis, and with Mexican, Indian, Thai, and Chinese foods that are filled with flavor and sting your palate. Make sure you consume hot foods as hot as you can take them.

Indian Wisdom

A *kapha* imbalance might make you feel heavy and sluggish, less than alert. So to change this, you need stimulation in all aspects of your life. Eat light foods (nothing deep-fried) with a lot of warmth and spice to them. You can take a cup of hot ginger tea with meals to sharpen your taste buds and can chew fennel seeds after your meal to speed digestion. Avoid sweets except for honey.

In your daily life, be sure to stay warm and avoid dampness. It's a good idea to start the day with a dry massage (Ayurvedic practice recommends raw-silk gloves, but you can substitute a loofah sponge). Give your limbs an invigorating rubdown to get your circulation going. Daily exercise is essential—select an activity you really enjoy, whether it's walking, dancing, martial arts, or racquetball. If you play a competitive sport, decide that you're going to win.

Breathe Alternately

Alternate nostril breathing balances the two hemispheres of the brain and tones the nasal passages. It is also reputed to facilitate neurotransmitter activity, which may help to motivate you. Place your right thumb on your right nostril and inhale through your left, then exhale left. Cover your left nostril with your pinky and ring finger and release your thumb, then inhale through your right and exhale right. Repeat for at least five minutes. (This therapy will also clear your sinuses.)

Determine to Dance

You can rev yourself up to high speed if you go dancing. The idea is not to travel languidly around the floor, but to really get down and boogie. Try partnered dance, and you be the leader, regardless of whether you are male or female. In a dance, you need to be alert to follow the rhythm and dynamics of the music, and without words, you have to transfer this awareness to your partner. Swirling, jumping, hopping, dipping, and jiving can be a wonderful way out of your listless state.

Get a Massage

An aromatherapy massage, using a stimulant such as Patchouli oil to lift anxiety, pine to clear the mind and alleviate mental fatigue, or ylang-ylang to stimulate the senses may help to strengthen your spirits. Use two or three drops of essential oil mixed with a carrier oil such as Almond or Jojoba oil.

LONELINESS

see also Aging, page 17; Alienation, page 28; Broken Heart, page 78; Depression, page 112; Grief, page 193; Hopelessness, page 226; Sadness/Despondency, page 375; Tearfulness, page 421

Being alone is beneficial to the soul; being lonely can kill. There is a sense of being stranded in your own world where you and only you speak the language and know the customs. You can see other people, but you can't relate to them. When you don't bond with anyone else and can't remember the last time you shared an intimate look with another, you may actually feel the pain physically. If you don't have someone in your life who cares, why should you get up in the morning or do your hair or see a doctor for your aches and pains? Loneliness is neglect and abandonment, and it carries with it a sense of shame and humiliation that nobody wants you.

What Happens When You Suffer From Loneliness

You are truly suffering, and you feel as though you are the last person on earth. You try to reach out to others, but even when you're in a crowd, you feel the same lack of human contact. You can't figure out whether you feel miserable because you have nothing to give to anyone or because you have no one to give it to. Loneliness can be worst when you actually share a home with a partner you feel disconnected from or with older children who live their own lives separate from yours.

People who feel isolated have three to five times the mortality rates from all causes when compared to people who don't feel isolated, and these rates do not reflect their cholesterol level, blood pressure, or whether they smoke. The rates do reflect a lowered immune system—as if loneliness itself made the body less able to defend itself against foreign invaders. In a recent Swedish study on social isolation as a cause of heart attacks, it was found that loneliness created specific neuroendocrine effects that led to atherosclerotic problems. Out of 150 men who smoked and drank minimally and were evaluated over a ten-year period, it was found that loneliness was an independent factor for death in 20 cases. David Spiegel's classic studies of women with breast cancer offer astounding figures: Women who belonged to a support group throughout their surgeries and subsequent treatment lived twice as long as the women who had no support group.

Joining groups and starting projects is the first step toward banishing feelings of loneliness. The proximity to the rest of the world is a prerequisite for joining it. But remember, being in a social setting guarantees only that you'll be around people—this does not necessarily lessen your feelings of loneliness. Only you can banish loneliness by presenting yourself honestly to others and accepting what they can give back.

Visualize Yourself as a Sharer

Although it may seem counterproductive to sit alone and meditate while you do a visualization, this can often be the first step toward understanding what it is that makes you feel so separate from the rest of humanity.

Sit comfortably in a quiet, dimly lit room and begin to concentrate on your body. It is one entity, all by itself, and yet it fits perfectly in the configuration of the floor or chair you're sitting in. It takes up just the right amount of space, and there is no break between it and the air around it.

Imagine yourself now with another person beside you. Feel the warmth of her proximity and look at the space between you as a link rather than a dividing line. Be aware of every aspect of this person—her smell, the way she breathes, the touch of her hand, her presence in the room with you. Enjoy the quiet the two of you have created, or speak a word to her and imagine her response. This person is more than an extension of your mind; she is a representative of all that you give out to others and receive back. Feel the blessing of this jointure between you, and as you open your eyes, understand that you can take the energy that you have just created with another into the world and share it with those you meet.

Play Ball

Do anything once a week—chess, cards, racquetball, a barbershop quartet—that gets you out and interacting with others. The regularity of a social event and something to look forward to keeps you healthy in mind, body, and spirit.

Get Support

If you ask for it, you are much more likely to get it. Call someone you know and make a regular date for exercise or food shopping. It's important that you set specific days and times so that both of you begin to rely on each other. If the weather's bad, be certain you keep your date by telephone, fax, or e-mail.

The Internet offers a world of people to communicate with even when you don't know them. Joining forums and chat rooms can be an adjunct to your real human contact during the week.

Be a Leader

Start thinking of yourself as someone with a lot to offer, someone that others seek out for advice and help. You may do this by becoming active in your church or synagogue, or by teaching a night course at an adult school. You will have to change your attitude in order to change your behavior, but if you take the first step, your interesting activities will provide you with the next step—and the next.

Volunteer Your Time

A friend in need, the saying goes, is a friend indeed. By offering your services—at a school, a hospital, an emergency squad, a literacy program—you will see the rewards coming back to you. The warmth of others' appreciation can get you out of the shell you've been in.

Play Like a Child

Children rarely feel lonely because they assume they're liked as soon as another child wants to play with them. (They also usually have a lot of imaginary friends!) Try taking a friend (child or adult) to a public park and use all the equipment available. A swing lends itself to cooperation between partners (one to push and one to ride), a sandbox is much more fun when two of you create the castle, and a see-saw can't even be used by one alone. Doing things that require physical give-and-take can point up the benefits of emotional give-and-take.

Get a Pet

Your best bet is a dog, since cats are terribly independent. You don't need a fancy breed—mutts are actually the best tempered and live the longest. (They're also widely available and all you need to pay for is their shots.) The comfort and unconditional love provided by a warm, furry creature is often the catalyst for being able to feel human love as well.

LOSS OF LIBIDO

see also Sexual Dysfunctions, page 387

Sigmund Freud was the originator of the idea that we are all born with an instinctive drive for sensual and sexual pleasure. As an infant, we are all id, the irrational and instinctive creature who thinks only about satisfying desire. Freud describes the libido as a sexual drive; however, the more important component is that id-based need for sensual pleasure.

As we develop an ego, a rational mind in an individual personality, and then a superego, the "policeman" of our actions, thoughts, and desires, the id sometimes goes by the boards. It is not uncommon for depressed, anxious, or traumatized individuals to lose the drive for pleasure they were born with.

■ *What Happens When You Lose Your Libido*

It's as if a veil had been cast over the world. Colors aren't as bright, smells not as sharp, images not as vivid. Because nothing gives your senses immediate satisfaction, you don't feel the same desire to explore and investigate your feelings and inner needs. The drive to be physically close to another human being is a reflection of our joy in life, and when one is gone, the other can't survive. Whereas before a whiff of a clean body or the sight of shapely legs might have excited you, now you look but don't see.

A loss of libido implies that you had one to begin with; however, many people are stunted before puberty by fears engendered by rigid parents, religious superstitions, childhood abuse or by some other negative experience, or some incorrect information. If your immediate reaction to a highly charged sexual situation is turning off, you can never feel the type of desire that would move you toward sexual union with another.

Other individuals, however, have lost the desire they once had, some because of rape or abuse, some because of chronic depression, some because of conflict and tension in a relationship, and still others because of changes of mood and temperament at different life stages such as pregnancy and menopause.

In order to feel sexual desire, we have to have certain physiological prerequisites: adequate gonadal hormone levels and good functioning between various centers in the brain, and adequate neurotransmitter production to send messages from the feeling brain (the limbic system) to the thinking brain (the cerebral cortex). Part of the preparatory work for feeling desire is recognizing triggers for fantasy and establishing the look in the eye and the openness in the body that takes place at the beginning of each courtship dance.

There are various types of desire-phase dysfunction. One is sexual aversion, a true disgust or fear of sexual intimacy. This often stems from rape or abuse as well as from family or religion-based guilt and shame. If you can't trust the other person—or you think your personal boundaries may be violated—you undoubtedly won't feel comfortable about allowing intimate physical contact.

A second type of problem is inhibited sexual desire (ISD). This may be physically based (low levels of testosterone, the hormone responsible for our sex drive), emotionally based (relationship problems, fear, guilt, and the like) or have a circadian basis (some women have no desire around the time of ovulation or menstruation, and some men have cycles of lessened interest at different times of the year).

A third type of problem, sexual desire conflict, occurs because of an imbalance of desire in a relationship. When one of you wants it much more than the other, it can be intimidating to the more reticent partner.

It is always possible to restore libido *if you want it back.* The problem is how to convince a person who has shied away from it that it will enhance his or her life and alleviate many mental and emotional problems.

Stimulate Your Senses

Part of the loss you have experienced is in your ability to experience the bounties of the world around you. First thing in the morning, lie in bed and examine the quality of the light in your room. Listen to the birds and traffic sounds; take in the scent of the sheets and blankets, feel the warmth of your own body. At each moment of the day, capture every sight, smell, sound, taste, and feeling. If you can, jot them down in a notebook. Not every sense will be pleasant, but all of them should stimulate your memories, dreams, fears, and hopes.

The more you become aware of your surroundings, the more excited you will be about greeting each day and the people you share it with. After several weeks, you may find your desire and interest sparked once again.

Try Sex for One

Very often, the pressure of performing with a partner gets in the way of desire. Masturbation, on the other hand, is something you do by yourself, to discover exactly what gives you pleasure. Although most people pleasure themselves when they feel desire, your assignment is to make a date with yourself even though you're not interested. Take an evening home alone with a bubble bath, a glass of wine or iced herbal tea, soft music, and a vibrator. Establish a setting that will put you in the mood to take good care of yourself and have a good time, whether or not it leads to sexual excitement.

The point of this evening of pleasure is to figure out what you like and to give it to yourself with abandon and delight.

Watch a Movie

It is said that men have visual sexual triggers and women have auditory ones, but sometimes both can benefit by watching other people make love. Most erotic films are genitally based—that is, the point is intercourse (usually hard, fast, and repetitive). However, recent films, many created by women, offer a total turn-on that transcends gender. The work of Candida Royalle, a former porn star turned producer, is an example of the extraordinary power of visual imagery to stimulate the imagination. Her movies are breathtakingly sexy and recommended viewing for anyone who has lost his or her libido.

Just Touch

Very often a person with a low libido gets out of the habit of touching because he or she fears it will enflame his or her partner. If you're worried that the other person will be "carried away" and unable to stop, this may be a reflection of your own inhibitions about sex. Touching isn't sexual, it's sensual. Talk to your partner openly about not wanting to consummate the act, but still wanting to be close. Cuddling, hugging, and stroking can all be done with your clothes on, which may make you feel safer about intimacy.

Talk It Out

If you are in conflict with your partner about any issue—from child care to the price of your new couch to whether your mother-in-law should come to live with you—it's virtually impossible to feel desire. Sit down and have an open talk without interruptions or criticisms. Being receptive to thoughts is similar to being sexually receptive; the more you and your partner can open your minds and really hear what the other has to say, the more likely you will be to relearn what it is that attracted you in the first place.

Practice Sensate Focus

This exercise is often recommended by sex therapists to balance the power in a relationship. It can also help to increase sexual desire.

One person is the giver, the other is the taker for 20 minutes, at which point you switch roles. The taker does nothing but lie passively on the bed or floor, receiving the touches, kisses, and other stimulation that his or her partner wishes to bestow. The giver is allowed to do anything sensual—no sexual contact is allowed. This means you should practice the exercise clothed at first, and you may not touch your partner's breasts and nipples, vulva or vagina, penis or testicles, or anus.

Whether you feel that this nonsexual touch is neutral, annoying, or pleasant, keep at it. After practicing for a couple of weeks, sensate focus exercises will probably start to trigger fantasies that can lead to sexual desire. The intimate touch of another that goes just up to but not over the sexual border is sometimes the best way to start those colored lights going.

MAGNETIC HEALING

Magnetic therapy is based on the electromagnetic properties of cells. The nucleus of each cell in the body has a positive charge; the exterior membrane has a negative charge. As the body's metabolism works hard to maintain itself—and possibly overworks when the body and mind are under stress—the amount of energy in each cell is depleted. Magnetic therapy increases the oxygen-carrying content of cells, removes lactic acid from injured muscles and calcium from injured joints, and increases blood flow to every cell.

If you're very anxious or depressed, the cells in your central nervous system have to work harder. Various problems such as anxieties, phobias, obsessions and compulsions, depression, and seizures may have an electromagnetic cause. As electrical stimulation rises, so does south-pole magnetic energy, which creates a pH imbalance in various bodily fluids. South-pole magnetic energy puts the body into an acidic state by increasing hydrogen-ion concentration. If you reverse the magnetic pull, however, you can bring the body back to a more alkaline state and alleviate many emotional and mental symptoms. North-pole orientation reduces hydrogen-ion concentration and reduces symptoms of addiction, toxicity, anxiety, and depression.

The relation of positive to negative magnetic fields is similar to that of the sympathetic to the parasympathetic nervous systems. In a positive field, the body's energy is evoked, similar to the "fight or flight" response of the sympathetic nervous system. The heart races, blood pressure rises, pupils dilate, and the body is ready for action.

But when we relax, our parasympathetic system calms the heart and the nervous system, and so does a negative field. Cells are oxygenated in the presence of this magnetic force, and the body can once again regain equilibrium. Negative magnetic energy also stimulates the production of melatonin and growth hormone (which are both activated when we sleep).

How the Magnets Work

The earth's magnetic field is 1/2 gauss, which means that both poles nearly balance (positive is only slightly more forceful than negative). When the gauss strength of both poles is applied at the same time and remains under 100 gauss, it is antistress. But in therapy, the distinction between the poles is exaggerated. Forces of from 2,000 to 5,000 gauss are used to heighten the effect of the antistress negative force, although these high levels may not be necessary for regular treatment.

Most therapy is performed with an 800- to 1,000-gauss north-pole oriented magnetic field with the patient lying for a half hour to an hour on a magnetic bed pad with magnets placed at the crown or back of the head, on the upper body and on the spine. The magnets can be an auxiliary treatment during chiropractic treatment or during craniosacral or myosacral manipulation.

Some therapists offer symptomatic relief of general tension with a variety of magnetic implements that can be used during the day—magnetic foot pads, insoles, hand-held devices, mats, and chair coverings. You can wear spot magnets on your sore wrist to speed healing or place one on your forehead to treat a headache. Anecdotal evidence indicates that magnetic therapy can work to relieve sleep problems, shingles, headaches, mental and emotional ailments, and a variety of physical problems as well. People with pacemakers and pregnant women should not use magnet therapy.

MANIPULATION (Chiropractic, Physical Therapy, Osteopathy, Naturopathy)

see also Craniosacral Therapy, page 104

The word "chiropractic" comes from the Greek *cheir*, or "hand," and *praktikos*, "done by." Most ancient civilizations used some form of manipulative technique in order to dispel pain and disease.

The formal therapy known as chiropractic came into being around the turn of the century, when Daniel David Palmer restored the hearing in a profoundly deaf janitor who worked in his building. Palmer believed that human health depended on a lack of obstruction in the central nervous system. He was sure that his patient's inability to hear was caused by a blockage in the transmission of nerve impulses. After his success with this one case, Palmer went on to develop his theory of subluxations, the condition where the partial loss of connection between vertebrae results in a pinching of the nerves in between and surrounding the obstruction.

Although chiropractic, and other allied therapies such as osteopathy and naturopathy attempt to fix physical dysfunctions created by vertebrae that are out of alignment and impinging on nerves, the mind, emotions, and spirit can also be helped by manipulation. Evidently, since the nervous system connects to the brain and chemical messages constantly pass throughout the system, any problem in the spine may affect the way we feel and behave.

In a healthy spine, there are three natural curves. The cervical vertebrae arch in an outward U-shape (a lordosis), then gently flow into the inverted thoracic curve (a kyphosis) and filter down to the lumbar curve (a lordosis), which ends at the sacrum. If you have had bad posture all your life, you probably get tired easily when you stand or sit, and in many cases, this is because your three curves don't align the way they're supposed to.

Emotional problems can cause you to hunch your shoulders, tense your neck, and thrust your hips out unnaturally. Over years of misalignment (possibly aided and abetted by car accidents, sports injuries, computer work, or high heels), you may throw all the various curves out of alignment. The more stress on the vertebrae, the more likelihood of pinching nerves. And as we age, the cushions, or disks, between vertebrae tend to bulge or flatten out, exacerbating already existing problems. When the vertebrae don't sit properly on top of one another, the opening between the bones that accommodates the nerve trunk (the *intervertebral foramina*) gets smaller, and hard bone presses on the soft nerves. The degree of pressure can be microscopic and still create undesirable changes in the entire nerve network. A subluxation in the middle of the back may cause pain or problems in an organ that is touched by the nerve that's pinched. Once this type of pressure is exerted, the affected area of the spine is sensitized and weakened.

The first symptoms that may clue you into the fact that you have a subluxation are headaches, tingling in the hands or feet, dizziness, or ringing in the ears. We may experience these symptoms when we are particularly stressed. Because the sympathetic nervous system is the overriding factor in our ability to relax, any type of blockage in the nerves surrounding the spine may cause increasing mental and emotional difficulties that we no longer have the resources to cope with.

Modern-day manipulation is as diverse as the practitioners in the field. Although there are still some old-fashioned "bone crackers" around, most chiropractors today rely on X-ray technology, ultrasound, and a deep knowledge of the organs and the web of fascia or connective tissue that joins structure to structure. There are practitioners who place no more than four ounces of pressure on the patient (Tofnis chiropractic, craniosacral therapy), those that do very light work until they feel a clear impasse in the body and then apply more force (Network chiropractic), and those who do the type of deep muscle work often associated with rolfing and shiatsu (applied kinesiology).

Although most critics of manipulative techniques claim that these therapies are too limited to treat successfully any ailment that is not directly related to the spine itself, it must be noted that any treatment involving the laying on of hands offers the benefit of healing touch. From the earliest studies onward, it's been proven that being touched externally makes us feel deeply (consequently, we say, "I was so *touched* that you thought of me"). It is indicative of the vast numbers of people who are treated by chiropractors in this country that we feel a need for someone to handle us—gently or roughly— while they attempt to heal us.

▪ *Manipulation and Mental or Emotional Problems*

More than a quarter of all those who go to a chiropractor come in complaining of stress-related problems rather than for an aching back. The headaches, nervousness, fatigue, dizziness, chest pain, and so forth, that has become intolerable may well be related to subluxations of the spine. Back in 1910, D. D. Palmer himself decided that chiropractic was useful for treating mental illness. He successfully alleviated behavioral and emotional problems in patients using chiropractic. During the period spanning from 1920 to 1960, there were six institutional programs in America devoted to treatment of abnormal behavior with chiropractic. Currently, there are therapists using manipulation who feel that subluxations in the neck and head can affect vascular and neurological nourishment of cerebral structures. As the practitioner works on various areas of the spine and is able to realign vertebrae, patients very often feel more than physical relief. It is then the secondary job of the practitioner to elicit some of the underlying reasons for the subluxation. By talking about the sensations we get when we hold and release tension, it's often possible to unearth the emotional bases of pain.

Then is the pain mental or physical? At least half of all patients with mental problems are misdiagnosed when they arrive on their doctor's doorstep with somatic complaints. It's generally considered okay to feel lousy if the pain is physical, but many people think it's a sign of weakness to say that they experience mental or emotional difficulties. The advantage of manipulation is that the practitioner is working on both the physical body and the mental state (via the central nervous system sheathed in the spine) simultaneously.

The Varieties of Manipulative Therapy

It should be mentioned that all methods of manipulation have specific approaches to the same goal, that is, freeing the nerves from vertebral pressure. Physical therapy uses massage, heat treatment, electrical and mechanical equipment, and water therapy for rehabilitation. Osteopathy, developed by a surgeon named Andrew Still in 1874, is not the same as chiropractic but can also be used to alleviate mental and emotional problems. Where chiropractic uses manual adjustments on various vertebrae to correct misalignments, osteopathy uses leverage, traction, and pressure to work on the entire structure—bones, muscles, fascia, organs, and skin. In addition to manipulation, osteopathy uses massage, stretching, twisting, use of water and heat therapy, and medication to restore nerves to normal functioning. Naturopathy, a more wide-ranging system of health care, believes that health consists of the harmonious interaction of four major factors: heredity; body chemistry; the physical structure of the body; and the mental, emotional, and spiritual attitudes that make us unique. A naturopath uses dietary adjustment, manipulation, and stress management techniques to deal with all four aspects at once.

MASSAGE

One of the oldest therapeutic techniques in existence, massage is a hands-on method of relaxing muscles, reducing tension, releasing toxins, and making the recipient feel nurtured and cared for. Massage—dry or with oils—is an integral part of traditional Chinese and Ayurvedic medical therapy.

A light massage concentrates on the skin, which is a major producer of hormones, and therefore can help to balance the endocrine system. The skin, of course, has thousands of nerve endings that connect with other parts of the body.

A deep massage works the muscles and fascia or connective tissue between muscles, tendons, and ligaments. As the therapist uses more forceful finger and hand pressure, you will find that it often stimulates different emotions. When we contain our rigidness or our misery in one certain area and it starts to break apart, it's impossible to hold onto that tension any longer.

CASE HISTORY

Jocelyn was exhausted all the time. She couldn't remember when she'd felt really okay; she couldn't remember a lot of things these days, and that frightened her. Her knees were swollen, she had a frozen shoulder, and every doctor she'd seen for the past six years said she was just overworked and tense. A new doctor, recommended by a friend, did a test for Lyme disease. Bingo.

"He put me on antibiotics right away, but they didn't do a thing for me—maybe it was too late, or maybe it wasn't the right medication for me, I don't know. I stayed bloated—all my joints were swollen, and I actually went up a shoe size. I thought a complete rest might help, so I went down to this spa in Mexico—a gorgeous place on the ocean. I had a massage every day and I started feeling like myself again. They worked me over like a big piece of putty—I could feel the fluids moving inside me, and that suddenly made me feel contented, relaxed. I think my lymph glands had kind of gone dormant, but the stimulation prodded them back to life. When I got back to New York, I kept up the massage, and I go now about once a month. I think it's vital for my mental as well as my physical health."

Massage can concentrate on certain muscle groups or be completely generalized. A typical Swedish (rubbing) massage covers the entire unclothed body, front and back. You are worked on by a therapist who rubs, pulls, and shakes one limb at a time, as well as your back, neck, and scalp. In a more directed clothed shiatsu massage, the fingers, knuckles, elbows and heels of the hand are used for deeper contact with the various layers beneath the skin.

Massage has been shown to reduce blood pressure, alleviate some headaches, increase energy, move fluids through the lymphatic system and thus rid the body of toxins, and has been used effectively in the treatment of depression brought on by trauma. A 1993 study at the University of Miami Medical School showed that depressed patients who received a 30-minute massage had consistently lower levels of stress hormones, were able to sleep better, and were more alert when they were awake.

Part of the benefit of massage is that there's nothing you can do. You are encouraged to let the therapist move you as you allow your body to go limp. By letting go and yielding up all your tension and anxiety, sinking deeper and deeper into the table, you can make some inroads into accepting whatever happens to you without trying so hard.

MEDITATION

There is nothing mysterious or foreign about meditating; probably the first meditators were our cave-dwelling ancestors who stared into a fire and put themselves into a type of trance state. They were able to create silence inside themselves as they obliterated all external stimuli and went within to calm their spirits.

As you meditate in the privacy of your bedroom or in a field under a starry sky, the goal is no goal at all except to be aware of the feelings and internal environment at that particular moment. When you practice, you simply exist. There are various types of meditation—prayer is probably the best known to Americans, but there is also TM (Transcendental Meditation), mindfulness meditation, and from the Eastern tradition, Zen meditation, Buddhist meditation, and Taoist meditation. They all focus and quiet the busy mind. The intention is not to remove stimulation but rather to direct your concentration to one healing element—one sound, one word, one image, or one's breath. When the mind is "filled" with the feeling of calm and peace, it cannot take off on its own and worry, stress out, or get depressed.

Herbert Benson, M.D., a professor at Harvard Medical School, describes the meditation experience as the "relaxation response." He discovered by studying various yogis and long-time meditators that the process counteracted the effects of the sympathetic nervous system—the one that wants to fight or flee. Whereas the sympathetic system dilates the pupils and gets the heart rate, respiration, and blood pressure up, the parasympathetic system, activated when we meditate, does just the opposite. Muscle tension decreases, blood pressure drops, and for some extraordinary practitioners, even temperature and basal metabolism rates drop during a prolonged meditation. Oxygen needs of the body are reduced when you are in a highly relaxed state, and brain waves change from the busy beta-waves to the blissful alpha waves.

How to Meditate

Meditation is also known as "sitting," and that's just what you do, nothing more and nothing less. If you can't sit cross-legged on the floor for 20 minutes without acute discomfort, you might also try a sitting cushion (or your balled-up sweater or a pair of sneakers) under your tailbone on the floor for support. You can also straddle a couple of thick pillows and kneel. If you can't sit with an unsupported back, use a straight-backed chair, with your feet flat on the floor. You can also stand, walk, or lie down and meditate (although it's hard for beginners not to drop off to sleep if they're prone). The important thing is to forget about your body, so you want to be as comfortable as possible.

Sitting meditation is not easy, particularly for impatient people. It's hard to just stay there and "do nothing," when your back rebels and your feet fall asleep and your brain wants to jump around and survey the mental landscape. But the more you do it, the more natural it becomes and the more benefits it conveys.

If you're in pain or feel uncomfortable, that's fine. Don't stop just because you've had enough. Instead, shift your concentration away from the pain to your breath. Let it take over and assure you that all's well and you're doing fine. Start to relax one body part at a time, directing your breath into tense joints and muscles so that they can let go.

Most Americans think that meditation is supposed to clear the mind completely. But it's virtually impossible for those of us brought up in a Western tradition to make the mind a void. You don't have to erase your thoughts, just don't let them linger in your mind. As you receive an impression, let go of it. Then the next and the next. The longer you sit and give yourself to the moment of just being there, the less you will feel impelled to pay attention to your noisy thoughts. Finally, once in a while, you will discover a wash of pure sensation that carries no concrete thought or mental images with it.

The easiest type of beginning meditation is the one where you simply focus on your breath. Keep the rhythm of your inhalation and exhalation as even as possible and imagine your mind and body as a bellows, with its sole function to pump in and out. You can also meditate on a single word, such as "peace" or "love" or even a sound such as "om."

The more you meditate, the more reliance you will have on the self inside and the less occasion you will have to get anxious, angry, or depressed.

MELATONIN

Melatonin is a hormone produced by the pineal gland deep inside the brain. A smaller amount is made in the retina of the eye. This substance not only gives us our awareness of when we should be active and when we should be dormant (waking and sleeping), it also controls the migratory patterns of birds and influences reproductive cycles. The amino acid tryptophan (present in milk, bananas, turkey, and many other foods that tend to relax us and make us sleepy) functions as a building block for melatonin. Melatonin is vital to our feeling of well-being because it is the precursor for serotonin (the brain hormone that makes us feel good and that is used to make Prozac and other mind-altering drugs).

Scientists have gone so far as to speculate that a decline in melatonin in our later years may be what triggers the degeneration process that leads to death. So if we supplement this hormone in midlife, is it possible that we could sleep better, have an improved sex life, a better memory, a stronger immune system, and even a longer life? Perhaps.

Melatonin's multiple benefits seem to center around the fact that this hormone acts as a powerful antioxidant—it is able to scavenge for wild chemical reactants called free radicals that destroy healthy tissue. Free radical oxidation is responsible for cataracts in the eye, plaque on the arteries, and a lowered immune system. But melatonin acts inside each cell of the body to protect the nucleus—the structure that has within it all our DNA. By keeping DNA intact, melatonin helps the cells to repair themselves, and this may help to prevent cancer, or at least prevent the proliferation of abnormal cells that may develop into a tumor.

How Melatonin Promotes Mental and Emotional Health

The amino acid glutamate is both a helpmate and a destroyer of nerve cells. This substance is essential to good communication between nerves throughout the brain and central nervous system. It sets up chemical routes through which dendrites can branch out and connect to axons of other nerve cells.

The activity of nerve cells takes place at the synapse, the gap between one neuron and another where electrical impulses travel along, directing the nucleus to release chemicals (neurotransmitters) that allow us to sense and feel the world. But as this process takes place, free radicals are released along with the neurotransmitters, which kill off nerves. Glutamate generates free radicals directly; however, melatonin protects the nerve cells and keeps the neuronal networks flexible, helping to direct neurotransmitter "traffic" to bypass routes that are less busy. This keeps the neurons from becoming overstimulated.

As we age, we produce less melatonin, which means that we have an overabundance of glutamate. Cells begin to die off more quickly, and confusion, memory loss, and abnormal behavior may result.

How to Get More Melatonin into Your System

The first rule of thumb is a regular schedule. The more you can regulate your life so that you get up with the sun and go to bed with the sun, the more melatonin you'll produce naturally. Staying in synch with your circadian rhythms—your innate sense of light and darkness awareness—is vital in your quest for good mental health. If you possibly can, avoid working late at night, traveling a lot—particularly to different time zones—or doing shift work.

Sleep in a dark room, try not to nap during the day, and be aware of times when you feel lowest; the slump around 3 P.M. is normal, but if you're unable to get out of bed in the morning because you feel exhausted, you may need to correct your light/dark scheduling. Individuals who get depressed only in the winter months are suffering from irregularity in melatonin production (see SAD, page 373, for a discussion of "winter blues").

You should also eat regular meals (your cycle of digestion and elimination also affects your moods) and avoid stimulants and sedatives such as caffeine and alcohol that can affect your sleep. Be particularly careful about taking over-the-counter antihistamines for colds and bee stings that might make you drowsy, and never take sleeping pills, which will also affect your cycling.

◼ *Should You Supplement Melatonin?*

The decision is still out on whether or not it's beneficial to supplement melatonin. Studies on laboratory mice indicate that low dosages of melatonin extend the life span and have no side effects other than drowsiness. Some preliminary evidence shows that too much melatonin causes light sensitivity, which means that giving yourself more than a minimal dose might be similar to staring into the sun for prolonged periods. There have been no controlled studies on humans, so it's impossible to say what long-term effects might be.

It is possible that supplementing tryptophan may be an optimal solution, since this amino acid works as the building block for melatonin production. If you decide to take a melatonin supplement, however, you should take no more than 1 or 2 mg. daily after darkness falls, ideally an hour or so before bed. (Higher doses will make you very sleepy, and the effects may last into the next day.) This supplement should always be used in addition to other lifestyle changes that enhance natural melatonin production.

MINDFULNESS

The practice of mindfulness is similar to that of meditation; however, your focus becomes whatever it is that you are currently doing. This is an easier practice for many novice meditators. You can be mindful about washing your face, signing your name, or sweeping the floor. Mindfulness can be done sitting, standing, moving, or lying down as long as you concentrate completely and fully on your activity. Ideally, each day should be an exercise in mindfulness; every moment should be explored to its fullest whether you are staring out the window, listening to music, or making love to your partner.

Jon Kabat-Zinn, director of the Stress Reduction Clinic at the University of Massachusetts Medical Center, suggests that you try being mindful about a very specific task—eating a raisin. This one is particularly good for beginners, since most of us take raisins for granted and would be more likely to grab a handful and throw them in our mouths than consider just one. (You can use one peanut or one section of orange if you prefer, although this experiment is excellent with foods you don't like as well as with those you do like.) When you eat mindfully, you first hold the food, feel it, sense its texture, think about where it grew and how it was picked. Then you bring it close to your face and smell it, place it close enough to your mouth so that you can begin to salivate as you anticipate eating it. At last you lick it, anticipating what the eating experience will be like. Then you can put it in your mouth (don't chew) and let the flavor blossom there. You can think about triggers for eating and whether you are eating because you are really hungry or because it's comforting to put food in your mouth and you enjoy the taste. At last you can consume the raisin and see how your taste buds react. Chew slowly, perhaps 30 or 40 times, letting the flavor flood your entire mouth. Postpone swallowing as long as you can, relishing the long, drawn-out process of eating this particular piece of food. Consider the physical process involved—how what is being mashed between your teeth will turn to a paste with liquid and go down your throat into your stomach and intestines. At last you can swallow, being aware of the remnants of food in your teeth and the flavor remaining on your tongue.

This type of therapy isn't useful only for eating disorders, but for many mental and emotional problems. As we develop more awareness and attentiveness to the routine daily chores we perform, we can more easily learn to fill the mind with comfort instead of worry and pain. If you can use each moment profitably, creating a meaningful event out of the smallest acts and thoughts, you can calm a panic attack or raise depressed spirits.

MOOD SWINGS

see also Bipolar Disorder, page 67; Blues, page 72; Depression, page 112; SAD, page 373

It would be positively boring if everyone woke up each day feeling happy and well adjusted. We all have normal fluctuations of mood that depend on the state of our physical health, our finances, our relationships, our creativity, our job, and dozens of other factors that cause anxiety, boredom, or elation.

When we are never on an even keel, however, it is disruptive to our sense of identity. If we can't rely on being the same person with a particular range of feelings and emotions, we may become so disoriented we can't function properly. Many mood disorders are due to lifestyle abuse—too much alcohol, caffeine, and nicotine will actually unbalance the psyche. Others are due to hypoglycemia—if you are particularly sensitive to blood-sugar levels, you may find your moods and behavior changing radically if you haven't had enough of the right foods to eat at the right times. Still others are due to food allergies, and others are due to fluctuations in daylight and darkness as the seasons change (see SAD, page 373). Another cause for women is their monthly cycle—PMS symptoms such as fatigue, irritability, and difficulty concentrating are most prevalent in the middle of the month when the level of the gonadal hormone progesterone rises sharply. Pregnancy and menopause also bring with them radical shifts in hormone production, which can upset the most sanguine personality.

Probably the most common cause of mood swings is stress, which can deplete the body of vitamins and minerals, particularly zinc and vitamin B_6, that help to keep the emotions on an even keel.

Mood swings can be a precursor of bipolar disorder, but they are more commonly a mixture of highs and lows that co-exist in time rather than a cycle that takes the individual from a manic state to a depressed one.

If you are a parent, it is particularly important to watch for mood swings in your children. Whether they are in preschool or high school, if you see that they are spontaneously irritable or despondent or are having academic problems or exhibiting disruptive behavior, it is vital that you arrange for them to see a professional. Early treatment is essential, since early onset places children at greater risk for mood disorders during their lifetime.

▦ *What Happens When You Experience Mood Swings*

You are up one day and down the next, or, even worse, up for a few hours, and then spiraling into a pit of oblivion. You feel tender and bruised, equally capable of crying or laughing at any moment. You may go through days when you are irritable and yell at everyone and then find yourself so down you can't get out of bed in the morning. It's very often as though you were wearing two heads, one of which can see clearly and ration emotions appropriately and the other which rages against life.

You may also experience a variety of somatic symptoms, such as headaches, stomach aches, tingling hands, heart palpitations, or extreme fatigue.

CASE HISTORY

Terri was a world-class rower in college, but it seemed that the more she worked out, the sicker she got. She had been a terrific student in high school, but just a couple of years later she couldn't concentrate on anything, and her moods were so erratic her friends didn't know how to relate to her. As her depression grew worse, she stopped rowing and put on 50 pounds.

"I went to doctor after doctor and was told I just couldn't handle stress. When they couldn't find anything, I started experimenting with alternative therapists—I used magnets, I developed muscle strength through kinesiology, I went to a homeopath to get chemically balanced again. But I still felt miserable and angry. One day I tore up an entire Sunday paper, section by section, to avoid throwing a chair at my husband.

"It was just by chance that I had a battery of tests for some job and someone discovered that I'd been carrying around parasites for almost 15 years. All that lake water spewing up at me when I was a rower—well, I'd contracted giardia and had never known. So I got to a specialist who gave me medication to get the bugs out of me, but then explained that my body no longer absorbed nutrients properly because of years of gastrointestinal dysfunction. She then gave me a special diet and had me take colonics (I now have them once every four or five months to clean out my system).

"The different nutrients really gave me back my old sunny personality. I take flaxseed, black walnut seeds, pumpkin seeds, garlic, and ginger. I also have to restrict the amount of starchy foods I eat, since the parasites changed my ability to process carbohydrates properly. But the nutritional adjustment has really worked! I've lost 25 pounds of bloat, I'm not depressed any more, and I have all my energy back. One of the biggest differences in getting the mood swings under control was starting tai chi. The practice really balances me and also gets my circulation working better. In addition to my daily practice, I get massages now whenever I can and see my chiropractor twice a year for a tune-up."

Stick to a Regular Eating Schedule

Food allergies are a common and often undiagnosed cause of mood disorders. You may have to do some sleuth work to find out what you're allergic to: Be aware when you get suddenly depressed right after eating and experiment with eliminating one food after another from your diet.

Hypoglycemia is another probable cause of mood swings. The brain needs glucose for energy, and if your blood glucose level drops sharply, you may find that you feel fatigued, dizzy, headachy, confused, and emotionally unstable. In order to avoid this, you can try eating six small meals throughout the day to keep your blood sugar as level as possible. If you can't manage six meals, bump up your glucose level when it's flagging with a high-energy snack (an apple, a banana, or a handful of almonds).

Don't follow a high-carbohydrate diet, which will bump blood sugar up too quickly, causing you to produce increased amounts of insulin and less of the feel-good neurotransmitter, serotonin. Get rid of white sugar and alcohol in your diet, both of which can make you feel depressed and miserable. You may also wish to experiment with eliminating egg whites from your diet. They contain a protein that binds to biotin, making this vitamin unavailable to the body. Biotin deficiency has been shown to cause depression.

Get Help if You Need It

Short-term counseling or therapy can do a great deal for you. By talking to a therapist, you may be able to release some of the emotions that have been blocked up or unrecognized for months or years. Talk therapy is sometimes aided and assisted by body therapy; you may wish to see a chiropractor or craniosacral therapist who can listen carefully to your body by gently palpating it and can release some of the restrictions you've been holding in your soft tissue.

Get off Drugs

Medications (both over-the-counter and prescription) cause millions of people to feel "not themselves." If you're taking an antihistamine for a cold, antihypertensive medication, corticosteroids, or oral contraceptives, you may be dosing yourself with the substance that leaves you prone to emotional rebounding. Caffeine and nicotine will produce the same adverse effects.

Keep up with Your Supplements

In addition to your daily multi-vitamin, you should take the following vitamins: B-complex (50 mg.), folic acid (400 mcg.), biotin (100 mcg.), niacinamide (500 mg. three times daily), niacin (50–100 mg. three times daily), pantothenic acid (500 mg. twice daily), pyridoxine or Vitamin B_6 (50 mg. three times daily), Vitamin C (1000 mg. daily), Vitamin E (400 mg. twice daily).

You should also take the following minerals: calcium carbonate or citrate (1000 mg. at bedtime), magnesium (400 mg. at bedtime), manganese (15 mg. three times daily), zinc sulphate (220 mg. twice daily).

Amino acids can also be helpful. Supplement tryptophan by eating lots of foods such as milk, bananas, figs, dates, and turkey. Another important amino acid that works well on mood disorders is DL-phenylalanine. Take 375-mg. capsules three times daily, 30 minutes before meals.

Omega-6 fatty acids have also been found helpful in treating mood disorders. Take 500 mg. three times daily of evening primrose oil to supplement these fatty acids.

The Herbs of Choice

St. John's wort (Hypericum perforatum) enhances the function of the essential neurotransmitters norepinephrine and dopamine. Take 2 to 4 teaspoons infused in a cup of water or 25 to 30 drops tincture three times daily to stabilize your moods. Avoid prolonged exposure to sunlight when taking this herb.

Try Massage with Oils

The essential oils Clary Sage, Jasmine, Neroli, and Rose may all be used in massage or a diffuser to calm your anxieties and keep your emotions on an even keel. Use 10 drops mixed with 20 ml. of a carrier oil such as Jojoba or Almond.

Go Run Around

Exercise triggers the production of natural opiates in the brain that restore us to that feeling of well-being we often seem to lose. Daily exercise is preventive against mood swings, and if you get up half an hour earlier for a brisk walk, swim, or bike ride, you may be able to maintain your good feelings throughout the day.

NEGATIVE ION THERAPY

Ions are particles that carry an electric charge, either positive or negative. They are found in gases, in X-rays, and in radium, under the influence of electrical charges, and are generally present in the atmosphere in a positive to negative ratio of 5 to 1. In natural settings—at the ocean or in the mountains—negative ions are in abundance; in polluted or environmentally hazardous settings—in a busy city or at a chemical-treatment plant—positive ions proliferate.

Studies have shown that different charges cause biological and behavioral responses in animals and humans. The lower the negative ion content, the more we feel fatigued, irritable, and sleep-deprived. We may actually be more at risk for certain infectious diseases. Just as we are affected by our circadian rhythms that help to produce melatonin and serotonin in appropriate amounts, peaking and dipping at appropriate times, so we are also susceptible to ion imbalances in the atmosphere.

In a study on patients with SAD (see Seasonal Affective Disorder, page 373), it was found that use of a high-density negative-ionizer was extremely beneficial in alleviating symptoms. The patients were treated for 20 days for 30 minutes each time shortly after they woke up. Their depressive symptoms diminished slightly at 10 days and were even better after 20 days. The rate of improvement was similar to that with a 10,000-lux light box (see Light Therapy, page 273).

It's possible to reap the benefits of negative ion therapy without special equipment. A day trip to the seashore, a walk in a wooded glade, or a hike up a mountain (preferably on paths without automobile emissions) will afford the same benefits.

*N*ERVOUSNESS

see also Agitation, page 21; Anxiety, page 43; Chest Pains, page 87; Dizziness, page 124; Hyperventilation, page 231; Panic Disorders, page 344; Stress, page 407; Tension, page 425

When you are overwhelmed and anxious and feel you can't cope, your body and mind react by tensing up. That jittery sensation is actually called "a case of the nerves," or nervousness. And in fact, the central nervous system and all the billions of nerves in it are responsible for this jagged-edge feeling.

◼ *What Happens When You Feel Nervous*

You may or may not know what's wrong, but regardless of whether there's a cause for your agitation, you feel jumpy and upset. Your mind is going faster than a speeding bullet, close to panic but not yet there. You may pace or tap a pencil; it's as if your cells are about to burst from your body. The word "antsy" truly describes your feelings, as though you had ants in your pants and couldn't sit still. You can hear your heart beat and your lungs expand; you can feel the hairs stand up on your arms. Your eyes focus right, left, center—on nothing and everything. You are fearful even when you can't put your finger on the cause of your anxiety.

Being nervous is understandable if you're about to go into a job interview or get married; the typical "fight or flight" reaction of the stress cycle gets us up on our toes, prepared for battling the unknown. The autonomic nervous system, reacting to a stimulus from the brain, tells the adrenal glands to secrete hormones (adrenaline, norepinephrine, and cortisol) that will allow you to act fast. The sympathetic nervous system goes to work and gets your heart pumping quicker, your lungs taking in more oxygen, your pupils opening wider to see the problem. So when you're nervous because something unsettling is happening, such as a car accident or a mugging, this is a healthy, protective reaction. The heightened physical and mental response allows you to function well in the midst of mishap or danger.

But when there is no stimulus and you still feel nervous, then you have a problem. Your mental tone is turned up so high, it's impossible to hear the rest of life's symphony playing. When you feel anxious all the time, this can result in fatigue, loss of concentration, foggy thinking, burn-out (when we use up too much energy too quickly), insomnia, and lessened muscular activity. You can't react as quickly as you should even in an emergency. If you're nervous about driving in general and a child runs out in front of your car, you may not be focused enough to act effectively, steering away and stepping on the brake. Being nervous leads to poor performance, whether it's physical, sexual, social, or mental.

When you're nervous, you are usually not dealing with what's on your plate at the present moment. You're either struggling with the past, reviewing problems you haven't been able to take care of, or leaping ahead to the future, anticipating all the awful things that could happen.

Heightened nervousness leads to panic, where you completely lose control of the situation because of your need to run away from disaster, even before there is a disaster. Panic brings with it symptoms such as shortness of breath, hyperventilation, rapid heartbeat, elevated blood pressure, dizziness, trembling, fainting, and a fear of dying.

The key to handling nervousness is to stay in the moment and quell the stress reaction right at the beginning, before its effect takes hold. What we need to do is use the parasympathetic nervous system, which elicits the "relaxation response" and calms the mind and body.

Breathe!

When we are nervous, we tend to take very shallow breaths and may start to hyperventilate. So it's useful to have an antidote that will calm you down instantly when you feel upset and panicky. Place your hand on your belly and inhale through your nose into your abdomen, keeping all activity out of your shoulders and neck. Feel your abdomen contract inward with the breath. Now exhale through your nose and mouth, pushing out against your hand. The strength of this type of qi gong ("breath work" in Chinese) fortifies your spirit even as it increases the amount of oxygen your blood can carry to all the internal organs, including the brain. You will be calmer and less prone to nervous tension when you control your breath.

Press the Calming Points (See pp 10–11 for acupressure charts)

For general tension, press

> L.I. 4: on top of the hand in the hollow of the muscle between thumb and forefinger
>
> U.B. 10 (where the skull meets the neck on either side of the spine)
>
> E.P. (extra point) Yin Tang: right between the eyebrows, third eye point
>
> Ht. 7: in the hollow next to the bone on the crease of the wrist in line with the pinky
>
> Sp. 6: on the inside of the lower leg, four fingers from the upper edge of the inner ankle bone, in the muscle just behind the edge of the shinbone.

Drink an Herbal Relaxant

There's a whole repertoire of herbs that act as relaxants and anti-stressors. You can take teas (2 to 4 teaspoons dried herb to a cup of water) or extracts (1/2 teaspoon) of scullcap, feverfew, hops, catnip, chamomile, motherwort, passionflower, valerian, rosemary, or sage. Juniper berries, ginkgo biloba, and chia seeds strengthen the nerves and brain. St. John's wort is also useful as a sedative. (Avoid prolonged exposure to the sun when taking St. John's wort.)

Calm Yourself with Oils

Aromatherapy and massage are a great combination for nervousness. The relaxing oils are Lavender, Geranium, Chamomile, Clary Sage, Marjoram, Eucalyptus, Jasmine, Rose, Ylang-Ylang, Mandarin, and Neroli. Use two to three drops mixed with a carrier oil such as Almond or Jojobe and let your partner massage every inch of you with them. Be sure to breathe deeply to inhale the essence of these potent oils.

Jump, Hop, and Run Around

Exercise is an excellent tonic for nervousness. It's particularly effective when you select an activity in which you're not in competition with anyone (especially yourself). You will not only get a good cardiovascular workout, you'll also start producing the endorphins in your brain that act as natural opiates to take away your internal pain. A brisk two-mile walk or five-mile bike ride each morning has lasting benefits—studies show that the parasympathetic nervous system (the part that calms us down) is still at work a couple of hours after exercise.

Supplement Your Mind

The B-complex vitamins are essential when you're nervous. You can take 100 mg. daily with pantothenic acid, 500 mg. twice daily. You should also take 1,000 to 3,000 mg. of Vitamin C with bioflavinoids and Vitamin E (400 IU daily). Your mineral supplements should include calcium (1,500 mg. daily) with magnesium (750 mg. daily) and zinc (50 mg. daily). Other supplements that offer additional support are the amino acids GABA with inositol and tyrosine, both of which act as tranquilizers.

Have a Homeopathic

A special combination remedy for nervousness is Calmes Forte, useful for reducing stress, calming down, and sleeping soundly. You can also use Ignatia, Magnesia carbonica, Pulsatilla, and Strychninum nitricum.

Touch a Pet

Studies in nursing homes have clearly indicated that holding a warm, cuddly cat or dog, stroking its fur, and receiving its unconditional love can lower blood pressure and heart rate, calm respiration, and reduce a variety of unpleasant stress symptoms. It also increases neurotransmitter production of melatonin and serotonin, the substances that make us relaxed and fill us with a sense of well-being.

Give yourself 20 minutes a day to sit quietly beside your pet (or borrow a friend's pet if you don't have one).

Ease Into a Tub:

Lying in warm water is enormously relaxing. Pour yourself a glass of wine or a cup of herbal tea (see list of recommended herbs, above) and soak. Bath salts are a relaxing addition to the warmth. Don't even bother to wash yourself—this is just a time to close your eyes and enjoy the sensation of being held and carried by the water.

Can the Caffeine

Eliminating caffeine will remove one whole level of stress from your body and mind. You may expect from three days to two weeks of withdrawal (if you currently drink at least three cups of coffee, tea, cocoa, or sodas) when you may experience headaches and a feeling of disorientation. But getting rid of this stimulant will prove a real benefit as you learn to relax.

Soothing Meditation

One of the healing aspects of meditating is that you are able to gain control over thoughts and feelings that tend to run away from you when you're busy with the activities of the day. By clearing your mind, you can start to settle in and enjoy the process of focusing on one thing at a time.

Sit quietly and comfortably and close your eyes. Concentrate all your energy on watching your breath. You don't need to make it fast or slow; it should be completely natural. Inhale and don't hold the breath, but allow it to expand throughout you. Think of the breath as being covered with a silk liner, and this smooth surface is coursing through you. As you exhale, leave a delicate core of silk inside, softly caressing your nerves and spine. Each inhalation and exhalation will leave you feeling more complete, more in tune with yourself and your environment.

Take three more easy breaths and feel how content you are. You can keep this comfortable sensation with you all day. Now allow your eyes to relax open.

Say an Affirmation When You Need It

You need to hear the words in order to believe that there's no cause to be nervous. Repeat these affirmations into a tape recorder and play them back to yourself as you're lying in bed, ready to fall asleep:

I am perfectly all right.
The world is a safe place.
There is no need to rush.
I have all the time and energy I need.
Right now, in this moment, I feel calm and relaxed.
A soothing peace has entered my soul.

NIGHTMARES

see also Posttraumatic Stress, page 353; Sleep Disorders, page 404

Nightmares are unconscious experiences with frightening or uncomfortable emotional overtones that occur during REM sleep. They are usually very visual and tactile and are generally so lifelike you can recall many details vividly.

The most common theme of a nightmare is being in danger—being chased, drowned, thrown off a building or mountain, being beaten, tortured, or raped. It is very often difficult to rouse yourself from sleep, even when you think you are about to die. (There are no confirmed reports in Western cultures of deaths due to nightmares, although certain other cultures, such as the Filipinos and Australian bushmen who believe in dream death, have documented deaths that occur during nightmares.)

We find the stuff of nightmares in everyday life, movies we see, people we stand next to on the subway, the effect of drugs we take, and of course, in the deepest recesses of our own minds. Both physical and psychological factors trigger nightmares. You may have bad dreams because you suffer from endogenous depression or you abuse drugs and alcohol, but you may also have nightmares because of psychological causes such as childhood abuse or a recent trauma. People who have witnessed or undergone violent experiences in the past often relive the horrifying moments in their dreams.

What Happens When You Suffer from Nightmares

You feel as though you can't escape. You're paralyzed and can't figure out how to move or to save yourself. When you finally wake up you're drenched with sweat, disoriented, and still shaking, half-willing to believe that your dream was a real experience. The remnants of the nightmare cling to your unconscious and make the frustrations of your waking life seem almost surreal.

It can be terrifying to go to bed at night if you think you're going to have a nightmare, and this can affect the quality of your sleep in general. As you sleep less, or sleep fitfully, and wake unrefreshed, the day ahead can turn sour.

This can become a vicious cycle, being exhausted when you're awake but unable to fall asleep at night because you're afraid of having nightmares.

Night terrors, which are far less common than night-mares, occur during Stage IV sleep and bring on overwhelm-ing physical symptoms such as panic, sweating, rapid heart-beat, and great emotional upheaval. Because the individual is in the deepest stage of sleep, it is very difficult to wake from a night terror. (Some individuals have gotten out of bed and acted out the scenario of the dream, sometimes injuring or even killing their bed partners while in an unconscious state.) Usually, however, the person undergoing this event has no idea that it has occurred and wakes the next morning without any recollection of the terrifying experience.

Talk to a Professional

Short-term therapy is often a good idea when you are pursued by phantoms that clearly affect your unconscious. A therapist will be able to guide you in a description of the dream's potent elements and will elicit information about your past and cur-rent fears that may be reflected in the nightmares.

Take Some Tryptophan

In order to get a good night's sleep, it's wise to supplement the amino acid tryptophan. You can add tryptophan-rich foods to your diet (warm milk with a banana is a proven relaxant before bed), or you can take supplements available at your health-food store. (L-tryptophan has been taken off the market; however, there are many nervine herbal mixtures that contain up to 100 mg. of tryptophan.)

Deal with Your Monsters

It's important to deal with the elements in your dream that you find terrifying. Be sure to keep a pad and pencil on your night table so that you can jot down all the important ele-ments of your nightmare as soon as you're conscious. Before you're really awake, take these disjointed elements and create a visualization that will help you through the fear. This way, you can take charge of whatever scared you and rearrange the pieces for a positive resolution.

For example, if you were being chased by a monster with a knife, you may wish to turn around and throw a stick in its path so that it trips and falls on its own blade. Or you can put up a wall between you so that it can't catch you.

Another way to deal with the terror is to ask the monster what it really wants. Perhaps the fearful creature represents some element of yourself that you have trouble dealing with. Allow the monster to get rid of its dream persona and assume the real meaning it has in your life so that you can deal with it directly.

Get off Drugs

Many medications, over-the-counter as well as prescription, can aid and abet bad dreams. Antihypertensive drugs and steroids affect neurotransmitter production in the brain (which can influence our dreams), and cardiac medications to control arrhythmias can affect the electrical activity in the brain.

Hallucinogenic drugs, such as LSD, can alter many brain functions and produce nightmares long after you've come off the high. You may also have unpleasant sleep problems because of reactions to cocaine, methamphetamines, marijuana, or hashish.

Sleeping medications—barbiturates, hypnotics, or benzodiazepines (anti-anxiety and muscle-relaxing drugs)—can also give you nightmares. It's quite common to develop a tolerance for these drugs so that you need increasing dosages to get the effect you initially got with a small dose. Many of these drugs have half-lives, which means that you are under the influence of the medication even after the time period for effective coverage has elapsed.

Getting off drugs can also give you nightmares. If you've been taking more than 40 mg. of any sleeping pills daily for at least three months, you'll have some withdrawal symptoms if you stop cold turkey. If you wish to stop taking any of the above drugs, as well as other drugs such as stimulants, sedatives, or anticonvulsants, you must have a doctor's supervision to be weaned off gradually. At the same time, it's a good idea to take herbal remedies (see below) that will help you drop into a sound sleep.

Smell an Herbal Pillow

Lavender blossoms can be sewn into a small pillow that you can refresh with lavender oil from time to time. This herb helps you sleep soundly and brings soothing dreams.

Let St. John Guide Your Rest

Tincture of St. John's wort (1/2 teaspoon in a cup of lemon balm tea or a tea made of 2 to 4 teaspoons of dried herb) will relax you and alleviate anxieties before you fall asleep, which should remove the threat of nightmares. Avoid prolonged exposure to the sun when taking St. John's wort. Other herbs you may wish to try for restful sleep are scullcap, chamomile, and valerian.

Eat Lightly; Dream Nicely

Changing your diet can change your mind. You should eat a good breakfast, a dinner-sized lunch, and a lunch-sized dinner. Try shifting the balance of nutrients in your meals so that you are eating 60 (or more) percent of your calories in complex carbohydrates, 20 percent in protein, and 20 percent (or less) in fats. Try weaning yourself off red meat and processed deli foods and concentrating on high-carbohydrate, low-fat meals, filled with fresh fruits, vegetables, and whole grains. Make sure you don't spice your foods too highly and avoid caffeine and alcohol completely. Don't consume any food within three hours of your bedtime.

Sleep in a Lab

If none of the natural treatments suggested stop your nightmares, it's a good idea to make an appointment to spend a night in a sleep lab. You will be hooked up to an electroencephalograph machine that will chart your brain waves while you're sleeping. Your blood plasma levels of the amino acids tyrosine and tryptophan—precursors of melatonin and serotonin—will be checked. If your levels are very low, or you have some neurological disturbance that could be causing the nightmares, it's important to get professional counseling.

NUMBNESS, EMOTIONAL

see also Alienation, page 28; Depression, page 112; Loneliness, page 277

The experience of not feeling is a common protective device that many individuals use, either consciously or unconsciously. When you're overwhelmed with what's going on, it's much easier to retreat into yourself and turn off the feelings of compassion, joy, anger, and sadness that threaten to engulf you. If you can't feel, you don't hurt. A common symptom of chronic depression, numbness allows people to carry on, to go through the days and nights doing their work, caring for their children, preparing meals, and appearing to be functional in every way. However, numbness is the tip of the iceberg—underneath is a looming, often frightening, set of feelings that eventually will come out.

What Happens When You're Emotionally Numb

Nothing is good; nothing is bad. You're turned off to life and whatever it might hold in store for you. Even if you fall or hurt yourself, you don't feel any pain, because you're protected by an invisible protective shield. You are sometimes amazed that you can be so efficient and competent. Other people can't get to you; previously annoying or bullying behavior just washes over you. You feel almost that you are floating, outside your body, watching what the other person inside your skin is doing.

Many children who are victims of incest and people who've been raped or abused survive by becoming numb to the horror around them. Even if you have not been through a similar trauma, you may feel so beaten down by life that this is your only recourse. And although emotional numbness can serve as a useful tool to keep you sane, it's important to work through it in order to reclaim your personality and your options for the future.

Yell and Scream

You won't feel like ranting and raging, but do it anyway. Get yourself near a railroad track or subway station or a police car with its lights and sirens going and wait for maximum noise. You can also practice this therapy near the crashing waves of an ocean, which would give you more privacy. Get the impetus of the sound and take it inside yourself, then let it out at the top of your lungs. It is a wonderful catharsis and may startle you into the realization that you do have something bottled up inside that craves to be released.

Work on Your Body

Any type of bodywork, from manipulation by a chiropractor, naturopath, or osteopath, to rolfing, bioenergetics, Alexander technique, or Feldenkrais therapy is a particularly beneficial treatment for numbness. For example, in bioenergetics you are encouraged to let out emotions as you bend backward over a stool and breathe fully from the diaphragm and lungs. Another useful bioenergetic exercise is beating a couch or bed with a bat or stick. The activity of physical release can often start the process of emotional release.

Visualize What's Inside and Outside

Give yourself half an hour in a quiet room with no distractions. Sit cross-legged or in a straight-backed chair and begin to breathe easily and rhythmically. Tell yourself that you are about to go on a journey and find out what is beneath the surface layer.

Start with thoughts about the people close to you. Imagine them forming a circle around you, protecting you from any dangers. If you feel uneasy about anyone in the group, you may ask him to stand outside the circle, but not to leave.

Give yourself up to memories of yourself interacting with these people. If they were pleasant, encourage the good feelings these recollections inspire. If they're difficult, don't shy away from them. This is the time to ask the people standing outside the circle to deal with these hard experiences— promise to stick by them and help them through the rough times. At the same time, you should extract a promise from them to allow you the freedom to be yourself and not be subjugated to their will.

Now tell your group to move away from you but not to leave. It's time to work on the numbness all by yourself. Take a big imaginary pin and stick it in your hand, then your leg—let it hurt as much as it has to. If you want to cry, fine. Now withdraw the pin and see that the tip is no longer sharp and pointed. Instead, it is cut like a beautiful diamond that shows you all the facets of your mind and emotions. You can put the diamond pin into your heart and it will not hurt.

Look bravely at the experiences you've been floating past lately. Catch onto them as they go by and take a bite out of them. It won't taste good, and it won't feel good, but don't shy away from these emotions. If you can, throw yourself into the midst of whatever feeling comes up strongest and tell yourself that you can take it.

When you are ready, take three deep breaths, and become aware of your surroundings as you open your eyes.

Challenge Yourself

Although you don't usually feel like exerting yourself or taking any risks, this is the time to do something really challenging. If you're in good physical condition, start training for a marathon, a hike up a difficult mountain, or taking a substantial swim across a lake. Push yourself to do better than you ever have. You might also internalize this exercise and motivate yourself to challenge your partner if you are in a relationship in which you feel beaten down and used up. Make a stand to be treated better or to do more activities as a couple or a family; show your true emotions and stand up for your rights.

You will find as you use this technique, at first, that it feels fake, as though you're just working hard at a job that you don't care much about. But as you get into the swing of your training, you will find that your mind begins to latch on to the goals ahead of you and pulls you out of the slump you've been in. Don't give up! It is essential that you finish what you start.

Get a Massage

Since numbness is often experienced as an inability to feel physically, a thorough massage is wonderful therapy. Ask your partner or a friend to set aside an evening or make an appointment with a trained massage therapist.

The idea is to feel something deep down in your bones. Ask the masseur to begin lightly, touching only the skin. Then, as you relax into the touch of his or her hands, the masseur can go deeper, into the muscle. When you feel comfortable with this amount of touch, give the signal for the masseur to get into the nooks and crannies of your body, reaching as far down as you can allow the pressure to go. You may find that this therapy releases memories and feelings that you have blocked for years. Don't be afraid of them even if they bring up sadness and tears. Give yourself permission to feel again.

Try a Homeopathic

Some of the following remedies may help to remove the mask of numbness:

For indifference in company or society: Argentum nitrate, Kali carbonicum, Lycopodium, Natrum mur, Platinus

For indifference to loved ones: Phosphorus, Sepia, Platinus, Aconite, Arsenicum album, Belladonna, Mercury

For indifference to the welfare of others: Nux vomica, Sulphur, Platinus, Arsenicum album, Lachesis, Natrum mur

For feelings of isolation: Anacardium, Argentum nitrate, Cannabis indica, Platinus, Pulsatilla

Flowers to Incite You

The Bach flower remedy for the indifferent and inattentive who mentally escape from reality is Clematis. Take 5 or 6 drops under the tongue or mixed in half a glass of water, as needed.

*N*UTRITION

see also Eating Disorders, page 139

The old maxim, "you are what you eat" does not portray the situation accurately—what actually happens is that you *become* what you eat. Over the years of three daily meals and snacks, the blend of macronutrients (protein, carbohydrates, and fats) and micronutrients (vitamins and minerals) you select, the amount and types of foods you eat, your predilection for spicy or bland meals, and the attitude with which you eat—picking at your food, relishing each bite, or gulping everything down—can formulate your character as well as your body. The field of nutrition has developed in many exciting directions in the past decade, and it is now clear that the nutrients you ingest daily have a great deal to do with your moods, your behavior, and your general sense of well-being. The field of orthomolecular therapy deals with preserving and restoring the chemical constituents of the body.

Eating for a Healthy Mind

The human brain isn't very heavy—it's about one fortieth of your total body weight, but it consumes one fifth of the calories you eat each day. Being an intellectually developed human is a mixed blessing because we naturally seek out rich, calorie-dense foods to feed our hungry brain. It's as if we're genetically programmed to desire lots of fat and protein, although the rest of the body suffers if we eat it.

The doyens of clinical nutrition initially recommended nutrients only for those with physical illnesses caused by vitamin and mineral deficiencies. Certainly, cutting down on fat and cholesterol protects us from the development of plaque that can block arteries and cause heart attacks and stroke. The antioxidants in fruits and vegetables may keep us from developing certain cancers. But healthful eating does a lot more than build strong bodies and prevent physical disease—we know that nutrients can powerfully influence emotion, behavior, and thinking. A wealth of scientific study on animals and humans has shown that the right mix of ingredients can prevent or treat aggressive behavior, anxiety, ADD and ADHD, bipolar disorder, depression, fatigue, insomnia, learning disabilities, and a variety of eating disorders such as anorexia, bulimia, and bingeing.

Most of us don't eat right—the balance of our nutrients is lopsided (most Americans consume far too much protein and fat), we eat huge quantities of food, we skip meals rather than portioning food equally throughout the day to keep blood glucose levels even, we avoid certain groups of foods because of taste preferences, and we systematically rob ourselves of nutrients we need to stay healthy. Teenagers are prime examples of bad eating, grabbing dense, rich, quick meals on the run, but so are the elderly, who may not be able to get out and shop or don't have the motivation or inclination to prepare well-balanced meals for themselves. They may also be on restricted incomes and may not be able to afford good food. In many cases, behavior that seems erratic or irrational can be directly traced to a lack or imbalance of appropriate nutrients.

Another reason that bad eating creates mental problems is that a deficiency of proper nutrients effectively blocks the production of brain chemicals that give us a sense of harmony and well-being. If you're on a diet and denying yourself food, you may feel depressed or anxious because you're experiencing a decline in both dopamine and serotonin, two of the neurotransmitters that keep you on an even keel.

Your attitude toward eating can greatly influence the way that you process food. If you see it as fuel, or comfort, or a necessary evil, you never consciously integrate the items you're putting into your mouth with the flesh, blood, and bone that they eventually become. Ideally, it's best to regard what's sitting on your plate as a part of you that just hasn't yet taken shape. The experience of eating can be filled with spirit—think about the rituals of bread and wine discussed in the Bible.

We can also approach eating as a kind of meditation. Jon Kabat-Zinn has structured an exercise in mindfulness (see page 296) for consuming one raisin. The eater is reminded that she always eats raisins by the handful or stuck in a muffin or cookie, but this time, she will experience the raisin all by itself. We need to appreciate the texture, the feel, the smell, the sensation—and finally, the taste—of this one morsel of food. If we ate all our meals this way, we would have a sense of what "nourish" in terms of eating really means. Just as we nourish a relationship or a new business venture, so we can nourish ourselves and eat to improve our mind, emotions, and spirit.

▓ *Am I Really Allergic?*

There is an ever-growing body of evidence that indicates we may be giving ourselves emotional problems by consuming food to which we're highly allergic. Although this allergy doesn't cause rashes or sneezing, it does in fact give us a chemical hypersensitivity that can cause headaches, pain, fatigue, or chronic depression. Usually the allergy produces a delayed reaction, so that symptoms don't appear until an hour to three days after eating the suspected food.

A food allergy produces an irritation or inflammation in the body because of the particular allergen to which we're susceptible. But the type of reaction is usually so minor at first that we don't really notice. Several signs that your emotional problems may be caused by the food you're eating are mental or physical fatigue, water retention, dark circles or puffiness under the eye, crying jags, restlessness, free-floating anxiety, mental confusion, and panic attacks.

The most commonly diagnosed allergic foods are wheat, rye, eggs, milk and other dairy products, soy, nuts, and some fruits and vegetables. If you think that you may be suffering from a food allergy, try eliminating these one at a time from your diet and see if there is an improvement in your symptoms and mood.

▓ *What Should You Eat?*

The controversy about the correct balance of nutrients will never cease. One year, the fashionable way to be healthy is to consume nothing but potato skins and bottled water; the next year, it's thick steaks and poached eggs. How do you make sense of this hodgepodge of nutritional nonsense?

The best advice is to eat the types of foods that make you feel good. This does not mean that you should eat whatever you like—a diet of candy bars and French fries may taste good, but in the end, doesn't make you *feel* good. Forget your mouth, and think more about the sensation of your body and mind half an hour after your meal. You should feel energized, alert, not hungry and not stuffed, and in good spirits.

The process of trial and error will make it easier for you. Given the basic American food pyramid (see below), you will have to adapt and adjust to your own needs. If you're at a business lunch and need to think fast and smart, a high-protein, low-fat meal is the ticket—one good combination would be turkey breast, green beans, and low-fat or skim milk. If you're racing around doing errands and want to calm down a little, stick with carbohydrates—have a bagel without the cream cheese. If you need to relax before bedtime and want to get sleepy, try foods containing the amino acid tryptophan—a warm milk and banana float.

Eating different foods for different purposes will allow you to trigger the production of dopamine, norepinephrine, and serotonin when you need it. Remember, however, that the body takes longer to process protein and fat than it does carbohydrate. The more work your gut and intestine have to do to digest your meals, the less blood and oxygen to your brain for a longer period of time.

If you crave protein and consume a lot of it, you're prematurely aging your kidneys by giving them too much work breaking down so many extra amino acids and excreting so many nitrates (toxic chemicals). If you crave carbohydrates and consume too many, however, you may be encouraging a depressive cycle. If you feel very low most of the time and feel that you'd rather go to sleep than get out and see people, you should see a professional for some nutritional counseling (see Resource Guide, page 00).

The more conscious your eating, the more you'll feel you're controlling the food instead of allowing it to control you. This in itself can give you an incredible sense of self-confidence and self-esteem.

▓ *Adjusting the American Food Pyramid to Your Needs*

The Surgeon General gives us general guidelines for healthful eating:

- Consume only enough calories to meet body needs (between 1,800 and 2,500 daily, depending on your size and weight). The calories will be apportioned between carbohydrate, protein, and fat (the macronutrients).

- Eat little or no saturated fat and cholesterol.

- Cut down on salt and sugar.
- Increase your consumption of fresh fruits and vegetables.
- Increase your consumption of whole grains and cereals.
- Eat less animal protein, more vegetable protein (legumes such as lentils, peas, and beans).
- Eat more lean poultry and fish than red meat.
- Avoid processed foods.

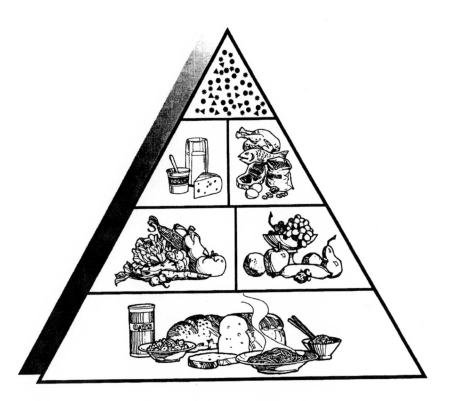

These recommendations are the basis for the American food pyramid, which offers a well-balanced diet that includes all food groups, laden with carbohydrates, vegetables, and fruit at the bottom layers, getting smaller with animal products, dairy, fats, oils, and sweets as we move upward. Unfortunately, this is a diet that calls for 30 percent of its daily calories from fat, which most experts feel is too high for optimum health throughout the lifespan. Reducing dietary fat will not just prevent atherosclerotic plaques from developing, but will also improve the condition of your arteries and may also help to reduce blood pressure and blood sugar and will allow more blood flow to the brain so that it can think and feel clearly.

It's not only the macronutrients we have to be concerned about, but also the micros. For good mental health and the best modulation of your feelings, it's vital that you get the vitamins and minerals you need (see Supplementation, page 409). Although you can pop pills for those essential B- (anti-stress) vitamins, A, C, and E (antioxidant) vitamins, and the various minerals such as calcium, magnesium, and iron that help you to think and balance emotions, it's generally acknowledged that you get more out of these micronutrients when you eat them. Citrus and other fruits, green leafy vegetables, yellow vegetables, whole grains, and high-fiber cereals contain all your required daily vitamins and minerals, which will give your brain the boost it needs.

A good menu plan contains the following amended pyramid:

Bread, Cereal, Rice, Pasta: 6 to 11 servings daily (serving is one slice or half a cup)

Vegetables (starchy and nonstarchy): 3 to 5 servings of half a cup daily

Fruits: 2 to 4 servings of half a cup daily

Legumes (peas, lentils, beans—soy, pinto, kidney, navy, white, pink, garbanzos): 1 one-cup serving daily

Soy Products: 1 one-cup serving daily (this includes tofu, tempeh, miso, and commercial products such as "No-Dogs." Soy products are not low in fat; however, they contain valuable phytosterols (plant hormones) that enhance the body's natural endocrine production and also encourage the production of high-density lipoproteins, the good, or HDL, cholesterol in the blood.

Milk, Yogurt, Cheese Group: 1 serving, one cup each, low-fat varieties. Select skim milk or 1 percent milk and no-fat yogurt. Soy cheese is an acceptable substitute for animal cheese. The lowest fat cheese is parmesan, which you'll use sparingly since you sprinkle it on.

Meat, Poultry, Fish: Try to cut down to 3 to 4 times weekly or less, in portions of 3 to 4 ounces. They can be used as "condiments" in vegetable dishes or stir-fries. Meat should be trimmed of all visible fat; poultry should be skinless.

Eggs, Nuts: Consumed once or twice weekly, depending on your general health. You can substitute egg whites for eggs in recipes.

Fats and Oils: Use sparingly and stick to olive and canola oil for cooking. Although real butter is high in saturated fat, it is still preferable (in small quantities) to polyunsaturated vegetable oils such as margarine. These oils have been partially hydrogenated so that they are substantial enough to spread on bread. The hydrogenation process creates trans-fatty acids that raise LDL and lower HDL cholesterol levels.

Sweets Group: Use sparingly. Refined sugar has been implicated in many mental and emotional disorders because it triggers excess insulin production. A little honey or brown sugar is a better bet for your brain.

Beverages: Stay away from caffeine, which has been shown to create mood disorders in most users. It's also a good idea to cut down on carbonated beverages, which contain phosphates that break down bone tissue. Drink plenty of pure spring water and fruit juices mixed with water.

▥ *What's Wrong with Dieting?*

Many people complain that they are depressed because they're too fat (very few complain of depression because they aren't heavy enough, since our society wrongheadedly believes that you can never be "too thin or too rich.") And because many people use food as a tool to comfort themselves when they're down, food and mood changes are often interlinked—you're miserable so you eat, then you gain weight and you get more miserable, so you eat some more to comfort yourself.

If you decide to go on a diet to lose weight, you are certainly not alone. More than 29 billion dollars are spent yearly in our country on diet foods, appetite suppressants, weight-loss programs, and diet books and cassettes. The problem with diets is that they work for a while, sucking you into the belief that you will be thin, and then, as you plateau and stop losing weight despite your best efforts, you get disheartened and give up.

If you're like most dieters, you begin with a flourish, starting by cutting back radically on calories, something your body protests against. As you starve yourself to get rid of the excess poundage, you feel deprived. Restricted eating makes you feel left out, as if everyone is having a good time except you. Your body demands more fuel to carry on, or you have a rough day and need something to make you feel better, and you break the diet. Over 95 percent of all dieters gain back every pound they lose (and sometimes more) within five years of being on a diet. Letting your weight yo-yo up and down destroys the equilibrium of your metabolism and also weakens bone tissue.

Dieting also takes away the pleasure we have in consuming foods that are particularly meaningful to us. The punishment of dictating that you will eat *only* low-calorie, low-fat items makes you rail against the process. Even the strongest motivation to be thinner doesn't overcome the rotten mood you get into when you diet.

So if you want to feel better and lose some weight, there's an incredibly easy solution. Use common sense and understand that there are no quick fixes—you must lose slowly to lose steadily. Eliminate junk food and high-fat, high-sugar products and continue eating everything else that you enjoy in moderation. Divide your portions in half (or if you can't manage that, eat two thirds of what you've been eating), and add an extra 20 minutes of exercise daily. This will effectively make you feel good about yourself and reduce your weight at the same time.

▨ *How to Eat*

Regardless of what you're eating, whether it's a snack of an apple and cheese and crackers or a multicourse banquet, it's vital that you make eating a comfortable and healing experience. The rules of thumb are

- Eat in a leisurely fashion, never in haste, standing up, at the refrigerator, or in front of the TV.

- Make eating a conscious experience—pay attention to the color, the aroma, the arrangement on the plate, the warmth or cold in your mouth. Use smaller plates, which makes the amount of food on them seem more bountiful.

- Eat because you've decided to eat—get rid of guilt. If you've selected a piece of chocolate cake (and every once in a while, everyone is entitled to one of these), really savor the experience of consuming it.

- Eat when you're hungry; stop when you're full.

The experience of eating used to be a family event. In the past, we fostered the communual spirit by preparing fresh-grown produce lovingly and eating it at a table with those close to us. Kids came home from school for the midday meal; everyone gathered for dinner and for holiday occasions.

These days, however, it is practically impossible to arrange schedules around mealtimes, and people rarely break bread together. The experience of solitary, often hidden, eating has driven many to overeating, bulimia, and anorexia. Even for those who have no eating disorder, enjoying food has become a guilty pleasure. In our schizoid society, one advertiser flaunts the importance of pleasure and abundance, and another gives you the Puritan party line that you should be lithe and lean and always deny yourself. In a culture where looks count, food is the enemy, and each meal is a battle to be won.

In order to change our attitude toward eating and nutrition, it's vital that we understand why and how we eat. If we're depressed, a whole box of cookies is comfort food; when we're angry, we may tear into a sandwich as though we want to hurt it, barely chewing, just devouring.

But if we can realign our sensibilities around food, we can use it for better mental health. Let us start with how much we eat. Most Americans consume more than they need of all macronutrients—we eat big portions of protein, carbohydrate, and especially fat.

The reason we eat too much is that we eat so quickly we don't give our brain time to catch up with our stomach. The hypothalamus in the brain controls two cell mechanisms that make up what is known as the *central sensations*. One set of cells controls hunger; the other controls the sense of satiety, or being comfortably full.

The stomach offers us peripheral sensations of hunger and fullness. When we feel hunger in the brain, we also feel it in the gut. Our satiety centers are not in synch, however, so there's a lag time of about a quarter hour after we've taken in sufficient food for our brain to record that it's satiated. Because we have stretch receptors in the wall of the stomach, it's always possible to eat past the point of comfortable fullness. And that's what most of us do. A binge eater, an overeater, or a bulemic eats as though this is the last meal and continues way past his or her limit. (See Overeating, page 331, for a hunger/satiety exercise that will give you a good idea of when your brain—not just your stomach—is satisfied.)

Once we have a handle on hunger and satiety and can liberate ourselves from the pressure of how much to eat, it's easier to make good judgments about what we eat. When you're really hungry and you pass a fast-food restaurant, you may have a yen for a greasy bacon cheeseburger and a thick shake. But when you think about how you'll feel after you eat it—logy, heavy, and often depressed about the calories you've ingested—you may be able to divert your hunger to a turkey burger or a salad.

The problem is, our food preferences aren't often determined by our body's needs. As a matter of fact, most of us wander through a supermarket completely unaffected by the promptings of our body, drawn on by the lure of marketing. It's a good idea to go food shopping when you're not hungry, and whenever possible go with a list of meals and their ingredients that you intend to prepare during the week. Make a conscious effort to bypass the aisles that contain nonfoods with great packaging and go directly to the outskirts of the market to load up on fresh fruits and vegetables.

When you're home, try and make the eating process as enjoyable as possible—a treat for eye, nose, mouth, and palate. Instead of filling your mouth, think of filling your spirit with nourishment. Try to have a beginner's mind about what you're eating and how it tastes. Pretend this is the first time you're eating an apple, or a plate of rice, or a bowl of cereal. Think about the nutrients going into you, making you more than you were before you began the meal.

The more you can absorb the essence of food—the stuff that gives you the energy to do your work, to care for your kids, to love your partner—the more you will reap the healing benefits of nutrition.

Use Foods for Moods

You can alter the way you feel with directed eating. If lately you've felt depressed, sad, fatigued, and lacking any get-up-and-go, try spicing up your life by spicing up your palate. Cook with unusual herbs and spices and experiment with chilis and hot foreign cuisines (Mexican, Indian, Chinese, Thai). Be sure your meal has lots of bright color—eat tomatoes, carrots, cantaloupes, squashes, avocados. Eat hearty soups and stews with lots of legumes (vegetable protein will give you a substantial meal with less fat than animal protein) and cut out sugar to keep your blood glucose level on an even keel.

If you've been angry and irritable lately, you need to tone down what you put into your body. Eat less, and consume it more slowly and deliberately. Try a three-day juice fast or vegetarian eating for a couple of weeks in order to balance your system. Eliminate any food products that bump your metabolism up and down, such as caffeine or sugar, which give you quick highs and then let you tumble into deep lows.

For particular mental and emotional problems, consult a licensed nutritionist for a complete diagnosis of your eating habits and preferences and suggestions on ways to make small but significant changes slowly for maximum overall health.

*O*BSESSIVE-*C*OMPULSIVE *D*ISORDER

see also Compulsive sexual activity, page 97; Hand-washing behavior, page 203

Obsessions are thoughts or images that invade our consciousness and distract our attention from work, relationships, duties, and activities. Compulsions are the things we do in order to reinforce our obsessions and usually involve secretive, ritualized, and time-consuming patterns of behavior. Some examples of this type of behavior are returning to the front door repeatedly to be sure that you've locked it, counting and repetitive movements, hand-washing behavior to alleviate a dirt phobia, or repeatedly calling or visiting the object of a sexual or romantic interest.

If you are nervous, tense, and apprehensive about life, you may be more prone to obsessive-compulsive disorder (OCD) than if you were an aggressive, forceful individual, or a laid-back, easygoing type.

One of the problems in treating this behavior is that the urge to resist the impulse causes a great deal of anxiety that is immediately alleviated by performing the behavior. There are two proven methods of beating it: One is flooding yourself with the experience you most dread, meeting the fear head-on. The other is distracting the mind and emotions with another interest, at least long enough to let the need for repetitive behavior pass. People who engage in ritualized counting or checking or thinking about a subject don't really want to are driven to it—so understanding that they can care for themselves comes as a great relief.

Desensitization and cognitive-behavioral strategies will help to resolve the behavior, but there are clearly more issues under the surface that must be dealt with. The most successful treatments also work on the underlying anxiety, inner

329

conflicts, and depression. (See Spencer, V.E., "Combined Therapies" in OCD, *The Journal of Psychosocial Nursing and Mental Health Services*, Vol. 34 (7) July 1996.)

CASE HISTORY

Alice never paid that much attention to the bruhaha over HIV and AIDS until her favorite cousin, Mark, died unexpectedly of a drug overdose. Alice adored Mark and had always accepted the fact that he was gay. But she was totally shocked when his doctor told her at the funeral that he had been sharing needles with his multiple lovers. Learning that he'd been a drug addict with AIDS brought out some long-suppressed fears in Alice. She became terrified that somehow he might have transmitted the virus to her. And if he hadn't, others might.

"At the beginning, I must have washed my hands and used a fresh towel maybe 20 times a day. If I was going to be away from home, I carried my own towel in a plastic bag. Then, touching stuff became impossible, so I started wearing several pairs of latex gloves. The washing escalated to 50 times a day. I was petrified that I'd be contaminated, even though I knew that's not how HIV gets passed around. I knew that antidepressants are often prescribed for this, but I couldn't take *any* drugs after Mark's overdose. I decided to treat my illness naturally.

"I decided to desensitize myself to dirt and germs. Revolted as I was, I threw myself into the therapies. Within a few months, I was down to washing ten times a day, and now, after a year, I can remember the behavior but not feel that overwhelming urge to do it."

Until recently, doctors always treated OCD with antidepressants, and it was considered the only really successful way to combat the problem. However, recent scientific investigation has shown that cognitive-behavioral therapy and other complementary treatments are just as effective as medication in changing brain patterns.

According to Dr. Jeffrey Schwartz, a psychiatrist at the Neuropsychiatric Institute of the University of California at Los Angeles, there are four key structures in the brain that become locked together in obsessive-compulsive disorder. But new findings indicate that it's possible to free these structures from one another by, quite literally, changing the patient's mind. With the reasonable, rational alternatives of cognitive-behavioral therapy in place, the brain produces different neurotransmitters that allow us to process our needs and desires differently.

Patients in Dr. Schwartz's study were taught certain behavioral techniques that allowed them to resist the urges they had previously succumbed to, and it was evident from sophisticated CT scans done on them that they had managed to unlock these essential brain structures so that they could operate independently. With this type of psychotherapy, patients are able to relabel their obsessive desires and talk themselves out of the feelings of dread and doom that occur around their behavior.

Treatments to try: Affirmations, page 16; Behavioral Therapy, page 55; Breathing, page 76; Cognitive Therapy, page 94; Desensitization, page 116; Exercise, page 145; Herbalism, page 216; Homeopathy, page 221; Massage, page 286; Meditation, page 292; Support Groups, page 414; Tai Chi Chuan, page 417; Visualization, page 442; Yoga, page 457.

OVEREATING

see also Eating Disorders, page 139

Many people overeat because of boredom, anger, anxiety, depression, and many other emotional triggers. The food becomes a substitute for love and encouragement, and in serious disorders can be a substitute for daily activities and relationships. Eating may be used as a mechanism to push others away—a person who gorges until she is fat and unattractive may be daring her partner to love her in spite of her looks. There's no way we can cram affection down our throats; however, a couple of slices of chocolate cake or a quart of ice cream goes down pretty easily.

Overeating leads to obesity, which is a big health risk, particularly in America where over one third of the population (approximately 58 million adults) are either overweight or morbidly obese, which means that they are in immediate danger of dying from the complications of their condition, complications such as cardiovascular disease, hypertension, diabetes, osteoarthritis, gout, and certain types of cancer. Ridding yourself of this behavior can actually save your life.

▨ *What Happens When You Compulsively Overeat*

There are compulsive overeaters who decide to consume everything they can, but this is more typical of bingeing behavior (see Bingeing, page 59). Overeating is more commonly unconscious; you realize at some point standing at the refrigerator eating a whole cake or finishing off the leftovers in front of the TV that you have lost control over your eating behavior. You might not even have had a hunger pang before you started eating, and yet stuffing your mouth seems like the only thing you can do. If you are going through a difficult time in your life and you feel that you have no one to turn to, food may be your only pleasure. You eat to stop the pain, and then, as you continue beyond your true capacity, you feel numb. You may feel that you have to turn off your eating control in order to manage the rest of your life.

Overeating is very often a concrete way of armoring the body. If you're padded, nothing can hurt you. Many women who were victims of incest or spousal abuse eat in order to protect themselves from anything that might happen in the future.

Overeating often prevents you from dealing with many challenges and hurdles that must be faced at some point or another. If you're too fat you may be excluded from many good jobs (discrimination in hiring fat people is rampant, though illegal), you may have trouble getting to appointments because seats in public buses, trains, and subways are often too small for you, and you may not have the energy to involve yourself in hobbies or creative endeavors.

Many people who overeat also try desperately to lose the weight they've gained. Dieting is a preoccupation in our country—unfortunately, it rarely works. People in weight-loss programs tend to regain two thirds of their lost pounds within a year and many gain back more pounds than they've lost. This yo-yoing up and down on the scale makes the former and future dieter feel like a failure, one who feels doomed to eat himself or herself into a stupor to forget that he or she can't succeed at getting thin.

The difference between overeating and eating is in the attitude you adopt toward food and hunger. Eating should be healthful and pleasurable, and what you want to put in your mouth should ultimately be something that makes you feel energized, positive, and ready to take on the challenges of your day. Sugary, salty, fatty foods (the ones that most often trigger binge eating or an inability to stop eating) won't taste as good when you begin to eat consciously.

Don't Eat Alone

Since overeating generally takes place alone, at occasions other than mealtimes, it's a good idea to have company when you eat. The support you'll get from family and friends works better when they are aware of your problem, but if you choose not to tell them, that's okay too. It's a good idea to eat with people who aren't overly concerned about diet, who approach food naturally and only when they're hungry.

Join a Support Group

Overeaters Anonymous, like Alcoholics Anonymous and other 12-step programs, has proven enormously successful in helping individuals with eating disorders. Understand that eating is not an addiction—we have to eat or we die—it's the behavior around eating that becomes problematic. The advantage of Overeaters Anonymous is that you are paired with a buddy or mentor, whom you must call daily with a report on what and how much you're going to eat. You set your own limits, but once you have decided, you cannot deviate from your plan.

Use a Structured Food Plan

Whether or not you join a group, you can use their designated food plan to help you over the hump. You will create for yourself a list of certain foods you will and will not eat. OA feels that all refined flour and sugar products and nuts, chips, and other salty foods should be eliminated because they trigger binges. You know better than anyone which foods you tend to overeat. At the beginning of your therapy, you should avoid any foods that will cause you to lose control.

Supplements Calm Cravings

Overeaters tend to be deficient in several vitamins and minerals. In addition to your regular multivitamin, you should take a B-complex daily (100 mg.), magnesium, (750 mg.), and chromium (200 mg. daily).

Modify Your Eating

An important lesson in cutting down on quantity is to use the hunger/satiety exercise. Satiety is what we strive for—that's the feeling of comfortable fullness (not being ravenous and not being stuffed).

Make yourself a regular-sized meal, possibly a lunch that includes a sandwich, a pickle, a few chips, a soda, and a piece of fruit for dessert. As you sit down to eat, consider the food and consciously ask yourself if you're hungry for it. If it's your usual eating time, you will salivate as you contemplate.

Eat half of what's on your plate. Now get up and walk around the block, make a phone call, send an e-mail transmission. In 15 minutes, you can return to the table and ask yourself whether you're still hungry. If you are, cut the remaining portion in half. Eat the next quarter of your meal. Once again, get up and do something. If you are still hungry after another 15 minutes, you may finish the meal.

This exercise will teach you that sometimes you aren't hungry, in which case it's okay to leave something on your plate. To curb overeating, you have to believe that you can really have food whenever you need it, and that, when it comes to big portions, it's perfectly okay not to finish what you started.

Think Before You Chew

Self-hypnosis can be used effectively to calm your eating frenzy. Sit quietly and prepare to relax. Roll your eyes upward, close your eyes, and hold your breath. Then allow yourself to feel that you are floating, that your left arm is raising by itself. You will give yourself the suggestion that too much food is bad for your body (not for you but for the corporeal house you live in), that you respect and are responsible for your body and must treat it well. You would not overfeed your dog to the point of obesity or heart-disease risk; therefore you must respect your own body at least as much as your pet's. You will relish each bite of food and think about stimulating your body with quality, not quantity.

Don't Start Smoking

Many women substitute smoking for food. A cigarette is something to put in your mouth when you're anxious, and its chemical properties assuage the feelings of loss and deprivation. Smoking is one of the worst health hazards around, for both mind and body. If you're currently smoking in addition to overeating, don't try to get rid of both habits at the same time—it's too difficult. You may have to continue this addiction until you have your eating under control. Once you've changed your eating habits, you'll have enough self-confidence to get rid of cigarettes as well.

Pray Over Your Food

This treatment is really an expanded version of saying grace. As you eat, be thankful for the nourishment that keeps you alive. Consider the miracle of ingesting these substances that eventually become part of us: the blood, sweat, and tears, the bones, sinews, and tissues that go into our ever-changing system. As you consider the miracle that brought you here and will keep you here in good health, you will come to the realization that you must nourish yourself carefully, not too little, but not too much either. And as you chew and swallow, pray that you will be strong for one more meal to put down the fork when you're full and take it up only when you're hungry again.

P_{AIN}

see also Abuse of Substances, page 1; Aging, page 17; Anxiety, page 43; Broken Heart, page 78; Chest Pains, page 87; Depression, page 112; Gastrointestinal Disorders, page 189; Headaches/Migraines, page 209; Stress, page 407; Tension, page 425

Pain results from nerve connections between the brain and other parts of the body that experience the sense of touch. We can also trigger painful feelings without a stimulus—you don't have to be hit on the head to get a headache. Emotional pain can produce the same type of neurotransmitter and prostaglandin production as physical pain and can feel just as bad. But the pleasure and pain centers in the brain are next to each other, and by stimulating one, you can effectively tone down the other.

What Happens When You're in Pain

You can't think about anything else. There is only that throbbing, stabbing, squeezing, aching, burning, strangling sensation that won't go away no matter what position you take or whether you move or remain still.

Pain can be acute (and this type of agony is more easily healed) or it can be chronic, which means that it goes on all the time, day and night. The question, of course, is how much of the physical pain has a somatic source and how much an emotional source. There are a variety of alternative therapists who state categorically that most pain stems from a misalliance of brain and body, which means that if you change the brain patterns, you can eliminate or at least reduce the pain.

| CASE HISTORY |

Leanne couldn't remember when her neck didn't ache. It sometimes felt as if she couldn't hold her head up, it was so bad. "I started seeing a chiropractor when I was about 20," she said, "and I'd get depressed every time I had a session. It was like I was in a hole, and I couldn't do anything to help myself."

Leanne, now in her early forties, had feelings that she had forgotten something vital, something that might help her put her finger on the reason for the physical tension she always felt, but she wasn't sure what it was. She tried hypnosis, and the therapist tried to regress her backward in time, but "there was nothing there, like I didn't have a past at all."

She began seeing a therapist and slowly was able to piece together the horrible history she had buried for so long. One afternoon, at home in the apartment she shared with another woman, she finally remembered that her father had taken her to bed with him and had an orgasm while lying on top of her when she was about eight.

"Then other things came back," she said. "I remembered me and my brother in the coal bin—he could get up the shute but I couldn't. My father was drunk most of the time, but that day, he let me go. My mother found my brother's underpants and they were full of blood (he was bleeding rectally), and she couldn't figure it out. I remember she demanded at dinner why his whole body was covered in coal dust and his clothes were clean."

Leanne's daughter had tried Network chiropractic, a form of manipulation that primarily uses pressure points. The therapist is attuned to the energy in the patient and does an adjustment only when the time is right. Leanne visited a doctor for months before she was considered ready for an adjustment, and then, she said, "it felt like something was leaving my body. It felt good that it was gone. Afterward, I went in the next room and huddled into myself and just cried for half an hour."

The physical pain was intricately tied to the emotional pain, and once she had allowed the memories to go, she had no further problems with her neck. When she began studying tai chi, she stopped going to the chiropractor. She is doing her own adjustments now, inside and out.

Erase the Pain in a Trance State

Pain has been called "an urgent call to action" from the body to the mind by Dr. Herbert Spiegel, psychotherapist and proponent of hypnotic trance for healing. The mind has the ability to process pain signals in a variety of ways. If it doesn't perceive pain as "painful," we have no trouble dealing with it. The severity of the physical injury often dictates what we do about the pain. If you fall down a flight of stairs, the pain signals that reach the mind through the nervous system are overpowering and must be listened to. If you are in the delivery room of a hospital and looking forward to having a child, however, the labor pains can often be controlled.

Roll your eyes up and close your lids, then take a deep breath and hold it. When you are ready, begin to breathe slowly and easily, sensing that your body is floating. If you try to hold your left hand on the arm of your chair, you will find that it won't stay but levitates up by itself. You will now give yourself the suggestion that you are baking a cake with your mind, working the dry ingredients through a sifter. The pain is one of these ingredients and you will filter it out of your mix and discard it at the end of this process. You do not need to keep your pain; you can choose to get rid of it.

You may also suggest that while your arm is in the air, it is getting colder. It is freezing up, becoming numb. You are floating in water, perhaps in an Arctic sea, with seals diving and penguins playing around you. The area of pain is becoming numb with cold, giving you a protective shield around the location so that it can heal on its own.

Dr. Spiegel also uses a series of exercises to control pain. You can practice these when you are not actually hurting.

- Make a tight fist and put your arm out straight in front of you. Use all the muscle tension you can muster; then open your fist and release it. See how much pain is alleviated when you relax.

- With your opposite hand, take a piece of skin between your thumb and forefinger. Create pain by pinching hard; then release it. Now stare at a painting on the wall. Focus all your concentration on the painting as you try the pinch test again. See how much less pain you feel when you are distracted by something very interesting.

- When you next get a headache or back pain, try and distract your attention by focusing on your fingers. Rub your fingers against each other and think about the sensation you feel, the temperature of your skin, the smoothness or roughness of the texture. Choose to pay attention to your fingers rather than to your headache.

- Give yourself a suggestion that the pain is decreasing. Tell yourself that you can no longer feel the sensation you had before.

- Relax completely. Believe that you have control over your pain.

Biofeedback to the Rescue

Since pain is both physical and psychological, it's possible to change one of these elements and alter the degree or intensity of the pain. For example, putting your hand in ice water may be excruciating after just a few seconds, but if you imagine that you are on a tropical beach with your hand in the warm ocean, you may tolerate the experience far longer.

Firewalkers and yogis who sit on beds of nails are able to control pain by generating alpha and theta waves in the brain—those slow-patterned waves we produce when we meditate or are going through a creative spurt. By hooking a patient up to an EEG (electroencephalograph) machine and placing electrodes on the scalp, it is possible to use biofeedback techniques to train the brain to produce these pain-blocking waves. Biofeedback is often used in conjunction with hypnosis to decrease or eliminate pain.

Visualize a Beautiful Scene

The next time you are in pain, you can try visualizing yourself on a tropical island, floating in the water. Or you might see yourself on a mountaintop, looking down at the green valley. Conjure up the warm air, the soft grass, all the details that will distract your mind from the pain.

Talk to Where It Hurts

If you don't know the reason for your pain, maybe you can find out. Ask different questions of your pain and wait a minute or so for a somatic response. You'd like to know:

- Do you hurt more when I move or when I'm still?

- What position am I in when you start up?

- What memories do you bring back?

- Can you come out a different way—instead of a stabbing sensation, can you produce an ache or a dull throbbing and then finally, a hypersensitivity that I can deal with?

- Wouldn't you rather go somewhere else?

When you treat the pain as though it were an adversary, you never resolve your conflict. But by treating it as though it were a companion in trouble, you may get better results.

Get Manipulated

Chiropractic or massage are two excellent, proven ways to deal with pain. A chiropractor will manipulate the subluxations that may cause pressure on various nerves; a massage therapist will work on the fascia, muscles, tendons, and joints that hold pain. There are many different types of touch, and only you can decide whether you benefit more from deep or surface pressure, or from fast or slow manipulation. Pay attention to the way your body relaxes or tenses when you're being worked on and give your practitioner feedback if you're not getting what you need from the session.

Touch the Pain with a Magic Glove

An effective means to dull what hurts is to imagine a magic glove that soothes effortlessly. All you have to do is put this glove on your own hand and touch yourself wherever the discomfort is. (It doesn't matter if you're having angina inside your body, since the glove reaches every cell.)

A similar technique is to develop a pain "switch" like a light switch that you can turn down or turn off whenever necessary.

The more you practice with these tools, the more quickly they will work for you when you need them.

Homeopathic Help

The homeopathic remedy most associated with pain is Chamomilla. The plant has mildly sedative effects and is an excellent remedy for a pain sufferer who is irritable, angry, and barks at others who offer help. This remedy is particularly useful for women and children.

Other remedies associated with pain are Aconite, Coffea, Hepar sulphuris Calcareum, Ignatia, and Nux vomica.

PALPITATIONS *(From Fear)*

see also Anxiety, page 43; Chest Pains, page 87; Panic Disorders, page 344; Stress, page 407

Palpitations are disturbances of the circulatory system generated by extreme stress or fear. Your heart rate increases (sometimes to an alarmingly fast 200 beats a minute), or becomes irregular, where you may feel your heart has stopped and then is jump-started. Palpitations are common in the midst of panic attacks, when you fear you've lost control over your bodily functions—you may really believe that you are having a heart attack. IF YOU COMMONLY EXPERIENCE CHEST PAINS WITH PALPITATIONS, YOU SHOULD SEE A DOCTOR AND HAVE AN ELECTROCARDIOGRAM TO DETERMINE WHETHER YOU HAVE HEART DISEASE.

The terror of the consequences of palpitations can increase the problem and even bring on arrhythmias that can cause real damage to the heart muscle.

What Happens When You Have Palpitations

You feel as if your heart is about to jump out of your chest, and you fear that you may die. You can actually hear your pounding heart and are sure that others are also aware of it.

There is generally a trigger for this terrifying lub-dub: You may be under extreme stress, in the midst of an argument, or suddenly frightened. Strong emotions and strenuous exercise often induce palpitations. They are quite common in women going through the menopause and may be brought on because of fluid loss from hot flashes or night sweats. They generally are accompanied by other symptoms of anxiety, such as hyperventilation, shortness of breath, dizziness, chest pains, sweaty palms, and a churning stomach.

The Flower of Your Heart

Rose is the Bach flower remedy to calm and steady the heart. Take 5 to 6 drops under the tongue or mixed in half a glass of water as needed.

Herbal Heart Balm

Try hawthorn, the best heart tonic available. Take 25 to 40 drops of extract up to four times daily. This is a very slow-acting herbal and may take a month or more to work.

Motherwort tincture also supports the circulation. Take 10 to 20 drops with meals and before bed. You can also take it as an emergency calmant—try one dose of 25 to 50 drops mixed with water.

Oat (avena) tea will make the blood vessels more elastic and is also a great stress-reducer. Take 2 to 4 teaspoons dried herb infused in a cup of tea daily.

Black haw (viburnum) has an antispasmodic effect on the heart. Use 25 drops of tincture or an infusion made of 2 to 4 teaspoons dried herb.

Supplement Your Heart's Needs

Take magnesium (500 mg. daily) between meals and Vitamin E (400 to 800 IU daily in two divided doses). Consult your doctor about the larger dosage if you have diabetes, hypertension, or rheumatic heart conditions, or if you take anti-coagulants.

Get off Drugs and Caffeine

The effects of certain medications, particularly decongestants, may make your heart race. And the same is true of caffeine, an addictive stimulant. Wean yourself off a cup of coffee or tea a day, substituting herbal teas (see above).

A Remedy in Time

The homeopathic remedies Aconite (for fear) and Stramonium (for terror and violent fantasies) may calm your palpitations.

Don't Diet

Restriction of your nutritional needs can cause major electrolyte imbalances that may trigger palpitations. Bingeing and purging will weaken and damage the heart muscle. It's important to eat regular meals made of whole grains, fresh fruits and vegetables, fish, seeds, and yogurt. Cut down or cut out red meat, marbled with fat, and eat only low-fat dairy to keep your heart plaque-free.

Breathe Steadily and Surely

When your heart is going like a house afire, sit down and take slow, steady breaths. Never try to inhale or exhale beyond your capacity. As you breathe, visualize your heart as a caged bird. At first you will see it flying madly from bar to bar, but as you fill yourself with oxygen and energy, you will see it settle down, lighting in one place and staying very still.

PANIC DISORDERS

see also Agoraphobia, page 24; Chest Pain, page 87; Dizziness, page 124; Fear of Going Crazy, page 175; Gastrointestinal Disorders, page 189; Hallucinations, page 201; Hyperventilation, page 231; Palpitations, page 342; Phobias, page 346; Shortness of Breath, page 397

Panic is a sudden onset of acute and frightening anxiety that seems to come from nowhere. It fills you with dread, a sense that if you don't escape fast, you will die. Panic brings with it a battery of symptoms such as palpitations and chest pains, shortness of breath and hyperventilation, dizziness, numbness and tingling, hot and cold flashes, trembling, and nausea. Worst of all, the attack usually makes you feel you have lost touch with yourself and with reality.

At least 1.6 percent of the population (about 3 million people) has experienced a panic attack at one time or other, and they often come in the midst of crises—when you're going through a divorce, going off to college, or when someone very close to you dies. A panic attack is not considered a disorder unless you have four panic attacks within a period of four weeks, or unless your anticipatory anxiety of the possible recurrence of this attack is so great that you avoid activities.

People who are likely to panic are also more likely to be perfectionists, always self-critical, always certain that they're going to mess up. Because they lack confidence, they have trouble taking risks and letting go of control. They also tend to have ongoing fears about their mental and physical health and the long-term implications of these disorders. For example, they may be certain that panicking implies they have some life-threatening illness such as a brain tumor or heart disease, or that they are losing their mind. The fear of repeated attacks can lead to complete avoidance of normal daily activities, and a development of agoraphobia (see page 24).

It is demoralizing to find that you have a hair-trigger reaction to life, particularly if there's no one element that sets off the attack. For this reason, at least half the people who are subject to panic attacks are also depressed.

It's vital to become aware of your coping behaviors that help you through a panic attack. Some individuals pace, some open a window to get air, some check their pulse, wash their face, or hold onto a chair. Although these can be comforting rituals, they add to the feeling of anxiety. It's as if you were saying, "Okay, here it comes, I'm girding myself for battle." Instead of doing anything to avoid the rush of fear, it's best to try to relax and breathe.

Because the attack itself deregulates breathing and heart rate, some of the best treatment involves learning how to monitor "involuntary" reactions. Any treatment involving systematic relaxation and breathing will be helpful before, during, and after an attack, and in preventing future attacks.

There are also a variety of preventive tactics you can use that may stop a panic attack in its tracks, but they all center on treating yourself differently.

First, you should keep a panic diary and chart each attack after it occurs. You should note the circumstances under which it started—whom you were with, where you were, what you were doing; the physical symptoms that accompanied the attack; what you did behaviorally such as pacing or hugging yourself; what thoughts passed through your head during the attack. Give the attack a rating from one to ten in intensity. Keeping this record will show you your progress when you begin to use various natural therapies as interventions.

Treatments to try: Affirmations, page 16; Autogenic training, page 48; Bach flower remedies, page 53; Behavioral therapy, page 55; Bioenergetics, page 63; Biofeedback, page 65; Breathing, page 76; Cognitive awareness, page 94; Desensitization, page 116; Homeopathy, page 221; Magnetic healing, page 285; Meditation, page 292; Mindfulness, page 296; Progressive relaxation, page 361; Self-hypnosis, page 383.

P*HOBIAS*

see also Agoraphobia, page 24; Fear, page 164; Fear of Animals, page 168; Fear of Failure, page 171; Fear of Flying, page 173; Fear of Going Crazy, page 175; Fear of Public Bathrooms, page 178; Fear of Public Speaking, page 180; Panic Disorders, page 344; Stage Fright, page 407

A phobia is a persistent and irrational fear of an object, activity, or situation that results in a compelling desire to avoid the fear.

Phobias can trigger anxiety and panic attacks, which can produce a battery of physiological symptoms such as racing heart, sweating, shortness of breath, and a need to flee the scene. There are three different types of phobias.

SIMPLE PHOBIAS: These phobias involve a fear of specific things such as snakes, dogs, illness, blood, heights, crowds, or storms. A person may suffer multiple simple phobias. Unlike social phobias or agoraphobia, simple phobias don't generally prohibit a person from living a normal life. Exposure and desensitization can work wonders on most of these phobias.

SOCIAL PHOBIAS: These involve a terror of a certain situation that may cause embarrassment. The trigger is having to perform and is apparent in phobias about public speaking, using a public toilet, being watched while eating, or a fear of sexual performance or of being touched.

AGORAPHOBIA: This is the most common and most debilitating type of phobic disorder. The outside world is so threatening that just being in it causes panic. This may mean that the sufferer can't stand crowds, but is also afraid of open spaces; that being confined in a tunnel is as great a problem as being out in the open on a bridge. This phobia involves fear of both objects and situations and is characterized by a terror of being trapped or caught in a situation from which there is no escape. Two thirds of all agoraphobics are women.

All types of phobias are hard to shake. As soon as your anxiety about dealing with an object or situation becomes a need to avoid that object or situation every time, it is with you constantly. The fear you have isn't just anxiety anymore; rather it is paralyzing terror, the kind that makes you feel like jumping out of your skin. Finally, in order for your fear to be phobic, it must seem as unreasonable to you as it does to others. You know perfectly well that there is nothing inherently dangerous about making a speech or standing on top of the Empire State Building, but the very idea makes you shake. (If you did not recognize that your fear was irrational, it would be classified as a *delusion*.)

It's hard to tell how common phobias are in the general population because many people don't disclose their fears. It may be too embarrassing to explain to friends and family why you can't go to a certain place or engage in a certain activity. It's been found, however, that the sooner the phobia is dealt with, the greater the chances of success in curing it.

Although one National Institutes of Health study indicated that one in nine people in American have some type of phobia, the real numbers are probably a good deal higher.

Do we fear a dog or an airplane because of some inborn chemical imbalance in the brain, or do we learn to fear? The answer may be that it is a combination of the two; however, the brain chemistry can change because of certain early situations that teach us about the terror. For example, if as a child you were always punished for your misdeeds by being locked in a dark closet, it would be likely that you would grow up fearing the dark because of its association with "something bad." We may fear public speaking because we are naturally shy, or because of an instance when our parents forced us to perform or recite and we felt humiliated and embarrassed as everyone stared at us. If we were also unprepared for the event and couldn't accurately perform the poem or piano piece, we were then judged harshly rather than praised.

Other fears may result from an association with repressed desires that we can't face up to. The avoidance of public toilets, for example, may be closely related to early childhood fantasies or getting caught while "playing doctor." Any instance in the future where nakedness or touching the genitals is involved can bring on a terror of discovery.

A phobia often develops in order to avoid the response to the fear: We're afraid of shaking, trembling, blushing, stammering, and looking silly, so we don't get up onstage. We're afraid of running away and looking cowardly, so we avoid dogs.

And the more often we shut down the possibility of confronting the object of our fear, the less we feel capable of handling it. If we never face the ultimate challenge, we can never survive the situation. For this reason, most treatment for phobias involves some degree of desensitization and "flooding," or being overwhelmed with the object or situation. Cognitive awareness and behavioral therapy are essential for social phobias and agoraphobia.

Treatments to try: Affirmations, page 16; Bach flower remedies, page 53; Behavioral therapy, page 55; Bioenergetics, page 63; Breathing, page 76; Cognitive awareness, page 94; Desensitization, page 116; Homeopathy, page 221; Magnetic healing, page 285; Meditation, page 292; Mindfulness, page 296; Self-hypnosis, page 383.

PLAY THERAPY

The concept of play therapy originated with child psychologists and psychiatrists who understood that the way to reach the deepest levels of a child's psyche was through the medium he was most familiar with. A six year old cannot tell you he is depressed or anxious, but he can draw you a picture, create a scenario with dolls and stuffed animals, use water pistols or pillows to release tension and get out aggression, and reconstruct family dynamics by using dollhouses and dollhouse figurines.

This therapy works wonderfully—sometimes better—on adults who haven't had recent "practice" with toys and games. Because the mind is surprised by the tools and techniques of play, it's hard to get stuck in old patterns and unproductive discussions. Play is just play, and it gets to the heart of the matter very quickly.

You can reenact problematic issues in a relationship by using dolls and stuffed animals. You can improvise with them or actually write a bare-bones script and then let your imagination fly as you transfer your thoughts and feelings to these inanimate objects. You should assume the various roles and play out the feelings as you perceive them.

Artwork is a particularly excellent method of dealing with emotions. Grief and despair can sometimes be more easily drawn or sculpted than expressed in words. A well-known therapeutic approach for individuals dying of cancer or AIDS is to use a sand table. The working area is covered with sand so that you can mold and shape the landscape as your feelings demand. Small figurines are sometimes stuck into the sand pits and placed on top of sand mounds to symbolize different feelings. You can do the same thing with clay; working the pliable substance with your hands can be a very therapeutic experience.

Legos and other building toys can be used to fabricate situations and feelings. Whatever you create out of these interlocking pieces can be a big clue as to why you've been feeling low or scared or agitated. Jacks and pick-up sticks, which require agile fingers and much dexterity, teach you about being careful and cautious. It can be enormously cathartic to pound your ball on the jacks, scattering them everywhere, or to lift your sticks so that they collapse all the ones underneath.

It is sometimes helpful to work out anxieties and fears by being very physical. You can go to a playground (preferably with a child who knows her way around) and use the equipment to shake yourself up. Hanging upside down on a swing with your legs wrapped around the chains can make you want to scream with fear, delight, and expectation, and this is an acceptable place to release those emotions. A seesaw (used with a friend of equal weight) is a great way to understand balance in a relationship. It's always uncertain as to whether your partner is going to let you drop abruptly, or hold you up—just as in real life.

Throwing yourself into an activity such as a pillow fight, a fight with soft bats, or a wrestling match is a great emotional release. Working with a partner this way is an advanced stage of play therapy and should be attempted only after you have worked solo with other media such as arts and crafts, toys, and dolls. It's okay to get physical, as long as you set limits for yourself and your partner. You should establish code words to use when one of you wants to stop ("no" can be interpreted as part of the play). You may find as you lock limbs with a partner or bat them on the head that you are able to tap into feelings you haven't been aware of. It's common to cry, yell, laugh, and even shake uncontrollably when you use play therapy. For this reason it should be done only with a compassionate and understanding partner who can support you when you most need it.

Positive Self-talk

see Affirmations, page 16

Postpartum Depression

see also Depression, page 112

Many women feel moody during pregnancy, but it is far more common to become depressed after the excitement is over and the baby is born. Of course, there are wild hormonal changes going on in the body that account for a portion of the problem. Certain studies have shown that women who tend to be depressed postpartum have higher levels of estrogen prior to birth and lower levels after birth than other women. However, hormones are only part of the problem. Stress and the overwhelming responsibility of taking care of this tiny, dependent being can bring on feelings of helplessness in many women, particularly if their own egos are slightly shaky. It's hard to suddenly metamorphose into a supermom if you really don't think you could possibly be counted on to bring up a child. Other factors that may precipitate this crisis are the lack of a support system, one or more other young children at home who become upset when their new sibling arrives, or the lack of a compassionate partner.

Postpartum blues are quite common; however, adjustment reactions to becoming a mother, clinical depression, a feeling of being trapped with no escape, and postpartum psychosis are relatively rare.

Postpartum depression is not necessarily limited to a new mother having her first child. Very often, veteran mothers who have had no problems after earlier pregnancies find that they suddenly can't cope. In this case, of course, it's vital that your other children get the care they need from other adults when you are in distress.

■ *What Happens When You Have Postpartum Depression*

You feel "blue" and tired and may not even have any interest in your baby. You may find that the work or hobbies that once gave you pleasure don't appeal to you at all. It's common to start crying at the drop of a diaper and to lose all interest in sex. You may feel agitated and anxious, or confused and hypersensitive. You may experience insomnia, feelings of paranoia, mood swings, hopelessness, obsessive or repetitive thoughts, and decreased appetite. More severe symptoms include a lack of interest in life, excessive crying, substance abuse, thoughts of suicide or of getting rid of your child. IF YOU SHOULD HAVE ANY OF THESE SEVERE SYMPTOMS, YOU MUST SEEK PROFESSIONAL HELP IMMEDIATELY.

Short-Term Therapy

If you cannot lift yourself out of negative thoughts and the fear that you might do something dangerous to yourself or your baby, your health-care provider can refer you to a counselor, a psychologist, or a therapist, or you yourself can contact your local hospital for a referral.

Get the Help You Need at Home

Ask your partner, your mother, your mother-in-law, or your sister to pitch in. You really need to be able to get adequate rest, eat right, and start exercising, and that means that you'll need assistance with child care. If you have no support system, hire someone to come in several hours a day to help out. If you can't afford a nurse or maid, perhaps you can barter with a neighbor, exchanging child care or help around the house for some skill or service you can perform.

Exercise

Getting out and getting moving will do three things: It will give you some time to yourself, away from the ever present responsibility of child care; it will start you back on the road to reclaiming your body and getting it fit and in shape; and it will give you regular access to the beta endorphins your brain produces that make you feel good.

- *Walking.* Not strolling the carriage, but brisk marching, preferably with some hand weights to get your upper body into action.

- *Swimming.* When you're postpartum, stretching your body in the water is enormously beneficial and will help heal tearing or episiotomy stitches as well. You can do laps or join a water-cise class.

- *Bicycling.* This is a great sport for the new mother because it lets her see the world. Riding a bike takes balance, and so does being a mother. This is an excellent activity for body and soul. Give yourself a set route that runs several miles, with gradations up and down hills. If weather doesn't permit, think about purchasing an exercise bike you can keep in the TV room.

- *Low-impact aerobics.* There are plenty of good videotapes for new mothers, or you can join a class at your local Y or health club. This will give you a social outlet as well as a physical one.

Meditation

Get your partner or a friend or relative to watch the baby so you can take 20 minutes each day to sit alone and breathe. This can help you to change your perspective on your role as a woman and a mother. You may listen to guided meditation tapes or simply let your thoughts and feelings focus in on the strength and quiet inside you. Try to stay in the moment and enjoy the feeling of your body and mind working together. (If you cannot find *any* time at all for yourself, you can meditate while your baby sleeps or nurses.)

Homeopathy

Try the following remedies for postpartum depression:

If you are depressed, irritable, want to be alone to cry, find the effects of grief and anger worse when consoled: Natrum mur

If you are anxious, guilty, hopeless: Arsenicum album

If you are nervous, sighing, sobbing, sad even after grieving, restless, anxious, fearful: Ignatia

If you are weepy, changeable, desire sympathy, irritable, jealous, suspicious, and have an aversion to smoke: Pulsatilla

If you are irritable, very sad, weeping, indifferent to loved ones and work, but the problem is better with exercise: Sepia

Rely on Chinese Wisdom

Acupressure or acupuncture may be helpful. Press the following points:

Pe. 6: on the midline of the inside of the arm, an inch and a half from the crease in the wrist, between the two tendons

Ht. 7: on the outside crease of the wrist close to the base of the palm on the side of the little finger in the hollow next to the bone

You may also try the patent formula *wu chi pai feng wan,* or "black chicken pills," which acts as a tonic for the Blood and chi, warms the uterus and nurtures yin energy. These can be purchased through mail order or at a Chinese pharmacy. Take one box daily.

Get the Support You Need

It will be easy to find a postpartum support group through your obstetrician, midwife, or local hospital. There are many women in your situation, and one of the best therapies is communal sharing. Postpartum depression is generally time-limited, and you will be able to see stages of "coming back" even within your group. This will reassure you for your own future. Most women come out on the other side of this problem much stronger in mind and spirit, which makes them better mothers and more integrated people.

*P*OSTTRAUMATIC STRESS DISORDER

see also Alienation, page 28; Anxiety, page 43; Numbness (emotional), page 313; Stress, page 407

Following a terrible event, such as the death of a loved one, a rape, a fight, or a natural disaster such as a hurricane or earthquake, we are generally in shock. We go about our business and may appear to function well, until we are caught up short by our proximity to danger—perhaps even to death. Often, posttraumatic stress occurs in people who are simply witnesses to tragedy. The brave rescuer of the child who was trapped in a pipe for days committed suicide years later; the survivors of the 1995 Oklahoma City bombing testified that it haunted them even a year afterward; and the brave fire-fighters and ambulance drivers who see death and destruction on a daily basis often cannot manage their personal lives and drink or abuse drugs.

▓ *What Happens When You Have PTSD*

You may feel a great deal of guilt as you try to puzzle out why you were saved and everyone else suffered. It's as if the experience had tainted everything else, because nothing in the world will ever seem as crucial as that moment when time stopped and the awful event occurred. You may experience anxiety, difficulty concentrating, recurrent dreams and sleep disturbances, an exaggerated startle response, flashbacks to the event and a withdrawal from your everyday life and those closest to you, a type of psychic numbing, or emotional anesthesia. Sometimes the flashbacks will involve a dissociation from real time, in which you actually feel as though the event is occurring again.

PTSD is not new. This stress syndrome was first identified by John Erichsen, who studied victims of train crashes in the mid-nineteenth century. In World War I, the syndrome was known as "shell shock." Physicians at the front line at first assumed that their patients suffered these symptoms because of neurological damage caused by their proximity to exploding artillery shells until they discovered that men who hadn't been under fire had the same problems. In subsequent wars, the syndrome was renamed "combat fatigue." Of course, it doesn't take a war to create posttraumatic stress. Unfortunately, we can go through experiences as horrendous as combat in our own homes.

The degree of damage done by this syndrome is extremely variable. In many cases personality determines how bad the effects will be—resilient, flexible people do better than rigid, controlling types. Some individuals are fine except when confronted with a situation similar to that which surrounded the trauma. Men who had survived Vietnam often had flashbacks the minute they saw tall, waving grasses or had to endure hot, humid weather. Other people develop phobias around the event—the driver in a terrible automobile accident who witnessed his passenger die might be unable to get behind the wheel afterward.

As might be expected, it's not the severity of the trauma that counts, but rather a constellation of experiences, feelings, and life events that make PTSD occur. Although hostages taken in Central America or Iran might have been uniformly tortured and deprived of the normal conditions of human existence, some recovered better because they were able to help a fellow prisoner or to accomplish some difficult goal when they were locked up.

Most cases of PTSD resolve themselves within six months of the event, but others last for years. The symptoms are usually worse if the individual has been physically abused or has witnessed someone else being physically abused. People with "doom and gloom" personalities, those who are shy and withdrawn, and those who are irritable and impulsive, seem to be more at risk for long-term effects of PTSD. Education and intelligence seem to be protective against it, because they can help you make sense of what's happened to you. The effects seem to be worse on civilians than those in the military, who after all, expect to weather danger as part of their job.

Imagine You Are Responsible Only for Yourself

Using self-hypnosis, you will re-create the success that is yours to own. Roll your eyes up and close them, taking a deep breath and holding it. Allow your breath to flow freely now as you see yourself as floating. Your left arm will raise automatically. Now you will give yourself the suggestion that you have the ability to change. If you have been depressed and angry, you can use this altered state of consciousness to concentrate on one thing about yourself that needs attention. If you have had a psychogenic wound from the traumatic experience, you will focus on that problem and heal it with the same success you had in coming out of the trauma in one piece.

Understand that you were not responsible for others who may have been injured or hurt, but that you *are* responsible for yourself and your continued well-being. Use this suggestion several times daily at first, tapering off as you begin to see a difference in your feeling state.

Desensitize Quickly

It's been found that the best recovery from PTSD happens soon after the trauma has occurred. The more quickly you get back on the "horse" that threw you, the better. In the desensitization process, you work your way up to being flooded with the terrifying experience. By confronting it again—this time in a safe context—you feel that you've accomplished a great deal. For example, if you're a woman who's been raped, you might take a self-defense course that ends with an all-out fight with a padded attacker. You will be encouraged to subdue the opponent with every ounce of energy you've got—screaming, biting, gouging, and kicking.

A person who has survived a terrible natural disaster might volunteer for the Red Cross after another earthquake or fire to distribute supplies to the victims. By "undoing" the past, you will be able to move ahead to the future.

Get in a Group

Support groups are almost essential for those who have been through a terrifying experience. The group helps by allowing you to get perspective on the event and also by encouraging your reliance on others, something that you may have lost at the scene of the accident or attack. Veterans' Administration Hospitals run such groups for PTSD; look in the Yellow Pages for the one nearest you.

Herbal Relief

The extraordinary anxiety that is engendered after surviving the trauma can be helped by using a number of herbs. St. John's wort is the herb of choice for anxiety (be sure you avoid prolonged exposure to the sun while taking it); chamomile or lemon tea are relaxants, and you can try oat tea, scullcap, or valerian as sedatives. It's a good idea to take a nerve tonic as well—dandelion, burdock, yellow dock, or nettle (singly or in combination) will strengthen your nervous system. Take 1/2 to 1 teaspoon extract daily or one cup of infusion made with 2 to 4 teaspoon of dried herbs.

Melatonin for Sleep

Because nightmares are such a common symptom, it may be a wise idea to try to regulate your production of melatonin and serotonin by taking a supplement. Consult with your physician before taking 1 mg. daily of melatonin an hour before bed.

Turn on the Radio

The right kind of music is often helpful in the treatment of PTSD. If you had a type of soothing sound that you enjoyed before the event, you can re-create your feelings when you listen to it again now. Sometimes songs that you remember from childhood or a tune you heard on your first date can bring you back to a time when things were good and safe. Start with favorite selections and experiment with similar music; then combine them to make a tape you can keep by your bedside or in your car.

No More Caffeine

Because caffeine is a stimulant and can cause symptoms of anxiety such as palpitations, gastrointestinal upset, and sweaty palms, it's best to eliminate it from your life completely. Wean yourself off a cup a day for a week or cut real coffee with decaf. When you're down to one cup of tea, coffee, soda, or cocoa, stabilize for a week before stopping. Understand that you may have headaches and a disoriented feeling for from two days to two weeks after you quit.

Trust in a Flower

Rescue Remedy is the Bach flower remedy to take for PTSD. Keep a bottle handy in your purse or pocket, and take 5 to 6 drops under the tongue or mixed in a glass of water if you are experiencing anxiety in order to forestall a flashback.

Homeopathic Help

The best remedy for fright is Aconite, and this relates to fright at the sight of an accident or the memory of that fear.

The second most likely remedy for terror and trauma is Stramonium, particularly if you are having violent nightmares.

Other remedies for fear are Belladonna, Causticum, Lycopodium, Phosphorus, Silica, and Pulsatilla.

PRAYER

Prayer means many different things to different people. At its most basic level, it is the manifestation of hope in human beings, our ability to say that we don't know everything, that there is something or someone larger and wiser than we are that can guide our lives.

Recent scientific investigation shows that prayer can be used as an alternative therapy as successfully as meditation, exercise, or herbalism. A 1988 study in San Francisco involved coronary care-unit patients who received prayers and had fewer medical problems than those patients who didn't. A study of 91,000 people in rural Maryland showed that weekly church attenders had 50 percent fewer deaths from heart disease than nonchurchgoers and 53 percent fewer suicides. An ongoing study from the University of New Mexico Health Sciences Center, funded by the NIH Office of Alternative Medicine; is looking into the success of prayer when used on individuals with alcohol- and drug-related problems.

Prayer really *does* work in mysterious ways, and on non-human controls. In an experiment conducted at McGill University in Montreal, sealed containers of water were given to a psychic healer to hold, and others were given to a depressed patient to hold. The plants watered with the healer-held water had an increased growth rate; the other plants had a decreased growth rate.

Spirituality has taken on a new meaning for many individuals who don't regularly attend church or synagogue. Many experts feel that the immune system is strengthened and nourished by a sense of peace, which can be transferred from one individual to another or used inwardly by an individual on him or herself. Of course, the ancient stories of the Bible and seminal works of Eastern religions link healing with faith. If doctors prayed with their patients before and after surgery or before administering a course of powerful drugs, it's possible that this treatment might assist in the patient's recovery. Thirty medical schools in America are now offering courses in faith and medicine.

It has been found that belief in a higher power can enhance the relaxation response we get when we're in a meditative state (which is, of course, very similar to prayer). This means that when you pray and really believe that you will derive benefit from it, your blood pressure lowers, your anger vanishes, and you are more quickly able to tap into your potential for healing. Sometimes, just calling on God in the way you've done countless times over the years can start the positive effects. Saying, "Our Father," or "sh'ma Yisrael," or "om" gets the mind ready to pray.

There are several factors that make prayer beneficial in the healing process. First, a deep faith tends to encourage discipline with lifestyle change, so that if you've committed to following a new holistic program, you'll stick with it. Second, people who truly believe that they can get well again seem to have a better memory of what feeling good was like before they fell into a slump. Finally, faith itself calms and supports these individuals, which gives them an extra boost every minute of every day.

Another factor, of course, is that you can alleviate mental and emotional problems with prayer. If you truly believe that you can be changed—through your own intercession or that of a divine being—then your possibilities are limitless. It's not easy to rid yourself of depression if you think that no one cares and that you are fighting a losing battle by yourself. But if you are encouraged by the thought that a friend is offering prayers for your increasing mental health and even more, if you feel that those prayers are reaching the "ear" of a power greater than your despair, you may be able to heal. The best co-mingling of mind, body, and spirit takes place when we direct our heartfelt energies to getting well.

CASE HISTORY

Sam had a mostly good marriage for 20 years. He and Patsy had two wonderful kids, and although their relationship was often rocky, it was pretty stable. "I thought I'd be married forever, even after I started having an affair. The fling with this other woman was strictly extracurricular, except when Patsy found out, she decided it was the most important thing that had ever happened between us. So she threw me out and filed for divorce. I pleaded with her, but she was like a rock.

"I had gone to church all my life, and this was no time to stop. I was guilty as hell, and I felt even worse when I realized that Patsy was turning the kids against me—they refused to see me. I got an apartment near the house and I went to their team matches and school plays, but it was as if I were invisible. So prayer became a way that I could reach out to them, even though it was indirect. I went to a men's group at the church and signed up for a retreat at a monastery in Vermont.

"That weekend was a turning point for me. It's funny because the place was very casual—the brothers all dressed like normal guys, and nobody gave any big sermons about how to live your life. But maybe it was this atmosphere that convinced me that God is everywhere and in everyone. I had hope again that I could patch up things with my kids. Before, I felt like the center of my lousy universe—it was all *my* fault, *my* guilt, *my* shame. But picking myself up spiritually has helped me see that I'm not alone in this—there's a higher power in charge who can help me."

If you can be reflective about the things that happen to you, you will be able to consider the bigger picture in a difficult situation rather than reacting spontaneously and emotionally. Instead of flailing out with anger when you feel you've been wronged, stop a moment and consider what the implications of your anger might be. In showing your rage, you may be perpetrating the same rotten situation you're reacting against.

You don't have to believe in a deity in order for prayer to assuage the most desperate or agonizing of your mental and emotional problems. If you think of yourself as part of a larger entity, for example, the cosmos, you can realize how small you and your responses are in the context of all of life, and yet, how important you are as part of the whole. One individual can really do nothing to fix what's the matter on earth; however, the conglomerate of energy we all belong to in some way may have a very powerful effect.

When you are really down, when you feel that nothing can help, that your friends and family have failed you, that you have little reason to get up in the morning, this is the best time for prayer. Those individuals who have been in real danger—for example, hostages who are completely at the mercy of their captors—have said that although they personally could do nothing to alter their circumstances, they knew beyond a reasonable doubt that they would be protected by some higher authority. If you can hold that hope even in your darkest moment, think what you can do on a daily basis with prayer.

If you have prayed all your life, you understand the true benefit of this practice. Use it well and wisely. If you have never prayed and feel self-conscious about perhaps borrowing a facility that you think you don't have, here are some useful hints:

- Prayer works best on your mind and body when it's cumulative. Daily prayer is a good idea, even if you think you have nothing to pray about.

- Pray for others as well as for yourself. This is not simply an admonition not to be selfish; rather, the force of your actions is too powerful to be directed inside only. By including those you care about in your prayers, you are solidifying the bonds between you.

- Try not to think consciously; rather, as in meditation, let the feelings flow inside you. You may find your prayer moving in a very different direction from the one you thought you'd take at the beginning of your practice.

- Over time, change the organization and location of your prayer. You don't need a church, synagogue, or shrine; your kitchen or the backyard will do just fine.

*P*ROGRESSIVE *R*ELAXATION

This exceptionally beneficial relaxation technique, developed by Dr. Edmund Jacobson, works because it teaches you how to isolate the smallest parts of your body and become aware of subtle ways in which you hold tension. Progressive relaxation is the basis of Lamaze breathing for natural childbirth, relaxation for hypnosis, and behavioral therapy. By breaking down your tension into workable units, you will be able to recognize it whenever it appears and let go of it quickly.

You can either make yourself a tape of the instructions and play it as you move through the exercise, you can have someone read it to you, or you can simply do a body inventory in your mind, thinking about each limb and muscle, as you alternately tense and relax it.

Lie flat on your back and let your knees fall open. Close your eyes and begin to breathe slowly and easily. Do a quick inventory of your body to see if you are holding any part of it stiffly and then attempt to release that tension by adjusting your position, breathing more deeply, or sinking your body into the floor.

Begin with your arms. Make a fist in each hand and hold it tightly, as tense as you can. Then, let go completely. Relax the hands. See how different the entire arm feels.

Now tense just the forearm. Tighten all the muscles, then release them. Relax the forearms. Now tense the elbow by drawing your lower arm up until your hand touches your shoulder. Make it very tense, then let the arm go. Relax the elbow. Tense your shoulders, drawing them off the floor. Then drop them. Relax the shoulders.

Continue contracting and relaxing, moving up the body and then down the back. From your shoulders, go to your neck, your head and jaw, and then your face and eyes. Work your way to your forehead and scalp. Then come over the top of your head and concentrate on your upper back, chest, waist, stomach, pelvis, hips, lower back, buttocks, thighs, knees, ankles, feet and instep, and toes. Make sure each body part is as tight as you can possibly make it before relaxing completely.

When you have worked each body part, lie still on the floor and feel yourself letting go completely. The whole body will now relax as one element. If you feel residual tension anywhere, bring your mind to that spot and consciously release it.

When you first start doing progressive relaxation, concentrate on only one area of the body. You may work on your arms, your legs, your head, or torso. As you get better, you can add more areas until you finally work the entire body in one session.

R_{AGE}

see also Anger, page 31; Impulse Control, page 246; Violence/Aggressive Behavior, page 437

Rage is the end of the anger spectrum. It is usually the result of suppressing negative feelings until finally, like a pressure cooker, you have to let off steam. Rage effectively stops thought so that you simply act on your emotions, unleashing the violence that has been pushed down inside. It is the terrible dragon inside that cannot be tamed, the unchained beast we fear we've become. Although anger can usually be subjugated, pushed down, repressed, or channeled elsewhere, there is generally no way to manage rage except to let it roar.

One attraction of succumbing to rage is that you know you can shock other people into submission. Since their level of commitment to the problem is usually not as great as yours, they often quietly move out of the way, just to get the unbridled anger to stop. Since this is not a great method of getting your way, it's best to learn how to use anger appropriately and keep rage from happening.

■ What Happens When You Feel Enraged

Giving in to rage is often aptly described as "losing your head." There is nothing and no one who can stop you, so you howl. It's as if your head were gone, and in its place is a raging volcano with lava pouring out, hurting anyone who gets in its path. There seems to be no end to your passion—you could go on screaming forever. It's as if your rational mind had shut off; your reactions are more instinctive, more animal than human. You see red, you hear the roaring inside you, you smell danger.

Count to Ten

Yes, it really works. There is something about the enforced delay that makes it possible for you to breathe more fully and think more clearly. If you can give yourself enough time, the rage will dissipate somewhat, giving you the opportunity to do something constructive with your anger.

Change Your Behavior

If you never express your anger and never get the opportunity to "vent," eventually you pass your threshhold for tolerance. Instead, allow yourself to get *moderately* angry whenever something seems really wrong to you.

You are going to select nine appropriate reactions to anger on a sliding scale of 1 to 10. The idea is never to arrive at 10, which is uncontrollable rage. As each episode presents itself, label it. A 1 might require an annoyed face and a comment about not liking what's going on; a 3 might require a confrontation and a debate about how to handle the problem next time; a 7 might allow you to yell, and then go off for a time to be apart from the person or event you're angry at. When you've determined that it's okay to be angry, you need never give over to the unpleasant explosion of rage.

Give Yourself to Your Breath

A directed type of yoga breathing has an excellent calming effect. The *ujjayi* or "ocean-sounding breath" is produced by closing the lips and imagining that you are fogging a mirror behind your teeth with air from the back of your throat. When you inhale, imagine that you are reversing the process and that the mirror is in the back of your throat. The stream of air should be drawn in and out very slowly, and you will find that you have a lot more space for inhalation and exhalation than you do with normal breath.

As you practice, close your eyes and allow the sound of the ocean to comfort you. Concentrate only on the air going in and out of your throat. The longer you can keep up the ujjayi breathing, the more stable you will feel.

Have a Tantrum by Yourself

If you have to act hysterical, do it alone and don't subject anyone else to your inappropriate behavior. Go near some train tracks and yell as it passes by; find a secluded place in the woods and smash dishes (cheap ones) against the trees. When you've accomplished this wild feat, go back and confront the person or situation that has triggered it and use your mind, rather than your emotions, to deal with the problem.

Let Someone Else Win

As an experiment, when you are about to explode see what it feels like to throw up your hands and yield. It won't feel good, and you may wish to rescind it later on when you're calmer. But acting "as if" you didn't have to win will allow you to see someone else's perspective even if you think it's wrong (see also treatments for Anger, page 31).

RESTLESS LEG SYNDROME

see also Sleep Disorders, page 404

The condition known as "restless leg" is most common in older adults when the legs twitch and dance within the sheets and the only solution to the problem is getting up and walking. Some individuals are awakened from a sound sleep with an excruciating cramp something like a charley horse. A disorder related to restless leg was originally named *noctural myoclonus* or "muscle twitching at night," which consists of twitches every few seconds, usually in the legs.

What Happens When You Have Restless Leg

This syndrome can drive you right out of your bed; you feel you simply have to walk around. Unfortunately, as soon as symptoms vanish and you crawl back into bed, the legs start twitching and cramping all over again. The frustration of not being able to sleep can lead to symptoms of sleep deprivation—anxiety, irritability, and mood swings.

Two categories of individuals suffer from restless leg. One group has an inherited predisposition because of an imbalance of the neurotransmitters dopamine and serotonin. There are also disease-based causes; for instance, nerve damage from diabetes or disk problems may bring on the condition, as can deficiencies of folate or Vitamin B_{12}. Many pregnant women get it, as do individuals with rheumatoid arthritis and people who consume too much caffeine or alcohol. It can also be attributed to a drug reaction—if you take lithium, beta blockers, anticonvulsants, or neuroleptics, you may be prone to restless leg. Some physicians feel that restless leg in children may be connected to attention-deficit hyperactivity (see ADD and ADHD, page 13).

Relax Progressively

This stress-management technique will sometimes work for restless leg, if it's not completely due to physical causes. Working from the toes up, you will alternately tense and release each body part. Starting with your toes, contract your muscles and hold your breath, then let it out and relax completely. Continue by contracting and releasing the feet, legs, thighs, torso, back, arms, chest, neck, and head—and every place in between. At the end of the sequence, your whole being should feel very loose and comfortable.

Cut Out Stimulants

Both caffeine and alcohol can trigger the condition. Try getting rid of both, and you may see an improvement in several weeks.

Clean Out Your Medicine Cabinet

Restless leg is sometimes triggered by stimulants or antidepressant medication. Diuretics are another cause of the condition. Go over your medications with your physician and, if possible, taper off.

Herbs May Relax Your Muscles

The antispasmodic herb of choice (used in the treatment of Parkinson's disease and for individuals who have seizures) is passionflower. The dosage is 1/2 teaspoon infused in a cup of water three times daily. Other herbs that relax muscles and improve sleep are scullcap (2 to 4 teaspoons to one cup water, 3 times daily), valerian (1 to 4 teaspoons dried root to one cup water, 3 times daily) and pasque flower (1/2 to 1 teaspoon dried leaves to 1 cup water, 3 times daily). You may also take celery seed and add celery to your diet, since it has a special affinity for the musculoskeletal system. The dosage of tincture is the same as above; for a tea, brew 1/2 to 1 teaspoon of dried herb in a cup of water.

Exercise Before Bed

Just a few strategic stretches may keep you asleep all night. To work the calf muscles, start with a runner's stretch against a wall. Stand about two- and -one-half feet away and press your hands into the wall, stretching your Achilles' tendons.

Now sit and stretch your right leg out in front of you. Place your left foot against the inside of your right thigh. Inhale and curl down over the outstretched leg, holding on wherever it's comfortable—around the knees, ankles, or the soles of the feet. Stretch and breathe in the position, then slowly roll up. Repeat on the other side.

Rub Down the Tension

A massage with the essential oil of Chamomile or several drops of the oil in a bath before bed can calm your muscles as well as your mind.

*R*ISK-TAKING

see also Impulse Control, page 246

The compulsion to take dangerous risks—to drive over the speed limit, to have an extramarital affair, to invest in an unproven venture—motivates certain people who claim that "they just can't help" what they do. The incredible high they get from taking risks is too exhilarating to give up, no matter how dangerous the proposition.

The downside of this type of behavior is that when you risk it all, you can lose it all—family and loved ones, home, job, self-respect.

The other side of risk-taking is a positive one, however, and allows you to see new possibilities where none existed before. Although it may be risky to move across the country for a new job, or to have a baby at 46, or to take early retirement so you can travel around the world, just think what you might have missed if you hadn't jumped off the high board. (More individuals have to be pushed into trying something new than be held back from squandering their future.)

What Happens When You Take Risks

The steep rock face is there, so you have to climb it. The game of three-card monte looks so easy to crack, so you bet. You just have to take a risk because if you don't try it, you'll feel like a failure. But when you take the risk and it works out all right, there is nothing like the high you get. It's as if you were always testing life to see whether you can beat it. When you do, you can laugh in its face; when you don't, it wasn't your fault, and there will always be another chance right around the bend.

Risk-taking involves a suspension of belief and a sense that you are invincible. It also supplies you with a fresh supply of stress hormones every time you plunge into a bad deal or spend an illicit afternoon with your married lover. So in addition to losing everything if you play the game wrong, you also risk a heart attack, stroke, cancer, or other stress-related disease.

Talk Yourself Down (or up)

Use a tape recorder to get immediate feedback on the conversation you're about to have with yourself. Make two lists, of the positives and negatives inherent in your decision to take this risk. Order them so that you see the best and worst consequences directly across from each other. You are now going to have a debate with yourself, first arguing the exciting, wonderful outcome of the risk you want to take, then arguing the disastrous possibilities if things go wrong.

Now sleep on it. The next morning, play the tape—several times, if necessary—before making your decision. This will keep you from a precipitous and spontaneous choice, but it will also strengthen your resolve to take a risk that may be a challenge for you.

Let Your Breath Show You the Way

Cool yourself down with your breath. The yogic "cooling" breath is said to remove excess heat, hunger, thirst, and desire for sleep. For "hotheads" who act rashly, this can be a beneficial treatment.

Curl your tongue into a tube and stick the tip outside your mouth. Draw air in with a hiss, and fill the lungs up as far as they'll go. Bring the tongue inside the mouth, close the mouth, and retain the air as long as you can. Exhale through the nose. (Do three rounds, then return to normal breathing.)

Visualize the Outcome

Sit quietly and give yourself at least 15 minutes for this visualization. Start by calming yourself, feeling all your energy going into your breath. As you enrich your inhalation and exhalation, you will find that you are more grounded, ready for this journey.

Imagine that it is just before dawn and you are climbing a very difficult mountain. It's still a bit dark, but you know the summit is close. You are looking forward to the incredible view you will get when you reach the top and the sun breaks out. You have never climbed this mountain before, but you know you can do it. The energy and excitement you feel is palpable. Each rock, each shrub seems to glisten, touched by morning dew. But the climb is getting harder. There are fewer hand-holds, and your boots slip occasionally, making your stomach lurch.

The sky has dark streaks of pink and orange now, and you know you are close. Just a few more laborious steps—you haul yourself up just as the sun appears on the horizon. You stand at the top, looking over the valley beneath, and you are suddenly aware of the fact that you have wings. Wouldn't it be exciting to try them out for the first time up here?

You don't know what you have to do to make them work, and of course, you're thousands of feet above sea level. If you fail, you could fall. But if you tell yourself that you've got the power and the ability, you may just accomplish the greatest feat of your life.

What is your choice?

(You must finish this visualization for yourself—on some days it may be necessary to draw back and climb back down;

on other days, you may want to try the wings even if you fail; and on other days, you may want to soar.)

Stand on Your Head

The yogic practice of the headstand is considered by some to be one of the most healthful of all. (It is not an easy posture, and SHOULD NOT BE ATTEMPTED BY ANYONE WITH CHRONIC BACK OR NECK PROBLEMS.) The headstand tones the nervous system and is particularly beneficial for the pineal, pituitary, thyroid, and parathyroid glands. In addition, the nature of standing on your head is to reverse everything. When you look at what you're doing from this totally different perspective, you may start to think before you act.

Kneel on a mat and lace your fingers, placing your elbows on the floor about a foot from your knees. Place your head in the cup made by your hands and angle your neck so that the back of your head touches your palms. Raise your feet up onto your toes and walk forward. Place the right knee on the right elbow, and when you get your balance, place the left knee on the left elbow.

Inhale and straighten your back. Fold the legs so that the knees rest on or near your chest, the soles of your feet facing up. Lift the thighs so that they are horizontal to the body. Finally, bring the knees all the way up so that you are one straight line from the neck to the knees. Then raise the legs, pointing the toes. Hold the headstand as long as it is comfortable and then slowly lower yourself in reverse, back to the mat.

Follow the Wisdom of the Chinese Sage

The great Taoist philosopher Lao Tsu gives advice in his great work, the *Tao Te Ching,* for those who would win a battle. He suggests that you allow "the water to rise and the mud to settle, so that the right action can arise by itself."

In order to practice what Lao Tsu teaches, you can do some simple tai chi push hands. Stand opposite a partner, your right feet parallel to each other, about a foot apart, your left foot angled at 45 degrees, about two feet behind the right. Cross your right wrists. Partner A will begin to move toward the center of Partner B's chest while Partner B retreats, sinking onto her back leg, offering no resistance. When A is almost touching, B switches her hips to the left, changing the direction of her partner's pushing hand. Then B comes forward, moving toward A's chest. If both partners are in harmony, you will continue this circle indefinitely, but if one decides to rush the action and take a risk at pushing, the yielding partner, just by waiting for his opponent to overcommit, is pretty certain to topple the pushing partner.

By listening to your partner's movements and staying in harmony, the two of you can learn exactly when "the right action arises by itself."

SAD *(Seasonal Affective Disorder)*

see also Death, thoughts of, page 109; Depression, page 112; Hopelessness, page 226; Light Therapy, page 273; Sleep Disorders, page 404

When the dark time of the year comes around, it's not unusual to feel sad, tired, uncreative, and just plain miserable. About 11 million Americans, or approximately 4 percent of the population, suffer from a clinical disorder that is characterized by winter depression. Most sufferers start to feel the symptoms at Halloween, and they generally last until the first crocuses are up in March.

If you notice that your moods are substantially different from fall/winter to spring/summer, you may have this disorder. Early diagnosis is the key—children as young as two have been known to suffer from this mix-up in circadian rhythms.

■ *What Happens When You Have SAD*

You have no energy to get out of bed in the morning; you feel listless and heavy, as though your body weighed a ton; you are sad almost all the time; you feel a need to sleep a lot or to nap during the day and then stay up most of the night; you have little control of your appetite and eat much more than usual.

SAD is caused by a disruption in the body clock, or circadian rhythms that constitute the cycle of day and night, waking and sleeping. The pineal gland deep inside the brain produces the hormones serotonin (the "feel-good" substance moderated by Prozac and similar drugs) and melatonin (the hormone that controls our sleep/wake cycle, our reproductive cycle, and also triggers hibernation and migration in animals and birds). When winter comes and it's darker for more of the day, we have higher peaks of melatonin that last longer, and this can cause imbalances in natural circadian rhythms. Melatonin affects mood because of its indirect suppression of a pituitary hormone called ACTH, which activates the adrenal glands and triggers the production of the stress hormone, cortisol. With melatonin imbalance, you have less serotonin (which makes you feel happy) and more cortisol (which makes you feel stressed out).

Simply getting outside more doesn't do the trick for SAD sufferers; it takes brighter than average daylight and several other therapeutic measures if you want to restore the "winter" body and mind to a healthy "summer" perspective.

Look at the Light

Daily treatment of an hour's exposure in front of a full-spectrum 10,000-lux fluorescent white light box (see Resource Guide, page 475) should be started by the beginning of November and continued through early spring (depending on your time zone). This can regulate your natural melatonin production. Most experts feel that you should be getting light therapy during your last hours of morning sleep in order for the treatment to be effective, so you'll need a timer to turn your lamp on at about 4 A.M. or 5 A.M.

Try a Little Melatonin

If you wish to supplement melatonin to alleviate your depression, you should consult your doctor to see whether this treatment is appropriate for you. If you do decide to supplement this hormone, take the lowest dosage possible—no more than 1 mg. daily taken one or two hours before bed. Although it would seem that someone with SAD needs less rather than more melatonin, the problem with this disorder is really an irregularity in cycling rather than an overabundance of the hormone. Careful and judicious supplementation can get the system working more efficiently.

Homeopathic Help

Try the following remedies for SAD:

If you are overworked and overtired and often think too much about your problems: Sulphur, Calcarea carbonica, Lycopodium

If you are a hardworking overachiever and very sensitive to the lack of light: Aurum metallicum (aurum is made from gold, which sheds its own natural light)

If you have general SAD symptoms—lethargy, listlessness, sleepiness: Nux vomica, Mercurius, Rhus toxicodendron, Phosphorus

Go Away to the Sun

It's a good idea to map out your vacation time for winter so that you can escape for a few weeks to the sun when you really need it. If you can, arrange business trips or family excursions to warm places with lots of daylight.

Exercise at Noon

Although most individuals comply better with a morning exercise program, it's more important for a SAD sufferer to be outside at the peak of the day when the sun is brightest. The more aerobic your exercise, the better, since this is another way to trigger the beta endophins in your brain that fill you with a sense of well-being.

Eat to Win

Your diet should be heavy on complex carbohydrates, light on fat and protein. You should eliminate all processed foods from your diet. Start your day with cereal and fruit, have a salad and whole-grain bread for lunch, and a hearty vegetable/legume stew for dinner. Be sure to drink at least eight to ten glasses of pure spring water or juices mixed with water daily.

SADNESS/DESPONDENCY

see also Depression, page 112; Hopelessness, page 226; SAD, page 373; Tearfulness, page 421

Sadness—in its more potent form, despondency—is the capacity we have as humans to mourn events or people. It is our response to loss and is certainly not a self-destructive quality if we have it every once in a while, when it's appropriate to the situation. Whereas the blues is a feeling we may get for no reason at all—just because we're down and out— sadness generally relates to a specific thing or individual we can no longer connect with. Despondency is a deeper feeling of discouragement, dejection, or depression; it lies just on the edge of hopelessness.

What Happens When You Feel Sad or Despondent

The world is a gray place, and you feel gray inside it. Your limbs and head feel heavy, and nothing you can do will rouse you from your mood. The pervasive sense of loss makes you feel like crying (although sometimes you're numb and can't get a tear out) and temporarily takes away your ability to feel joy in everything else. Although you can see an end to this cloud hanging over you, you feel snug inside it, as though being encased in your mournful feelings protects you from having to deal with others. There are times when you just want to sit and sigh, and that's a helpful release for the anguish that has built up inside you.

Sadness is often triggered by memory. We can dredge up an event or a loss—or something we wanted to happen that never did—and re-create the feelings we had years before. We can have great nostalgia for something that was inconsequential at the time and feel terribly sad (in the present) as we re-create the past, but just the way we'd like to remember it. Way back then, we didn't feel sad; we were too young or immature to "get" it. But the realization of what we missed explodes our old innocence, and we mourn the self or the experience it's too late to recapture.

Sadness can be an overlay on a personality that never goes away. Certain people just feel sad about everything, from bad reports on the TV news to not making enough money to going to the zoo and thinking about the plight of endangered species. We call such people "sad-sacks," and they are generally the butt of jokes. If you always see the glass as half empty, and nothing is ever very good, then you can't get out of the ruts you have put yourself into.

Real loss, however, *should* make you feel sad. The death of a loved one, the breakup of a relationship, a fight with somebody you care about, a lousy tax bill—these are all good reasons to sigh and moan. Sometimes, we just want to get into our sadness and wallow in it. There's nothing wrong with that as long as it has an ending and you can move on.

Get the Sighs Out

It's therapeutic to sigh, so do it as much and as often as you want. There's a quality to sadness that makes you feel stuck inside your feelings, so by taking a deep breath and letting it out with a long sighing sound, you can expel some of the stale air and toxic carbon dioxide that help to make you feel miserable. Crying is another way to take deeper breaths and flood the body with healing oxygen, which in turn can help to trigger the release of "feel-good" neurotransmitters in the brain, so give into your feelings and express them.

Use a Bioenergetic Release

The therapeutic process of bioenergetics recommends body-work that stretches your mind and emotions. The traditional exercises of bending backwards over a stool and pounding a bed with a bat or your fists can be enormously helpful for dealing with sadness. Very often, if you're not aware of why you're feeling this way, the release of the exercises under a therapist's supervision will give you some clues. You may be astounded (or perhaps a little frightened) at the explosion of emotions that can come from bioenergetic treatment. It's possible that your feelings of despondency may be part of a bigger problem—clinical depression or bipolar disorder—which you haven't been able to face until now.

Rent a Funny Movie

When you are feeling sad about real life, it's sometimes hard to see your actual problems logically. But fantasy and fiction have nothing to do with you, and as you stand outside yourself looking at someone else's trials and tribulations, it's easier to get perspective.

Norman Cousins first recommended watching comedies in order to take his mind off the disease that left him in excruciating pain and nearly killed him. His "laughter" therapy has been used time and again with great success by those with physical and mental ailments. When you watch the Marx Brothers or the Three Stooges, there's no way you can concentrate on your sadness. And the action of laughing about problems too ridiculous to take seriously can often turn around your rigid thinking about your own difficulties.

Run Around Your Pain

Exercise is one of the best ways to beat depression of any type. As we get aerobic, raising our heart rate, respiration, and blood pressure, we also trigger the release of endorphins, the natural opiates in the brain that make us feel better. The runner's "high" not only provides a flush of good feelings, it also appears to clear the mind so that you can think about things you might not consider when you're sedentary. Many individuals who run daily say that they always come back from a workout refreshed, and with one or several plans of action for a problem or issue that's been troubling them.

Eat Right for a Brighter Outlook

It's crucial that you avoid junk food, caffeine, sucrose, and particularly alcohol (which is a depressant and will only make you feel sadder). And even though you may lose your appetite when you're low, it's vital to keep up your strength and have a well-balanced diet rather than grabbing a snack here and there when you think about it.

Concentrate on whole foods, including lots of carrots (for Vitamin A and beta carotene), green leafy vegetables (a good source of folate and calcium), citrus and other fruits (for Vitamin C), and whole grains and cereals. (You might want to cut way down on red meat and dairy products while you're feeling sad because they are harder to digest and a lot of your body's energy is now being expended on your emotional needs.)

Many sad individuals crave carbohydrates and consume great amounts of candy (particularly chocolate), cookies, and cake. These are not the kinds of carbohydrates that supply your needed energy, however. If you feel a craving coming on, eat a bagel with no spread on it, or have a bowl of pasta.

Deficiencies of folate and Vitamins B_6 and B_{12} are common in many types of depression; these are two micronutrients you should supplement when you're feeling low. Take 200 to 400 mcg. folate, 200 to 400 mcg. of B_{12}, and 100 to 200 mg. of B_6. Other vitamins and minerals that may reduce feelings of sadness and depression are B-complex (50 mg. in a multivitamin tablet), niacinamide (500 mg. three times daily), niacin (50 mg. three times daily with meals), pantothenic acid (500 mg. twice daily), pyridoxine (50 mg. three times daily), Vitamin C (1,000 mg. daily), Vitamin E (400 IU daily), calcium (1,000 mg. daily at bedtime), magnesium (400 mg. daily at bedtime), and zinc (22 mg. zinc sulfate twice daily).

Get Support

Sadness is not always sharable, but others who aren't feeling sad can be a good barometer of your feelings. When you talk to a friend, a group, or a counselor about your loss or your pervasive sense of mourning, you have to articulate what it is that's getting to you. Sometimes, making sense of sadness for another helps you to organize your feelings and see how they've gotten out of hand. Then, too, others may have been through the same experience you have and can give you perspective on how you might feel in the future when this wave of despondency has passed.

Go Dancing

The whirling dervishes understood that dance can put you into a trance where it may be easier to deal with deep feelings generated from within. When we truly let go in a dance and give ourselves to the rhythm and momentum of the beat, we are transported onto a different plane, where daily troubles become just a part of the bigger picture.

Whether you do this exercise at home in your living room with the rug rolled back, or in a club at night, with lights blinking and music pounding in your chest, you can derive a lot of benefit from letting your body take over. Be sure to include lots of bending and swaying (which serve as the type of self-comforting postures that babies do when they rock forward and back). Whirling around in circles is disorienting in a good way—you have to trust that you'll land back where you started—and this is also an important lesson to learn about your emotions.

It can be calming and soothing as well as cathartic to dance with a partner who holds you tight so that nothing can happen to you. Stop pushing yourself and let someone else lead; this may help you to let go of the need to control your emotions and rectify your depressed state. When you stop trying so hard and just stay in the moment, you can effect real change in your feelings and behavior.

Let a Flower Cheer You Up

The Bach flower remedy for despondency and dejection is Gentian. Take 5 to 6 drops under the tongue or mixed with half a glass of water as needed.

*S**ELF-ESTEEM*

If you like and trust yourself, you can like and trust others. But most people are either unsure of themselves and their effect on the world, or they devalue themselves at every opportunity, and this can lead to a lowered self-concept. The concept you have—that is, the image you develop of yourself—is in great part based on the feedback you get from others about things you do and ways you act, and most important, on the way that others gravitate toward you or shy away from you.

We are all indoctrinated at an early age with thoughts about how "good" or "bad" we are from usually well-meaning parents who make common mistakes in developing their children's self-concept. If our parents are always critical and point out our weaknesses, how can we disagree? If our parents are always praising, and never offer a correction even when we need it, how can we ever gain perspective on who we are and what we're worth?

Self-concept includes self-awareness, self-worth, self-love, self-confidence, self-respect, and self-esteem. Although most people think of this last feature as the one that counts when we're feeling low and can't give ourselves proper due, the truth of the matter is that self-esteem is based on the other facets of self-concept.

Awareness: We have to see that our being here makes a difference. When we're aware of ourselves, we see the impact we have on others.

Worth: We are given the right to life, liberty, and happiness at birth, and no one can take those inborn rights away from us. We are born and we die just as "worthy" as anyone else on the planet.

Love: We are born with the ability to forgive ourselves and have compassion for our faults. Self-love is a way of saying this is me—imperfect, perhaps, but at least for now, that's okay.

Confidence: We must learn to deal with the world, taking it on or backing away from it. The more self-confidence we have, the easier it is to achieve goals and see our plans come to fruition.

Respect: We must be able to honor our own personality and emotional makeup and make no apologies for our reactions to life.

Esteem: We earn compassion for ourselves through our actions. The more we attempt, the more potential for success we have in the world, and the more self-esteem we develop.

The problem with self-esteem is that external successes are a shallow way of measuring one's achievements. You may be great at sports when you're young, but if you can't play in later life because of age or disability, how can you have good self-esteem? You may excel in school, but after you've graduated, no one gives you credit for getting all A's.

This means that self-esteem must be built from within. Because you are given a sense of worth and love, and because you can develop an awareness, confidence, and respect for who you are as well as what you do, it's possible that self-esteem can grow as you mature.

In order to feel that you are a person worthy of esteem, you have to be honest with yourself, you have to learn how to get perspective on your real strengths and weaknesses, you must trust your intuition, and you must think positively about your life and everyone in it. These are not always easy goals to achieve.

When you feel anxious or depressed, self-esteem is usually the first part of you to go. The fear of failure, the conviction that others don't care about you or are out to get you, a codependency on others who abuse or criticize you, can wipe out your motivation to look at yourself differently. And of course, this leads to a vicious cycle of feeling rotten about yourself and therefore accepting depression as your due.

It's been found that those with low self-esteem who expect to do poorly in relationships, jobs, or life in general get their prophecies fulfilled. In fact, they don't perform as well socially, creatively, psychologically, or physiologically. They tend to take things personally and have a big backlog of anger and hostility to deal with all the time.

Lack of self-esteem may figure prominently in the way we handle chronic illness. Some studies show that many cancer patients tend to be helpless, hopeless, self-hating, and pessimistic. (It must be noted that this is a blame-the-victim view of a disease with many components, only one of which is personality.)

On the other hand, people with high self-esteem are far more able to survive trauma and recover more quickly from major and minor illnesses. People who are unafraid of change see a setback as a fleeting problem rather than an omen of continuing misery. They use their difficult change in circumstances as a means of enhancing their self-esteem; they challenge themselves to get better so that they can prove to themselves that they're worth the effort.

A useful suggestion about building your own self-esteem is to paint two different pictures each time you are confronted with a problem. Let's say you've been offered a promotion at work, but it's going to mean a stressful schedule, a demanding boss, and a team of individuals (with many, varied personality quirks) to supervise.

First, do the low self-esteem picture. You may first visualize turning down the job, convinced that you can't hack it. Those who've put you up for the promotion start to think less of you, and eventually you are ignored, even at the Christmas party. Or perhaps you accept the job, but it's way over your head. You feel the tension rising as you sit in a boardroom, about to make a presentation you're uncertain of. You can feel all eyes on you, and you're sweating freely.

The projects you start all fizzle, and your staff loses respect for you. Eventually, you're demoted or even asked to leave the company. You can't get a good reference for another job.

Now do your high self-esteem picture. You can visualize your new office, your high energy flowing, the respect you gain from your colleagues, and the completion of projects you've generated. You ask for feedback from your staff and can weigh the positive and negative comments dispassionately because you have good self-awareness. You learn each day how to turn adversity into triumph. How do these successes have an impact on the rest of your life? Can you see your personal relationships flourishing, your sense of confidence deepening, your monetary resources increasing?

It requires work and determination to pick the good scenario. You have to deal with problems instead of claiming you can't possibly try; you have to dig in your heels and keep at it even when everything looks bleak.

But the more you work at it, the more self-esteem you have. It is hard to undo years of damning yourself and give yourself a pat on the back when you deserve it, but the rewards can be greater than you think and will undoubtedly be a great asset in your mental and emotional health.

SELF-HYPNOSIS

The word "hypnosis" conjures up the picture of a cheap stage trick performed by a master of the con job with a swinging watch. But this is not really hypnosis. What actually happens when you go into a trance state is that you are brought to a level of consciousness not unlike that in meditation or prayer. If you can hypnotize yourself, you can calm your mental scene and put yourself into a quiet place where it is possible to give yourself suggestions for different attitudes and behaviors you might not accept while conscious. Hypnosis allows you to reevaluate your reactions to difficult situations with an open mind.

When you're hypnotized, you use your right brain—the intuitive, imaginative side—while keeping the left brain quiet so that its analytical function is put on hold. More alpha waves—those brain waves present during meditation—are available to the practitioner. Just as yogis can walk across a bed of hot coals and not be burned, or whirling dervishes can spin themselves for hours without falling, so can a person in hypnotic trance go inside to use emotional resources he cannot tap when he is in left-brain, beta-wave mode.

Certain personality types cannot be hypnotized; these are individuals who are highly rational, orderly, and analytical. People with addictive problems also have trouble being hypnotized, because they generally lack the concentration to stay with the process. Self-hypnosis requires an ability to let go and give into a nonlinear type of thinking.

A common self-hypnosis exercise is used by women in childbirth. The Lamaze and Grantly Read courses teach a kind of mental focus that changes the relationship between pain and comfort. Women who claim to have had moderately easy birthing experiences say that it wasn't that they didn't feel pain, but rather, that they were able to control the pain while it was going on. Also, that they were looking forward to holding their babies and could therefore temper pain with pleasure.

Hypnosis works splendidly to alleviate physical symptoms with emotional causes. A patient with asthma who is unable to breathe may be having respiratory problems because of some underlying anxiety. Once in a trance, it may be much easier for that person to get in touch with the terror that makes her hold her breath. A person with posttraumatic stress, who was unable to see after a rape experience, might allow herself to revisit the horror of the rape under hypnosis and resolve her revulsion about seeing her attacker.

Self-hypnosis can also be used as a preventive technique: When you feel that depression, panic, or a phobic reaction loom large, you can quickly put yourself into a trance and give yourself positive reinforcement to take care of the problem before it hits.

The Value of Being Hypnotized

If you have never been hypnotized, you probably think of this process as a scam, something you'd never let yourself in for. Or, perhaps, you have watched someone else fall easily into trance in a stage show or on television and wish that you were that suggestible and easygoing. The truth is that you have no idea about your own aptitude for this healing technique until you try it. If you really want to use self-hypnosis as a tool for better living, you must first change your attitude about what you can gain from this experience.

The psychoanalyst Dr. Herbert Spiegel, who created the format for most hypnosis used in medical and psychiatric treatment, determined that there are three basic principles that define the scope of hypnotic trance:

- Alterations of awareness are occurring in us from moment to moment, whether we are asleep or awake. Our brain waves are always fluctuating, taking in information from the outside world and processing it internally. This means that we all have a wide range of consciousness to borrow from.

- Hypnotic phenomena occur whether or not we think of them as such. The fact that you can suddenly stare off into space, unblinking, and clear your mind of all extraneous thought means that you have the capacity to induce trance and come out of it on your own.

- Hypnosis doesn't accomplish any miraculous healing that would not occur in a conventional state of consciousness—it just speeds up the process. You can more easily get in touch with the subtle workings of your mind-body in a hypnotic state, and this can allow you to take care of certain mental and emotional problems you may have been blocking or denying.

At least 70 percent of all individuals are able to use self-hypnosis for healing. About 25 percent may be biologically capable but their personalities won't allow them to utilize this ability; and 5 percent have such severe mental or emotional problems, they are not able to concentrate enough to enter a different state of consciousness.

It's clear that hypnosis can be an extremely effective way of dealing with certain traumas and conditions. But how do you get yourself to the point of being hypnotized? If you can find a therapist or social worker who is trained in using hypnosis, it's a good idea to have one session with a professional as your guide. Hypnosis is no longer considered quackery to much of the medical establishment and is in fact a benefit to a patient who may be too anxious to give a reasonable health history or to describe symptoms accurately.

Once you've had a professional check out your ability to be hypnotized and run a hypnotic induction profile on you (see below), you can do the same for yourself.

How to Hypnotize Yourself

The most telling trigger of a trance state, discovered by psychotherapist Dr. Herbert Spiegel, is called the "eye roll." He discovered that if you can see the whites of someone's eyes easily when he rolls the pupils upward, he can enter a hypnotic state. The idea behind this is that the longer you look up, the heavier your eyes get and the more they want to close on their own. Dr. Spiegel categorized people in levels from zero to four, four being the state where only the whites are visible. The person who can roll her eyes this far up is the easiest to hypnotize and the most receptive to using a trance state productively.

The reason the eye roll is effective in hypnosis is that it is the best way to get someone to close his eyes and relax. By concentrating directly on keeping the eyes up, you are allowing the brain to reverse what happens when you fall asleep—in fact hypnosis lets you pay attention in a way you cannot otherwise.

After experimenting with the eye roll, ask a friend to check and see how far up your eyes rotate. You can't yet make a definite statement about your ability to hypnotize yourself until you have tested out the hypnotic induction profile.

- On the count of one, allow your eyes to roll up.

- On the count of two, take a deep breath and hold it.

- On the count of three, relax as you close your eyes, and imagine yourself floating. Allow the breath to come quietly and easily now.

(This three count takes you into the trance state, and then, when you are ready, you will use the three count backwards to come out of the trance state.)

Now continue to experiment with your hypnotic control:

- Think of the floating feeling extending into your left hand. Touch the middle finger of your left hand with the middle finger of your right hand. Tell yourself that you cannot possibly keep your left hand in your lap—it is floating upward by itself like a balloon.

- Open your eyes and attempt to push the left hand down with the right. You will find that it floats back up again by itself. If you are ready, begin the backwards count:

- On three, you will close your eyes and allow them to roll upward.

- On two, you will take a deep breath and hold it.

- On one, you will open your eyes and come out of trance.

The goal of self-hypnosis is to teach yourself to master your symptoms rather than futilely expect that they will vanish by themselves. You have to take charge of your trance and of your commitment to change elements in your life that need attention.

SEXUAL DYSFUNCTIONS AND DISORDERS

see also Anorgasmia, page 38; Compulsive Sexual Activity, page 97; Impotence, page 241; Humiliation, page 228; Loss of Libido, page 280; Shame, page 393

We all spend a lot of time thinking about sex and desire a good sex life, yet many people are either terrified or frustrated by their sexuality. It is conceivable that we are all born with a perfectly healthy orientation toward our gender and our passion; yet somewhere along the way, usually in the first six years of life, we meet with family, society, or personal stumbling blocks and begin to develop fears that can lead to sexual dysfunctions.

■ Overcoming Our Sexual Past

Everyone is born a sexual being and begins to explore his or her own sexuality during the first year of life. Unfortunately, however, this healthy inclination to learn about one's body (and the various feelings that trigger its pleasures), is often thwarted by family, peers, school, and religious belief. Those children who are punished for masturbating, or told that they will "go to hell" for having touched another child's genitals, may be stunted from normal sexual growth. The other, and even more horrible side of the coin, is being introduced to the world of adult sexuality via the forbidden door of incest or abuse. The kind of shame that we carry with us—often a lifetime burden—can cut us off from the belief that our bodies are beautiful and that we have needs with reasonable outlets that we should be able to explore and invent on our own. Rape and abuse in adult life also thwart healthy sexual feeling.

The myths that keep us from healthy sex ("Homosexuality is a perversion." "The only acceptable sex is that which leads to reproduction." "Men are attracted only by big breasts." "Women are attracted only by large penises.") can bring on periods of real despair, particularly if we don't have enough self-esteem to correct the misimpressions society has handed us. People who grow up thinking that they are "bad" may be unable to have orgasms, may crave multiple but anonymous sex partners, or may give up on sex altogether.

A good love relationship—between a man and woman if they are heterosexual, and between two men or two women if they are homosexual—generally has a sexual component to it. And most, although not all people define "good sex" as that type of intimacy that mixes affection and fondness with physical passion. If we don't get that the first few times we hook up with a partner, we start to think there's something wrong with us, something that needs fixing. It's depressing if you don't want sex with the person you love, or you don't fall in love with the person who desires you sexually. It's also depressing if you really care for each other and really desire each other, but anxieties, depression, and miscommunication have kept you from developing a decent sex life.

Many people think they can "fix" what's wrong with their relationship by fixing their own personality. And one particularly thorny way of approaching this process is to take drugs that you hope will make you a warmer, deeper, sexier person. In fact, medication may do just the opposite.

Drugs and Sexuality

It is curious that one of the most popular antidepressants on the market, Prozac, is a chief culprit that robs people of sexual satisfaction. It has been found that fully one third of those patients who take this mood-altering drug lose all interest in sex and ability to orgasm. In clinical studies, sexual dysfunction developed at the lowest dosage of the medication (20 mg. daily). So many people have been so upset by this unexpected side effect that they stop taking the drug, and their depression and anxiety return full force (which, in turn, have an impact on their sex lives). Although other serotonin reuptake inhibitors like Wellbutrin and Effexor seem to be less harmful to the libido, they don't work on symptoms exactly the way Prozac does, so they may not be an efficient replacement.

The same neurotransmitter found in Prozac—serotonin—is released naturally when you're involved intimately with another human being. And as long as your sex life includes affection and respect for the other individual with whom you're involved, it's far better to get this "feel-good" substance at the source, right in the mind and body.

Moving Onto a Sexual Future

So what do you do if you're anorgasmic, if you have compulsive sexual fantasies that you act out, if you feel shame and humiliation every time you touch yourself or you take your clothes off in front of a lover, or if you are numb sexually and can't even remember what it was like to feel desire?

The first goal that transcends your sexuality and your dysfunction is to find out what you like about yourself as a person. You cannot be vulnerable with a partner until you feel comfortable about your body, your mind, the way you approach others, and the way you accept pleasure.

You have to awaken your sensuality before you can become a healthy sexual person. Sometimes a simple experience like having a massage, taking a sauna or steambath, or lying in a field and listening to the birds as you smell the grass around you can change your outlook on what turns you on.

Next, you have to feel secure with a partner doing things that aren't sexual. The biggest clue to whether or not you'll get along in bed is if you can talk and laugh and be quiet together. It's vital that you trust this individual with secrets and funny habits you may have. If you can cook a meal with this person, or if you can go dancing and keep the beat together, there's a pretty good chance that you'll enjoy sleeping together.

If you have been having sexual problems for a long time, don't expect natural therapies to cure them overnight. Reclaiming sexuality takes time. You need to talk to your partner, establish ground rules that will make you feel comfortable, and work together on achieving balance together. Try to be forgiving of your own weaknesses; if you get to the brink of your difficulty and can't go any further, that's fine, too. Make a little progress slowly, and eventually you will conquer the dragon.

Healing sexual dysfunction can be a vital step in mental and emotional well-being. When we truly like ourselves and feel the joy bursting out of us, that's when we are the most erotic and playful. Understanding our needs and fears will bring us closer to the harmony we all strive for in every part of our life.

Treatments to try: Aromatherapy, page 46; Ayurvedic medicine, page 49; Chinese medicine, page 90; Drug rehabilitation, page 135; Herbalism, page 216; Homeopathy, page 221; Massage, page 286, Support groups, page 414.

SEXUALITY

Sexuality has rarely been explored as a therapy for mental or emotional health, but in fact, it can be one of the most beneficial treatments available.

Our sexuality is strongly bound to our sense of ourselves. When we are first held close by a parent, that touch becomes the chief focus of our nourishment, caring, and sense of well-being. And over the years, as we figure out just what it is that makes us appealing to ourselves and to others, that primal desire to be held and cared for becomes a vital force in our development as healthy adults.

Harry Harlow's landmark experiments with monkeys deprived of their mothers have been re-created many times and show us the impact of maternal touch. The baby monkeys who were given only a wire figure to represent their mother refused to eat, defecated where they slept, and became hostile and territorial around other monkeys. But those animals who were given a padded surrogate strung up with a bottle they could nurse at, played with, groomed, and petted the creature as though it were real and turned out socialized and well adjusted.

It's been shown that gentled rats and rabbits injected with pathogens remain healthy and active much longer than those animals who are not touched and cuddled. Studies on orphaned children show astounding progress from nearly sociopathic behavior (head banging, rocking, slowed cognitive and social development) to perfectly normal as soon as they are picked up and carried several hours a day.

Why is touch so vital to our existence? One reason is that our muscles relax when we are touched appropriately (by ourselves or by another), and since anxiety and stress produce huge amounts of tension in the body, this therapeutic effect works on the mind as well as the body. The skin itself is a superconductor, with nerve endings all over that connect to the spinal cord and brain. Warmth, pressure, wetness, vibration, and tingling are all important messages conveyed through the skin that make us feel good and let us know we're being taken care of.

Touch is the physical part of sexuality, and it's usually what draws us to a partner in the first place, but the benefits go far beyond this first dimension. Our sexuality has advantages that can be extremely therapeutic, particularly when we think about how we feel and think about ourselves and a partner. Mentally, we have to be aware and attuned to our needs; emotionally, we have to trust that deep well of feelings; spiritually, we need to rise above the daily concerns that keep us bound to old patterns, depressive tendencies, and anxious reactions.

■ *What a Healthy Perspective on Sex Can Do for Us*

Healthy sensuality and sexuality inform our relationships with rich possibilities. They also teach us a great deal about our sense of self. When we like the person we see naked in the mirror, we radiate an effectiveness and an excitement that is positively infectious. When you're at your best sexually, you are more creative, more spontaneous, and able to see the bigger picture. The petty problems that occasionally drag us down take on less urgency when we embrace another and for a brief time, become "one soul in two bodies."

Boosting the Immune System—and Other Benefits

Our sexuality affects every part of us: the endocrine system, the brain and nervous system, the cardiovascular system, the musculoskeletal system, the respiratory system, and quite possibly, the immune system.

The endocrine system pumps hormones that interact with brain neurotransmitters to give you a sense of well-being. The nervous system puts out serotonin and dopamine (in addition to other neurotransmitters), both of which stimulate significant emotional reactions. The cardiovascular system keeps the heart and circulation healthy, and all the exercise you get from sexual activity keeps the bones strong and the tendons and ligaments flexible. The respiratory system is greatly stimulated—when we're excited, we breathe more heavily, which sends oxygen through the tissues and releases carbon dioxide from the body. There are several interesting studies on the immune protection of sexuality as well. It's been found that women with breast cancer who describe their sex lives as "excellent" have higher numbers of T-cells (white blood cells that fight pathogens) than those women who have no sex life or consider their sex life unsatisfactory.

When all these systems are working at peak performance levels, we are in balance. We feel and look better, and these advantages make us more resilient and better able to handle adversity.

How Sexuality Fights Depression and Anxiety

It's been shown that sexuality can be a partner in the battle against depression. Those individuals who are afflicted with this condition often talk about the fact that they feel physically numb, as though they were paralyzed. They have difficulty "feeling," whether it's emotional or physical. But a loving partner who will stroke, kiss, caress, and cuddle can sometime be the key to a breakthrough. By opening up the body and the various energy centers sexually, it's often possible to clear away the heavy curtains of doom, mistrust, and hopelessness.

People who are sexually comfortable tend to be better leaders and better followers. They can let go and be vulnerable; they can also take charge of a partner and initiate different activities. Their bodies respond in the same way—when they're involved, they are as awake and aware as they can be; when they're relaxing in the afterglow of a sexual encounter, they can fall asleep quickly and get down to deeper levels of sleep that restore and refresh the body.

A committed sex life with a loving partner also alleviates loneliness, which is a major factor in many cases of depression and anxiety. We can be surrounded by crowds of admirers and still feel isolated; but when we are bonded to someone who knows us and cares about our needs, we know for certain that we are not alone.

Perhaps because sex is one of the most primary and instinctual of human forms of expression, we can use it to join minds, emotions, and spirits, and lift ourselves out of our everyday concerns. The exchange of body fluids is not a necessary goal—the real sexual healing takes place when we acknowledge our true commitment in life to pleasure and joy. A touch, a kiss, a firm embrace can renew our faith in ourselves and in those we love.

S HAME

see also Anxiety, page 43; Sexual Dysfunction, page 387

Shame is the introspective quality of judging and censuring ourselves for something—real or imaginary—that we have done. It is also a weapon that can be used on another individual if we want to cast blame for some real or imagined fault. Shame often accompanies humiliation (see page 228). Parents often shame their children in a wrongheaded attempt to develop a "moral, ethical" individual. But this type of psychological abuse serves only to make a child feel like an outcast. No matter what he does—from masturbating to taking another child's toy to not cleaning his dinner plate—he is bad. And to a child, there is no cure for badness. It's a quality he fears he'll never shake, no matter how hard he tries. So he hangs his head in shame.

Over the years, we internalize the blaming parent and develop our own moral "policeman" who can do the job of inflicting guilt and inspiring shame just as efficiently as our mothers and fathers ever did.

■ What Happens When You Feel Ashamed

You are mortified and want to hide. You feel as though you're in deep disgrace, although no one knows about it. In a way, the internal punishment is worse than public humiliation, because you have to live with this feeling of being dirty and unworthy every minute of every day.

Shame, therefore, goes deeper and has more destructive psychological ramifications than guilt, which is generally a feeling of being sorry for some concrete thing you did or didn't do. Shame, on the other hand, doesn't necessarily have a hook; you can be ashamed of standing up to speak in front of a group (because you think you're unworthy), you can be ashamed of your large breasts or small penis, you can be ashamed because you survived a terrible earthquake in which many friends and relatives died.

Shame is generally apparent to others, even when they don't know what it is that's wrong with you. When you walk with your head down, your shoulders hunched and your feet dragging along, you are trying to hide from yourself, and become smaller and less significant until, finally, you vanish and your embarrassment vanishes with you.

But when you acknowledge that you may be punishing yourself unduly, and you start to hold your head up, you can deal with the issues that have caused you to feel so guilty and unworthy.

Tell Yourself You're Good

No matter what you're ashamed of, it can't be as awful as your perception of it, particularly if this is a longstanding belief of yours. Record the following affirmations into a tape recorder and play them to yourself before you go to bed at night and when you wake up:

I have a great deal to offer the world.

Regardless of the way I've thought about myself in the past, I can change.

I deserve to feel happy and comfortable with myself.

I feel proud when I hold my head high.

If someone were to write my epitaph tomorrow, they would find a great many good things to say about me.

Get Rid of Someone Else's Shame

If it's too difficult for you to banish your own shame from your mind, you may find it easier to pass the buck to a person you don't know. Think about some policeman who took bribes, or a person you read about in the paper who abandoned her baby, or a politician who's been sued for sexual harassment. Think not about the act this person has committed, but about the various problems that might have driven her to do something she'd regret later. Then find it in your heart to forgive this person.

If you can forgive a stranger for doing something at least as bad as what you've done, can you possibly have the compassion to forgive yourself?

Look at It Logically

Using cognitive therapy, you can see more clearly what it is you've done and find a solution.

Let us imagine that you are a married woman, and you are ashamed of having lustful feelings toward a friend of yours who also happens to be a woman. Think about the irrational beliefs that make you feel ashamed.

If my husband knew I felt this way, he'd divorce me.

Homosexual love is disgusting and degenerate, which means that I am disgusting and degenerate.

If I have these unrequited feelings my whole life I'll always be unfulfilled—and ashamed.

Now see how you can deal with these thoughts in a rational way: You really have no idea what your husband thinks about. He may have homosexual fantasies, too. Just because you have a fantasy doesn't mean you have to act on it, nor does it mean that you are abnormal if you desire something out of the mainstream. Second, homosexual relationships can be true and constant, or fickle and perverse, just as heterosexual relationships can. Finally, these feelings may be part of the stage of development you're currently in, and as you move along in your marriage and in your friendship with this woman, everything may change.

Stay in the present instead of jumping ahead to possibilities that may never happen and you will be able to retain a sense of well-being about yourself and your life.

By getting rid of false beliefs, you can begin to understand yourself better and create a more appropriate view of reality.

Try a Flower Remedy

The Bach flower remedy for those who feel unclean or ashamed is Crab Apple. Take 5 to 6 drops under the tongue or mixed with half a glass of water as needed.

Homeopathic Help

Try the following homeopathic remedies for shame:

For self-blame: Aconite, Arsenicum album, Aurum, Hyoscyamus, Ignatia, Natrum mur, Pulsatilla, Thuja

For humiliation: Pulsatilla, Sepia

For humiliation and shame, being put down: Aconite, Argentum nitrate, Aurum, Colocynthis, Ignatia, Lycopodium, Nux vomica, Pulsatilla, Sepia, Silica, Staphisagria, Sulphur

For embarrassment: Ignatia, Sulphur, Colocynthis, Platinus, Sepia, Staphisagria

Take a Deep Breath

When you feel worthless, you tend to contract physically—rounding your spine, lowering your head—which makes it harder to get a full breath. The yogic three-level breathing is ideal for anyone feeling shame or embarrassment.

Lie on the floor with your hand on your stomach. Inhale and expand your belly until it is completely full. Exhale, letting the belly deflate. On the next inhalation, fill your belly, then continue the breath into the chest. Exhale, first from the chest and then the belly. On the third inhalation, fill up the belly, then fill the chest, and finally, open the throat, which will bring more oxygen and energy into your head. Exhale, letting the breath out from the throat, the chest, and then the belly.

If you practice this nine times daily—three rounds lying down, three rounds sitting up, and three rounds standing—you will find that you feel more in touch with your body. You may also find that as you open your throat, you have a desire to make a sound. Go ahead and sigh, moan, or scream if you like. This is a great outlet, particularly if you have kept your shame hidden for years.

*S*HORTNESS OF *B*REATH *(Dyspnea)*

see also Agitation, page 21; Anxiety, page 43; Hyperventilation, page 231; Nervousness, page 304; Panic Disorders, page 344; Stress, page 407

A lack of air, or "air hunger," is a common symptom of stress, and the feeling, which is tantamount to being strangled, can be terrifying. Shortness of breath is the prelude to hyperventilation (see page 231) and may accompany other uncomfortable stress symptoms that come with panic attacks such as chest pains, racing heartbeat, butterflies or knots in the stomach, and a feeling of impending doom.

One of the primary reasons for shortness of breath is the tendency to take shallow breaths from the upper chest, mouth, and nose. When you don't get a full breath from the belly, from which you can fill up your back and lungs, you are severely deprived of oxygen. When you are gasping like a fish out of water, you may actually feel as if you're going to die. (You can rest assured that if you do black out from lack of oxygen and throwing off too much carbon dioxide, your breathing when you're unconscious will immediately revert to normal.)

▣ *What Happens When You Get Short of Breath*

It feels as if there's not enough air in the room, or if you're outside, that there's not sufficient air in the atmosphere. You suck in, inhaling as much as you can, then not exhaling properly but rather, inhaling again. It's as though you were breathing through a thick mask. You fill up much too soon, and the results give you no relief. The terror of never again getting enough oxygen inside you can make your heart start beating wildly. You clutch at your throat, certain you're about to have a heart attack.

If your breath is "short," you have to lengthen it. As soon as you realize this, you won't progress to hyperventilation, and you'll be fine.

Learn To Relax

Three different relaxation techniques will help you to regulate your breathing. The first, autogenic training (see page 48), asks you to sit quietly and concentrate on the quality of warmth and heaviness in your limbs and body. First, imagine your right arm being warm, heavy, and relaxed, then your left arm, then your two legs. You should spend some time thinking about the lungs and the belly and feeling how relaxed and open they are.

The second technique, progressive relaxation (see page 361) has you alternately tense and relax each part of the body, starting with the toes and progressing up the back of the body and head and down the front of the body. The third technique, visualization (page 442), can be used on its own or as an accompaniment to either of the other two techniques. In this type of exercise, you will imagine the breath as a steady, constant stream, effortlessly passing through your belly and lungs. See the interior of the lungs as infinitely flexible, allowing room inside for as much oxygen as you need.

Daily practice of one of these therapies will stand you in good stead when you are rushed or panicked and need a reminder so that you can calm down quickly.

Breathe for the Sheer Joy of Breathing

Play with your breath and find out its limitations. You'll want to practice lying down, sitting, and standing. First, don't make any conscious effort to alter your breath. Pay attention to the miraculous way in which your chest inflates and deflates without your doing anything at all. Remember that your brain stem controls breathing *even when you are not conscious.* If you tell yourself that you don't have to lift a finger to inflate an alveolar sac, you may feel more reassured. This process will go on whether you try to help it or not.

Then experiment with different types of breath: Do some fast belly breathing, muscularly moving the abdomen in and out. Now take some long, slow breaths in your chest. Then move up to your throat and see how restricted you are when you take air in only through this narrow column. Do some panting (like a dog on a hot day) and get out of breath; then allow your breath to return to normal and see how quickly you get back full function. Get on your hands and knees and breathe into your back, rounding it like a cat when you inhale and flattening it out when you exhale.

Feedback Some Information

Using biofeedback equipment, you will be able to monitor what happens to your breath when you are anxious. You will be hooked up with various electrodes attached to different parts of your body to a machine and asked to breathe normally; you'll be able to see the pattern on a readout screen in front of you. Then you'll be asked to imagine a horrible scenario (being in a traffic accident, getting fired, getting divorced), and you will undoubtedly see lights and hear bells as the machine reacts to your erratic breathing. As you practice one of the relaxation techniques mentioned above, you'll see the pattern on the screen revert to normal.

Press a Point

The acupuncture point that will calm your breathing and alleviate heart palpitations is Pe. 6, one and a half inches up from the crease of the wrist on the inside of the arm. You can also press the two *ding chuan* points on the back—they are one and a half inches out on either side of the cervical spine, parallel to the bone in the back of your neck that projects out farthest when you bend your head forward.

Laugh a Lot

When you laugh, you naturally take in more oxygen. So reading a funny book (try the short stories of Robert Benchley or the hilarious books by Dave Barry) or watching a funny movie can put you in stitches. Make sure that you notice how your breath feels when you're in the midst of a big belly laugh—how easy it is to get enough air when you feel happy and relaxed.

Breathe Like a Flower

The Bach flower remedy for panic is Rescue Remedy. It's a good idea to carry this in your purse or pocket at all times if you're prone to shortness of breath. Take 5 or 6 drops under the tongue or mixed in half a glass of water as needed.

SHYNESS

see also Anxiety, page 43; Fear of Public Speaking, page 180; Phobias, page 346; Stage Fright, page 407

Shyness is a fear of oneself as well as of other individuals. It can be minor (if you find it hard to make witty conversations at parties where you don't know people) or crippling (if you can't go out of the house for fear someone might speak to you) or anywhere in between. This social difficulty is extremely common in children, and some people grow out of it naturally, though others find it a lifelong challenge. Social phobias that develop after puberty can be more difficult to treat than childhood shyness, because when it occurs later in life, avoidance of people becomes a protective barrier against every unfamiliar, unpredictable turn and twist of life.

▓ What Happens When You Feel Shy

You cringe when you feel you're being made the center of attention, which seems to be nearly all the time. You feel conspicuous, as though you had all your clothes off in the middle of a busy street. When you're spoken to, you know you have to respond, but the words and ideas stick in your mouth. You may nod or murmur something vague (although you know the answer perfectly well) and move away quickly. If you're called on to speak—in a classroom or at your job— you may blush and stammer, your heart beating wildly, and find that your mind has gone completely blank with fear.

Shyness is usually a manifestation of one's personality— some people naturally feel more comfortable out of the lime- light and find it painful to be pushed forward. Shy people are usually introspective and enjoy their own company. It's only when your temperament is in conflict with your needs or desires or those of the family or community in which you live that you'll have a problem with being shy.

Shyness can be manifested as hostility, and many shy people appear to be brusque and unfriendly because they don't want the hassle of dealing with others. In an attempt to quell the extreme anxiety they feel in social situations, they often turn other people off with bad manners, rude com- ments, or piercing stares.

Some shy people—certainly not all—also lack self- esteem. They think so little of themselves it's hard for them to understand why anyone would bother to spend time with them. It's vital for these individuals to set goals for them- selves and achieve something of which they can be proud.

Get Desensitized

Many psychologists feel that the best cure for avoiding social interaction is to interact with as many people as possible. Volunteer to make a speech at school or work; audition for a play and take the part if you get it; find out about possibili- ties to be interviewed in your specialty on radio or TV; work for a politician and canvas the neighborhood, going from door to door to convince everyone to get out and vote. Using your social skills on a regular basis won't necessarily make it easier or more comfortable for you to be gregarious. But real- izing how well you accomplish your incredibly difficult task will fill you with self-worth and a new appreciation of your abilities.

Sit Down and Meditate

When you are completely alone with your thoughts and feelings, you can allow the most significant parts of yourself to emerge. Allow yourself at least 20 minutes a day to meditate and to sit quietly with no expectations. Begin by concentrating on your breath and sense the strength and power inside you. Imagine that your shyness is a small, young bud, tightly wrapped in your heart. You may want to admire it, leaving it just as closed as it is now; you can always come back to it another time.

As you practice daily, you may become curious about the scent of the flower inside, the color and shape of the petals, the arrangement of the stamens and pistils. You will have to agree to let go of your tight control in order to allow the flower to start its natural process of opening. Let the process take as long as it needs to. You will find the way as you look inside and trust your own gentle resources.

Meditation makes us more aware and alert to the possibilities around us. By practicing, we give back to our souls the peace that is often hard to come by in our busy lives.

Try Some Body Language

If speaking aloud is difficult, express yourself in body language, but do it in a big way. Shy people sometimes strive to make themselves disappear because they fear being seen. But this attempt to vanish makes you only more conscious of the body you're trying to hide. A good therapeutic technique for shyness is bodywork. You might want to try a few sessions of Alexander technique (see page 27) or Feldenkrais (see page 181) and experiment with the way you feel when you release various muscular blockages that have held you back from exploring the world more fully. You may be surprised and delighted to find that it feels good to move around and be seen.

Hypnotize Yourself

People can take suggestions during a trance state that they cannot accept when they're conscious. In order to hypnotize yourself, first sit quietly and allow your eyes to roll up. Take a deep breath and hold it. Then close your eyes gently, telling yourself that you are completely relaxed.

While you are in a trance, you can suggest that you are gregarious and affable with friends, that you enjoy sharing thoughts and feelings with those you are close to, and that you would like to be more socially active in the future. You might assign yourself a project under hypnosis. This should be something that you do have some interest in—like planning a party or running for your school board but have avoided because of your social phobia.

When you are feeling comfortable and determined, come out of trance. Inhale and hold your breath, open your eyes, let your breath out, and allow the feeling of contentment to wash over you.

Use the Aromas That Stimulate

If you're feeling stressed and need to relax in social situations, try Neroli or Lavender. If you're not feeling very brave and need uplifting, try Tangerine, Orange, Cedar, Spruce, Pine, or Rosewood. You can carry an essence in a vial in your purse or pocket; put some on a cotton ball and carry it in a plastic baggie for a quick inhalation when you feel you need it.

Although it's hard for a shy individual to get used to the touch of another, a professional massage can restore a sense of completeness and a feeling that you are connected to others, despite yourself. You might ask the massage therapist to use a soothing oil such as Geranium, Chamomile, Clary Sage, or Ylang-ylang.

Join a Group

One way that people cope with their shyness is to make their social circle increasingly small. If they're married, they don't socialize with friends; they may work for themselves or may select a profession (such as writing or research) in which they can be on their own a great deal of the time. In order to find out what the world is really like (maybe it's not so bad!), join a group that does something you're interested in—a hiking club, a great books discussion group, a martial arts class. Make sure you get out every week to meetings and work your way slowly into participating in talks and activities.

SLEEP DISORDERS

see also Drowsiness, page 130; Fatigue on Awakening, page 163; Falling Asleep, Difficulty, page 155; Insomnia; page 248; Interrupted Sleep, page 251; Nightmares and Night Terrors, page 309; Restless Leg Syndrome, page 365

The body has natural rhythms that are essential to the maintenance of the entire system, from the brain to the heart to the skeleton. Our circadian rhythms (from the Latin, meaning "around a day") tell us how to respond to light and darkness and when it's time to let go of our tensions and thoughts and drift off to sleep.

It is during this seven- or eight-hour interval of subconsciousness that we are able to replenish and restore the cells and energy lost during the day, consequently boosting our immune system so that it can keep us healthy. When we're overly worried or depressed, our brain waves tend to become unbalanced, and this can affect our sleep cycles, which, in turn, will affect our feeling and performance when we're awake. Because sleep is restful to the central nervous system, when we get enough of it we're able to be more relaxed, alert, and able to concentrate.

We know so little about what makes the brain do what it does, but we know that there are four stages of sleep and, in addition, a wakeful stage known as REM (rapid eye movement) sleep when we dream. During each night, we complete about four or five cycles of these various stages.

Waking brain waves (beta waves) are typically quick and irregular, whereas when we begin to relax and become drowsy, the patterns become more elongated. Stage I sleep is light and easy to break apart—occasionally the sensation of falling (which is actually a blip in brain wave activity) will bring us back to consciousness. But as we gather random images and breathe more deeply, we enter Stage II, and brain waves become larger and slower. Alpha waves, which are those we produce during meditation and which typically give us a feeling of well-being, may be seen in this stage, but they shift to delta waves about 20 minutes after falling asleep, when we are in Stage III. A few minutes later, we drop down to the deepest Stage IV, from which it's difficult to wake. It's at this time when the body can do the necessary work it's unable to accomplish when we're awake and functional. In Stage IV, when we don't need to digest food or process thoughts and feelings, we produce the greatest abundance of human growth hormone. This assists in the restoration of the mind and body. After remaining in this stage for about 10 or 20 minutes, we drift back up to Stage III and then Stage II sleep. When we are at the brink of waking, we enter REM sleep and are able to dream. During this sequence of sleep, the eyes dart around, the body twitches, and we are ready for action (even if it's the bizarre carnival of dream action).

Adults stay in Stage IV sleep for far less time than children do, and older adults may spend most of their sleep time in Stages II and III. But it is the REM and Stage IV sleep that is apparently the most beneficial, and if we're deprived of these our waking life may be severely disturbed. In laboratory studies in which volunteers were awakened just as they began to dream, they began the next day irritable and anxious.

It is thought that REM sleep is a type of survival mechanism for the body and mind—if we were back in the days of having to run from wild animals, this would be the stage closest to waking, in which we could get up and protect ourselves. When we sleep, our pulse rate slows, becoming lower than it has all day. This offers a rest to the circulatory system. During sleep, as the body rests and restores itself, the brain produces growth hormone and melatonin (which is the trigger for serotonin, the "feel-good" neurotransmitter).

REM sleep is a time when the nervous system is supremely active, yet the brain is relaxed in a subconscious state. At this time, also, the body produces steroids that help to bolster the immune system, assisting in our resistance to infection and also regulating our metabolism and energy output. So if we don't end up in REM sleep several times a night, we don't get the hormonal activity so vital to our good health.

Sleep patterns do change in middle and old age, and experts aren't yet sure whether this is the normal course of events or is caused by various disorders that occur at this time of life, such as sleep apnea (suspension of breathing for short periods) and leg cramps. Adults between 20 and 60 should get about seven to nine hours of sleep in order to reap all of its benefits; people over 60 can get by with six and a half to eight hours. Teenagers should get about nine hours and children between nine and twelve hours.

There are several types of sleep disorders:

- Difficulty in falling asleep, which is usually a simple problem of learning to relax and calm the mind.

- Insomnia (poor sleep), a more significant problem that may be caused by depression, anxiety, or stress and also may involve an inability to move smoothly from one stage of sleep to the next. Most poor sleepers are able to reach Stage IV only in the early portions of the night and tend to be more aroused during sleep. They have higher pulse rates and body temperatures than good sleepers. They may drop off to sleep easily and then awaken in a couple of hours, unable to get even a few moments relief for the rest of the night.

- Narcolepsy, a hair-trigger sleep mechanism that may spring into action at the most inappropriate times, causing a person to drop into deep sleep in the midst of regular activity. It is characterized by a continuation of REM sleep throughout the waking hours.

- Fatigue on awakening, which seems to be an indication that the body is not following its natural sleep patterns and may be running through the stages too quickly, or skipping some.

Most adults run through one cycle of all the stages in 90 or 100 minutes. We *need* this much time to discharge some of the instinctive drives that accumulate during the day: We get rid of unused energies involving sex, aggression, hunger, and fear as we sleep. If our sleep is disturbed, either internally because we are feeling miserable or excited, or externally by a partner's tossing and turning or noisy garbage collectors in the street, we don't get the opportunity to finish the important neurological chores of the day. Once or twice a month, this kind of disturbance is merely annoying; on a long-term basis, it can be damaging to the psyche and the physical body.

Treatments to try: Autogenic training, page 48; Ayurvedic medicine, page 49; Breathing, page 76; Dream analysis, page 127; Drug rehabilitation, page 135; Chinese medicine, page 90; Exercise, page 145; Herbalism, page 216; Homeopathy, page 221; Light therapy, page 273; Massage, page 286; Melatonin, page 294; Progressive relaxation, page 361; Self-hypnosis, page 383; Sexuality, page 390; Supplementation, page 409.

*S*TAGE *F*RIGHT

see Fear of Public Speaking, page 180

*S*TRESS

see also Agitation, page 21; Anger, page 31; Chest Pains, page 87; Distraction, page 121; Dizziness, page 124; Fatigue, page 158; Feeling of Impending Doom, page 238; Gastrointestinal Disorders, page 189; Headache, page 209; Hyperventilation, page 231; Insomnia, page 248; Jitteriness, page 260; Overeating, page 331; Palpitations, page 342; Panic Disorders, page 344; Rage, page 363; Sexual Dysfunctions and Disorders, page 387; Shortness of Breath, page 397; Tearfulness, page 421; Tension, page 425; Trembling, page 428

Stress is probably at the root of most difficulties you may experience throughout your life and includes a vast range of symptoms. We can't eliminate stress, but we certainly can learn to manage it without medication.

Stress is the feeling of being overwhelmed, under pressure, compelled to be or perform a certain way. It is generated by our perception of a situation, for example, you may feel incredible stress to meet deadlines at work, whereas your colleague, a laid-back, easygoing type, is never worried by them. We can be stressed externally by circumstance and environment, but most assuredly, our internal stress—the type we lay on ourselves—is the most damaging.

Stress stimulates a gland in the brain known as the hypothalamus, which is the master turn-on switch for all the other glands in the body. The hypothalamus, in turn, sends messages to the brain's pituitary gland, which sends chemical messages (hormones) to the nervous system and adrenal glands that something is wrong and needs immediate attention. The adrenals produces *stress hormones*—adrenaline, noradrenaline (or norepinephrine), and cortisol. These "fight-or-flight" hormones can severely tax the body's resources and the mind's ability to cope. Over time, as we continue to pour out these killer substances, we may develop chronic ailments such as cardiovascular disease, cancer, a lowered immune system, depression, and allergies.

CASE HISTORY

Janice set herself up for a stress crisis. She was the type of person who couldn't do anything halfway: She had to be a sexy, efficient, wonderful wife *and* be the employee of the month—every month—at her job as well. She was a great friend and daughter, too, tending her buddies and her aging mother like hothouse flowers. She was available, accessible, always eager to be as perfect as she could be in whatever setting she found herself.

And for many years, she juggled pretty well. As a clothing buyer for a major fashion designer, she was on the road half the year, which made coming home to Tim a wonderful, romantic adventure. They talked about kids, but tabled the notion every time the subject came up. Janice said, "I'm not cut out for baking brownies—or chaperoning Brownies."

On her thirty-ninth birthday, she woke up at 4 A.M. in a panic. Maybe she should quit her job and get pregnant; maybe she should ditch this killer career and become a massage therapist. Each day, the 4 A.M. reveille got more frantic. She started developing headaches, stomach aches, chest pains, and palpitations.

On a stress-related high, she gave her boss notice, then told Tim that night at a candlelit dinner. His panic about their suddenly reduced income caused a lot of friction between them, and their arguments escalated to an operatic pitch. Their sex life, which had been middling to good, was now nonexistent.

"Marriage stress on top of job stress was like a 500-pound weight on my shoulders. But quitting somehow doubled the load. The sensation was like crawling up smooth walls, with nowhere safe to land if I fell. My body was literally falling apart, and it made me feel helpless. First came the insomnia, then the headaches and chronic diarrhea. I thought sometimes that I was going out of my mind, and that was the scariest part, like Alice falling down the rabbit hole, that I'd never get back.

"I'd heard a lot about TM, so I took a course at my local adult school. I cut up my cigarettes one by one and flushed them down the toilet. I stopped buying junk food and turned on an exercise videotape every morning. In a couple of months, I felt okay enough about myself to buy some sexy lingerie (I set myself a $20 budget) to win Tim back in bed. The next thing is figuring out how we up the income again. But I've learned a lot—you have to take it one day at a time."

In order to learn how to cope with stress, you have to learn how to relax. But if your idea of relaxing is watching TV, going out to dinner, or playing golf, you are fooling yourself. These activities may be enjoyable, but they aren't teaching your mind to unfasten the various locks that hold you to your stress. Relaxation involves altering brain patterns by using practices that involve focus, centering, and concentration.

If you are under pressure, if you're ill, traveling a lot, or overly worried about something, you may notice that you cannot function as you usually do. Your relationships may suffer; you may be distracted at work, snap at strangers, and lose your sex drive—all for no apparent reason. You may begin to feel that life is unfair, that you aren't good enough to make it, and these feelings of lowered self-esteem can lead to depression.

Remember that happy incidents and thoughts, like being in love or having a baby, also produce stress, but this type of good *(eu-)* stress is challenging and strengthens us physically, mentally, and spiritually. The flip side of stress—*dis*-stress or stress beyond the ability of the person to adapt—is what causes disease. Stress is a part of life and therefore impossible to avoid; however, it can be *managed* in a systematic and positive way.

Treatments to try: Affirmations, page 16; Aromatherapy, page 46; Bach flower remedies, page 53; Behavioral therapy, page 55; Breathing, page 76; Cognitive awareness, page 94; Dancing, page 107; Drug rehabilitation, page 135; Exercise, page 145; Herbalism, page 216; Homeopathy, page 221; Meditation, page 292; Mindfulness, page 296; Negative ion therapy, page 303; Nutrition, page 316; Play therapy, page 348; Prayer, page 358; Self-esteem, page 380; Self-hypnosis, page 383; Sexuality, page 390; Supplementation, page 409; Tai chi chuan, page 417; Visualization, page 442; Yoga, page 457.

S UPPLEMENTATION

The average American diet supplies a modest amount of vitamins and minerals and keeps us nourished and almost healthy. However, there is a great deal of documentation that indicates we can improve our health and heal certain specific illnesses and conditions by supplementing particular vitamins and minerals.

A daily multivitamin is now considered a must for all adults, but if you want protection from mental and emotional problems, you will have to learn some specifics about what the various supplements do. They are most helpful as part of an overall program, including a good diet, a daily exercise regimen, and other natural remedies you will find in this book.

CASE HISTORY

When Meg's mother complained of chest pains at 91, Meg flew across the country to see her. She arrived in time for her death and pulled herself together enough to relocate her ailing father to her brother's house. Still dealing with her mother's death, Meg went for a routine gynecological exam and almost didn't believe it when the doctor told her he felt a lump in her breast.

"I couldn't get sick—I just couldn't afford to. I'd told my mother that I would fly out to see Dad once every six weeks, and I had to keep that promise. He was so distraught he'd fallen and broken a hip, and I was too worried about him to even think about my cancer. All I needed was a lumpectomy and radiation; but then in a couple of months, I had to have my ovaries removed. I never told my Dad about any of it, and within another month, he was dead, too.

"I felt very lost at first—no parents, and this awful scare hanging over me. I'm a Quaker, but when I heard I had cancer, I said, 'This is *war.*' So I went to a nutritionist who put me on 18 different vitamins, as well as lots of European and Chinese herbs—ginkgo, echinacea, astralagus, burdock root, and shitake. I was taking these before and after the surgeries, and I'd never felt better. I was exercising a lot—I even walked laps in the hospital, much to the amazement of the staff—and I got regular massages to get some of the toxins out of me and to relax me, too.

"I think I made my body strong so my mind wouldn't fall apart—and it didn't. I think the combination of elements—supplements, herbs, exercise, massage, and most of all, my will—was what got me through it."

▨ Vitamins for Better Mental Health

A vitamin is an organic substance that can't be created in the body. We ingest vitamins with our food, but some must be taken in a precursor form and converted to the active substance within the body.

The B-vitamins, in particular, have been long associated with good mental health, and in fact, are often called "the stress vitamins." They are necessary for optimal functioning of the nervous system, and a deficiency could easily bring on depression or irritability. Vitamin B_6 (pyridoxine) is particularly important in the synthesis of serotonin (the "feel-good" neurotransmitter). Supplementing B_6 can work wonders in the treatment of insomnia, irritability, obsessive-compulsive disorders, and depression. Several studies on B_1 (thiamin) and B_2 (riboflavin) have indicated that they are both useful in the treatment of nervous-system disorders—mental confusion, memory loss, and fatigue. Folic acid has also been tested on patients with depression, with good results. One additional compound known as SAM (S-adenosyl methionine) has been found to be as effective as antidepressants in the treatment of depression.

Vitamin C is also essential to ward off stress. If you are having a particularly stressful time, perhaps around the holidays or during exam week or before a big crunch on a project at work, extra vitamin C may reduce the harmful effects of the stress hormones and improve your body's ability to handle the fight-or-flight reaction.

Vitamin E is a fat-soluble vitamin and has been tested on children with neurological problems who had difficulty absorbing fats and fat-soluble vitamins. But their degeneration improved greatly with supplemental doses of Vitamin E.

Minerals for Better Mental Health

Minerals are inorganic substances that remain after living plant or animal tissue is burned off. They work together with enzymes, hormones, and vitamins to assist with nerve transmission, muscle contraction, cell permeability, tissue integrity and structure, protein metabolism, blood formation, energy production, and fluid regulation.

Minerals can do their work in the body alone or in groups; but on the other hand, they can also compete with each other for absorption.

When you're under a lot of stress, your tissue stores of magnesium are depleted and you excrete more of this mineral in your urine. Magnesium is also important to ensure good sleep patterns with less waking during the night.

Zinc is also related to stress-induced problems. If you're zinc-deficient, your body will not be as able to repair damaged tissues, and your immune response will be lowered.

Iron can be essential to good sleep. Studies show that people with low iron intake are subject to fatigue (see page 158) and interrupted sleep (see page 251) and that they need longer total sleep time. Iron has also been given to improve cognitive function in children with behavior disorders such as ADD and ADHD (see page 13).

Supplementing Amino Acids

The 22 amino acids are the building blocks of protein—the body actually manufactures all but eight of them—and they can be recombined and recycled once you've taken in the requisite amount.

Tryptophan, found in milk and other protein-rich foods, is the precursor to serotonin. Taking more tryptophan (a gram a day) into your system just before bed increases blood and brain levels of this useful neurotransmitter, and studies have shown that this reduces the time necessary to fall asleep by 50 percent in many individuals. Overdoing the tryptophan, however, may bring on liver toxicity and other side effects. The product, L-tryptophan, was taken off the market in health food stores several years ago because of contaminated batches, but you can still supplement this amino acid by taking combination herbal stress formulas that include up to 100 mg. of tryptophan.

The Best Supplements Are the Natural Ones

Of course synthetic supplements are available (and cheaply bought) in the supermarket and drugstore, but it's best to use natural brands with no additives. A health-food store or mail-order catalogue (where you can buy in bulk and save money) is your best source. The products they offer contain no sugar, salt, preservatives, artificial colors, flavors, or sweeteners.

They also offer plant-based gelatin capsules as opposed to animal-based gelatins.

The delicate balance of what you put into your system does affect mental as well as physical health. This means that it's best to use natural products, and this is particularly important if you're treating a child with a condition such as ADD or an eating disorder, where what goes into the body is so essential to good, effective therapy.

Antioxidants Can Clear Your Mind

Antioxidants are helpful scavengers that roam the body sweeping up "free radicals," the harmful byproducts of oxidation that occur in the course of millions of different chemical reactions. Free radicals are found in air pollution, tobacco smoke, and rancid fats and are also spun off in the normal breakdown process of the body's metabolism. They are the culprits in destroying tissue elasticity (which causes wrinkles) and harden the lens of the eye, forming cataracts. Many mental conditions are aided and abetted by antioxidant damage in the body—the memory loss, confusion, and irritability we sometimes see in the elderly can, in many cases, be traced to atheromatous plaques, which form on the insides of arteries as cholesterol is oxidized in the blood and brain.

But if you supplement your diet daily with antioxidant vitamins, you are striking a protective blow against this process. Vitamins A (and its precursor, beta carotene), C, and E are the vital antioxidants that attack the free radicals and move them out of the body. They are able to shield the blood vessels that become increasingly susceptible to oxidation over the years. Antioxidants deactivate free radicals and stop them from branching out and destroying the molecular structure of cells. They also add an extra barrier against free radicals by strengthening cells walls so that they cannot invade.

RDAs and Dosage

The Food and Drug Administration set the "recommended daily allowances" of vitamins and minerals to establish what level you'd have to have in your system so as not to have a deficiency. However, these RDAs are much too low to effect any change in your system, particularly when you're working to improve mental and emotional health. Vitamin and mineral dosages are designated as *mg.* (milligrams), *mcg.* (micrograms), or *IU* (international units).

Keep in mind that you can go overboard in your supplementation and begin to have side effects or adverse reactions if you take too much of particular supplements. Vitamins A and D can be toxic in large amounts, and megadoses of Vitamin C can cause gastrointestinal upset, particularly in those who aren't used to such high supplementation. The following are daily high dosages of the various mind-friendly vitamins and minerals up to safe levels that have been suggested in the current scientific literature. Children under 12 should receive one third to one half these dosages, depending on body weight:

Folic acid	400 to 2000 mcg.
Iron	10 to 50 mg.
Calcium	1000 – 1500 mg.
Magnesium	400 – 700 mg.
Zinc	20 to 100 mg.
Vitamin A	10,000 mg.
Thiamin (B_1)	10 to 200 mg.
Niacin (B_3)	100 – 4000 mg.
Pyridoxine (B_6)	10 – 200 mg.
Riboflavin (B_2)	10 – 50 mg.
Vitamin B_{12}	10 – 1000 mcg.
Vitamin C	50 – 10,000 mg.
Vitamin E	100 to 1000 IU

If you intend to change your nutritional status by supplementing daily, it's a good idea to consult your physician or a certified nutritionist, particularly if you have a specific mental or emotional condition.

SUPPORT GROUPS

It has been widely reported in the medical literature that groups provide positive support for anyone going through difficult change and make it possible for the one struggling with a problem to lean on others. Being a member of a group means that you are not alone and also means that you have the responsibility to help others as well as to receive help yourself. Groups bond in exceptionally strong ways; the enormous success of Alcoholics Anonymous and other 12-step organizations is indicative of the power of the many to buoy up one in trouble. Groups exist for every possible purpose: from the support of cancer survivors to those overly concerned with their weight to those who have kids in jail to those whose children are dying of AIDS.

Groups are bound by a common experience—in other words, the members know their problems (and possible solutions) far better than any counselor or therapist can. When you get together with a group of peers, you can really explore your own feelings of isolation and loss of control in a safe setting. A group situation reminds us that we are not alone in our pain or fear, that there are always loving looks, hands, and words to comfort us.

Dr. David Spiegel, a professor of psychiatry and behavioral sciences at Stanford, has reported extraordinary results of women with cancer who formed support groups. These women were able to let out all their feelings and discuss the difficult issues such as death and facing pain, issues they weren't able to talk about with spouses or parents or children they might have hurt or who might not have understood. The women in groups tended to live twice as long after their cancer diagnosis as those who had just chemotherapy but were not in groups. They had to be there for one another; they couldn't let go of life when they had so many counting on them. The atmosphere of complete trust among the group members actually altered their stress and immune responses.

In order for anyone else to truly grasp a situation we are going through, they must "walk in our moccasins," as the Native American saying goes. In a support group, everyone wears those shoes, even if they're not the same size or color. According to Carl Jung, when we share sorrows or difficulties we become "wounded healers." We are experts who can mutually console one another because we have intimate experience with that particular wound and its manifestations.

In order to find a group that will address your problem, start by calling the public relations department of your local hospital to see if there is a group already established. You can also check the "community resources" section of your local

phone book. If no such group exists, think about starting one
yourself. You can put up notices at your supermarket or on a
church or synagogue bulletin board, or if you're computer-
savvy, you can start or join a forum on the Internet that
addresses your problem.

*T*AI *C*HI *C*HUAN

Tai chi chuan, or *taijiquan* as it is sometimes transliterated, is a
Chinese form of moving meditation. It offers a calm awareness
of the spirit, a relaxed, alert mind, and a flexible, strong body.
The word *chi* means the same thing as the Hindi (Indian)
prana, or life force. When you practice the various tai chi exercises, called "forms," you move the energy stored in the body
to promote good feelings, both internal and external.

Tai chi is used to improve health and to increase longevity, as a martial art and as a meditative art. It does require a
good deal of memorization—you have to learn the choreography of the "forms" before you can begin to apply the general principles to your daily life. But the real benefit of the
practice comes when you get out of your mind and into your
spirit. When you know the exterior motions better than you
know how to walk, you can stop criticizing your arm positions or the height of your kicks and instead, begin to concentrate on the feelings that motivate you to move. Tai chi is
the perfect combination of internal and external—you cannot
move your body until your life force moves you.

The movements of tai chi develop strength, endurance,
and elasticity in the practitioner, as well as an ability to relax
and release tension while moving. The breathing that accompanies your practice moves oxygen and energy, just as it does
in yoga. The type of breathing associated with Chinese medicine, known as *qi gong,* or *chi kung* (translated as "breath
work") has been used for centuries as a therapeutic technique.

Tai chi is based on the Taoist philosophy of nature that
divides the universe into a balanced set of opposites. The *yin*

energy represents the earth and is said to be yielding and responsive. The *yang* energy represents heaven and is said to be strong and untiring. Together the two teardrop shapes form a circle, the tai chi, but each has within it a dot of the opposite color. There can be no yin without yang, no yang without yin. Tai chi is based on circular patterns that mimic the cycling of human energy with that of the cosmos. Although you learn one form at a time, the goal is to combine many forms into one spiraling, coiling, circulating whole.

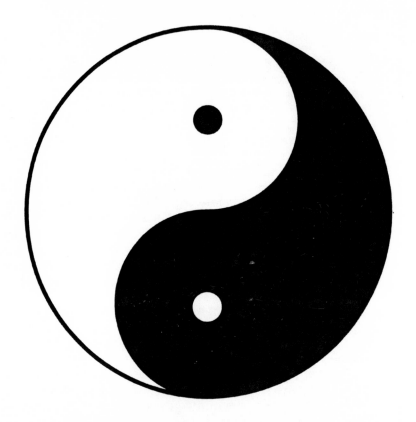

When we take the concept of yin/yang as a basis for healing, we are giving the highest priority to balance and symmetry in the body and mind. You cannot feel relaxed if you are pushing too hard; you cannot be effective if you give in all the time—it's got to be an appropriate mix of the two. And the less you try, the more the Tao (the "Way" or "Path") moves you. Eventually, your goal is no goal at all. When you have no particular intention, anything is possible.

How do you send energy from one part of the body to another? As you move through the choreographed forms, you are stimulating a variety of pressure points, alleviating stress, and working through blockages. As you calm your mind and body in practice, you can lower blood pressure and heart rate and develop excellent breathing habits that afford more oxygen flow to your brain and other organs.

Although tai chi may appear to the uninitiated as a type of graceful dance, it is actually an internal martial art. Each form has a defense application, and many practitioners find that the health benefits of tai chi are amplified by the knowledge that they can protect themselves with these movements. You might never use the slow, gentle forms to throw an opponent across the room, but knowing you have that power does a lot to improve your self-confidence and, thus, your whole mental and emotional state. As your mind becomes more flexible and yielding, accepting what you can and can't do physically, your body becomes softer and stronger, ever more resilient to handle the problems you encounter in your daily life.

The key to relaxation in tai chi is the idea of *sinking* your weight. You must feel so bound to the ground that you are one with it; as you practice, it should feel as though your feet have put out roots that extend as far down in the ground as your body reaches up in the air. If you can master the mental idea of getting rid of all tension in the limbs and torso, you can achieve a loose, relaxed body that is both substantial and flowing.

Tai chi can be used as a moving meditation. In giving up the body to your forms, your mind can be free to focus on breathing or on filling all the space around you. There are forms as short as 24 postures and as long as 103 postures. It requires patience to get through them, regardless of length, but this teaches you not to anticipate and jump to conclusions. And as in tai chi, so in life. The more we can relish each moment for just what it is, the better we can meet adversity and pain and move through it. Tai chi is one of the finest natural therapies for mental and emotional problems because it is a microcosm of life—a long form, or a long day, is just as good as we allow it to be.

CASE HISTORY

Maria went back to school at the age of 42 to get her bachelor's degree in sociology. She was working a full-time job and taking care of a family, but she was determined to finish school. The pressure and high stress of a college campus for this shy South American woman, for whom English was a second language, was almost too much to bear.

"I had incredible PMS for the first time in my life," she said, "and these mood swings nearly destroyed me and my family. I felt angry all the time, for no reason. I started tai chi about a year ago because I heard it was a good way to relax. I go to class once a week, and I'm constantly amazed at how, for that 90 minutes, I can concentrate so well. The rest of the world just goes away as I focus on myself and what I'm doing. I think it helps in my daily life, which is so fragmented—this practice brings everything together.

"I've noticed recently that my cramps are not as severe. I think it may be because tai chi has improved my circulation (I'm also taking a B-vitamin supplement, which may help too). But my practice also makes me feel very strong, and I really need that to keep up with those young college kids."

Tape Recorder, Therapeutic Use

Listen to yourself. It's not easy to hear the sound of your own voice, which you will discover when you use the tape recorder as a therapeutic tool. But it's very effective. In fact, replaying what you have said and hearing the *way* you've said it can teach you worlds about your personality, behavior, and predilection for emotional imbalances.

There are two ways to use a tape recorder effectively: The first is as an improvisational diary. This method takes note of the random thoughts that come into your head and allows you to hear them when you're feeling better. You may rant and rave at will into the recorder when you are depressed or agitated, feeling heartbroken, or about to go on an eating binge. Then, the next day, you can listen to what was going through your mind and process it logically. Just hearing yourself blow up in anger or wallowing in the depths of despair is usually enough to make you laugh (humor is also a therapeutic tool) at how intense you were, or figure out logically how you can avoid such a tantrum the next time something goes wrong.

The second use of the recorder is as a prompt for a new behavior you are trying to adopt but aren't yet comfortable with. If you are attempting a behavioral change, it can be helpful to hear your own voice telling you to accomplish certain things in certain ways. You can use affirmations (see page 16) to reinforce your ability to follow through with your intentions. This method requires you to write a set script and stick to the precise words that will influence you the most. If you are attempting to curb addictive behavior or overcome a phobia, the tape recorder will guide you through rocky moments when you think you can't stick to your resolve.

Most people don't recognize their voice when they first hear it; this is because we sound different in our own head from the way we do when our voice is broadcast to others. The discrepancy between what you think you sound like and what you really sound like can work well to assist in this therapy; it's as if your better half were telling you what to do. So you might as well listen!

T EARFULNESS

see also Blues, page 72; Depression, page 112; Grief, page 193; Hopelessness, page 226; Mental confusion, page 100; Sadness/Despondency, page 375

Sometimes we cry when we're sad, sometimes we cry when we're joyful, and sometimes we cry for no reason at all. Women, more than men, are often accused of being hysterical because they "leak" when something difficult, traumatic, or wonderful occurs. Every season, Hollywood puts out at least one good "tearjerker," a movie that literally pushes all the buttons of nostalgia, lost love, found love, bad guys gone good and good guys gone bad—not to mention a few tragic diseases of the week that kill off the character we have just bonded with. It's considered normal to cry at situations in films because those aren't our problems—they're someone else's, and anyway, they're fictional. But many in our society think that too many tears in real life imply a lack of stability and that it's important to exert control when you find yourself nearing that watery release.

Actually, tears are a cathartic expression of emotion that has built up and festered for some time, and it can be very therapeutic to cry. In many cultures, abundant tears are expected to commemorate deaths, births, weddings, and tribal ceremonies. Those who do not or cannot cry are considered hard-hearted and not very evolved individuals.

What Happens When You Are Tearful

There is a rush of saliva in your mouth and a tight feeling in the throat. The tears well up, sometimes staying precariously perched on the rim of the eyelid before overflowing and cascading down the cheeks. You can feel sobs welling up, and if you are really upset, the sounds that emanate from you may sound inhuman. The keening noise that sometimes accompanies forceful crying can be a rhythmic chant or a discordant, arrhythmic set of hiccups. Very often, we feel overcome by the impetus to cry; it seems impossible to stop, no matter how much we pat our eyes with water and no matter how kind and consoling our friends or relatives may be. The gush of tears is like lava pouring out of an active volcano, and it can have the same burning, ravaging feeling as it lays waste to our previously calm soul.

After the tears, we are completely dehydrated. Our eyes and face are red and puffy, and our voice sounds as though we had been shouting into a tunnel for hours. But we generally feel calmer after a good cry, as though we had been in a battle and come out the other side.

Go Ahead and Cry

It's really okay to indulge once in a while. If you're having your period or going through menopause or you've been fired or you've just recovered from an illness and can't believe how beautiful the sunset looks, a good cry is appropriate and wonderfully healing.

Drink Up

It's essential that you replace all the water you've lost. Although a little sniffle might be worth only a few teaspoons, true grief and crying jags that go on and off for hours can take away a pint of liquid. You're also losing sodium (tears are salty, remember), so you may feel very weak after you've finished crying. Pure spring water—at least 32 ounces within the next four hours—will help you feel better faster. You might also want to stock up on one of the sports drink products that are loaded with additional minerals.

Keep a Journal

If you are extremely aware of the triggers that make you cry, you can start recording them and making note of whether you simply allow your buttons to be pushed every time because crying is a habit, or whether you are actually responding deeply to some other issue to which you haven't yet given a great deal of thought. The underlying reasons for your tearfulness will probably come out if you write a little each day, vowing to be honest with yourself (no one else has to see this) and trying hard to express your feelings in words. You don't have to be a great writer to keep a journal; you don't even have to be particularly perceptive about your emotional life. When you start to set down events, you'll find that you want to embellish the facts with a variety of impressions and feelings that accompany each experience. By reading over several months of your journal, you'll grow to understand and, it's hoped, like yourself more.

Homeopathic Help

The homeopathic remedy for sadness is Stannum.

For melancholia: Aurum metallicum

For never smiling: Arsenicum album, Aurum metallicum

Herbal Relief

St. John's wort has been shown to be effective in dealing with mood swings and emotional instability. Take 20 to 30 drops of extract four times a day; or three capsules three times a day; or one teaspoon of dried herb to one cup water—take two cups daily. It will take about two weeks to feel that the herb is working. Avoid prolonged exposure to sunlight while you are taking this herb.

Use the Wisdom of the East

An Ayurvedic physician would diagnose tearfulness as a vata imbalance. Vata controls the nervous system, and therefore any trauma—grief or panic—can exhaust vata dosha. In the first stage of this imbalance, you will weep a great deal and be unable to sleep, with racing thoughts, shakiness, and restless behavior. If the stress proceeds and worsens, you may be unable to act and become apathetic and numb.

If you are prone to tearfulness, you may also notice some other vata disturbances: You react to stress with high anxiety; you abuse nicotine, caffeine, and alcohol in order to cope; you eat a lot of cold, raw, or dry foods and iced drinks; you diet or skip meals.

In order to stop the tearfulness, you must correct the imbalance. This means you should start doing everything in moderation— staying warm, eating regular meals (preferably of warm foods and drinks), getting enough rest, exercising lightly, and having sesame oil massages in the morning (you can do these yourself or ask your partner to massage you). You should avoid overstimulation and stay away from loud music, violent movies, and too much TV. You may notice that you are most stressed (and most prone to crying) in the late afternoon; give yourself a hot herb-tea break (gotu kola tea is excellent for calming the nerves).

The meditative practice of staring into a candle flame is thought by Ayurveda to be good for the eyesight, but it can also steady your mind as you use your eyes to concentrate, rather than allow them to give way to tears.

Press a Point

Use the acupressure points on the Lung meridian that sit on either side of the chest in the hollows formed by the collarbones and the tops of the ribs. Press these points and massage in a circular motion.

*T*ENSION

see also Agitation, page 21; Anger, page 31; Anxiety, page 43; Gastrointestinal Disorders, page 189; Hyperventilation, page 231; Irritability, page 253; Palpitations, page 342; Shortness of Breath, page 397; Stress, page 407; Trembling, page 428

Being tense is almost a given in our stress-filled, overstimulated environment. Most advertisements for tropical-island resorts invite you to stay at least a week because it takes that long to get rid of the tension.

Tension is caused by rigid muscles and stiff joints, combined with an inflexible mentality that makes us want to shield ourselves from harm. By stiffening up, we think we're making ourselves invincible, when what really happens is that we just load on the tension. Holding the muscles over time is terribly painful, because a partially contracted muscle closes the blood vessels and keeps the tissues from getting their full complement of blood. Tension also overexerts shortened muscles and tears their fibers or pulls overly hard on joints. When in this uncomfortable state, the body reacts with tension headaches, gastrointestinal disorders, and improper alignment of the head, neck, and spine, which can lead to serious back conditions.

What Happens When You Get Tense

You feel a vein pulsing in your forehead, and your whole body begins to harden like concrete. You feel rigid, and though you want to relax, it's impossible because you're encased in this coffin of steel. You are wound tight like a spring, and you feel that at any minute, the last crank will break the mechanism and you will fly—in pieces—all over the place.

If you can reduce physical tension, you can relax. (This is not as easy as it seems, since trying too hard to relax can tense you up.) First, your brain has to let go of its own type of "contraction" before the muscles of the body can release. Once you've cleared your mind, it's possible to get rid of the defensive need to stiffen your posture. By ridding yourself of tension, you can avoid dozens of different muscle-based aches and pains and start feeling better about your general health.

Learn the Difference Between Tension and Relaxation

Lie on your back and let your legs and arms fall easily away from your body. (You may find that this is difficult to do, since you'll probably be tense at the beginning of this exercise.) You are going to make a systematic tour of your body, tensing and then releasing every part of it. Begin with your toes—curl them tightly under, hold them in a hard contraction, and hold your breath, then suddenly let go. Now tense the arches of the foot, hold the contraction and hold your breath, then let go. Work your way up, from the foot, to the calf, the knee, the thigh, the hip, the buttocks, the lower back, middle back, upper back and shoulder blades, neck, back of the head, scalp, forehead, eyes, mouth, whole face, chin, shoulders and collarbones, ribs, waist, stomach, internal organs, genitals, then your upper arms, elbows, forearms, wrists, hands, and fingers. Finally, tense the entire body—it should feel almost as though it has lifted in one piece off the floor. Hold your breath, then suddenly, release everything. See how different your body feels now from the way it did at the beginning of the exercise, almost as though you had poured yourself into the floor. Enjoy the sensation of complete relaxation.

Press a Point (See pp 10–11 for acupressure charts)

The acupressure points for general irritability and tension are:

> L.I. 4 (on the top of the hand, in the hollow of the muscle between the thumb and the index finger)
>
> U.B. 10 (where the skull meets the neck on either side of the spine)
>
> G.B. 21 (in the center of the trapezius muscle, midway between the base of the neck and the tip of the shoulder)

Get Some Feedback

Biofeedback is a good teaching tool to make you more aware of your body and how it functions. You will be hooked up to a machine with a monitor by means of electrodes attached to your forehead, fingertips, and several other locations, depending on where you hold tension. Lights, sounds, and the level of a readout on a screen will give you a lot of useful information about your body's tension.

The machine will perform thermal measurements on your skin: If you are highly tense, you may have very cold fingers without much blood flowing through them. As you learn to relax, your fingers will warm up. As you squeeze your skeletal muscles, the machine will record the degree of contraction, pinpointing muscle tension before it reaches the uncomfortable or painful stage. Your brain waves can also be charted, to see how your conscious mind helps or hinders your ability to relax. As you work with the machine in your sessions and practice progressive relaxation, you will learn how much pressure elevates your levels on the screen, and you can then teach yourself how to let go and get the lights or sounds to turn off.

See Yourself Loose

Visualization can teach you what you need to do to relax. Sit quietly and begin to concentrate on your breath. Inhale and warm the inside of your body; then let all the old tension escape with each exhalation. Now notice that the floor beneath you is melting, becoming a jellylike mass, and you are floating on top of it. It has a wonderful, resilient quality that springs back each time you put weight on it. As you see yourself getting up for a walk, you too have assumed this looseness of limb. You look and feel like Gumby, your arms and legs stretching and bending effortlessly in every direction. Have a completely open mind as you look down and see your boneless body moving smoothly across the floor. You feel at ease, as though you had always moved like this—you have nowhere to go, nothing to do but enjoy the sensation of lightness and comfort in every cell. Play with your steps, throw your arms into the air, and sit down and roll onto your back, letting the floor carry you.

When you are ready, sit up again with your legs crossed and begin to solidify, returning to your everyday body and mind. As you open your eyes, you will retain the good, loose feeling you had during this visualization.

Dance Fever

One of the best ways to reduce tension is to abandon your body to the pulse and beat of music. You don't have to be a Gene Kelly—all you have to do is turn on the radio to a station that moves you and start to dance. You can also grab a friend and visit a club, where you have the additional stimulation of incredible amps that pound away in your chest, removing the ability and necessity to talk or think. Because most of us aren't professional and don't whirl, jump, sway, hop, and boogie every day, our muscles can't revert to old patterns. They have to stay loose to perform differently from the way they ordinarily do.

The next morning at the office, when you start to get tense, try to re-create the feeling you had on the dance floor and use it constructively to release tight muscles.

North-Pole Attraction

While lying on a massage table for half an hour with a 2,000-gauss strip magnet under your head, your central nervous system will be able to "tune down" and relax. North-pole energy appears to be a major influence on emotional conditions and may trigger parasympathetic reactions that can calm body and mind. The temporal lobe and metabolic function are also influenced by magnets. You can seek treatment from a massage therapist who uses magnetic strips on the massage table, or you can purchase special magnets for spot treatments; there are insoles, hand-held devices, mats, and chair coverings. (See Resource Guide, page 475.)

TREMBLIN

see also Agitation, page 21; Anxiety, page 43; Fear, page 64; Gastrointestinal Disorders, page 189; Hyperventilation, page 231; Jitteriness, page 260; Nervousness, page 304; Palpitations, page 342; Panic Disorders, page 344; Restless Leg Syndrome, page 365; Stress, page 407; Tension, page 425; Violence/Aggressive Behavior, page 437

Trembling is the most obvious physical manifestation of fear or anger. We have literally lost control of our arms and legs; we are all over the place. The feeling that you can't stop moving adds to the panicky sensation. Some trembling is invisible to an onlooker's eyes, but severe trembling is quite evident to everyone else, which adds a certain amount of embarrassment to your distress. This type of psychomotor agitation is normal when you're in a highly anxious state—what's happened is that a rush of stress hormones has actually set off an alarm system that unbalances the motor coordination of the body. When we're really scared or filled with rage, we have an instinctive push to move ourselves out of the path of danger. Trembling may be an involuntary method of keeping the body in motion so that it is more difficult for an attacker (animal, human, or imaginary) to pin it down.

What Happens When You Tremble

An earthquake has been set off inside you, and you're powerless to stop it. Your arms and legs vibrate, your teeth chatter, and you may be unable to hold anything without dropping and breaking it. Your skin is cold and clammy, and your stomach churns with anxiety.

When you think of the stereotypical sight of a victim cowering in front of a bully and quaking with fear, you have the quintessential impression of impotence. You can also turn the picture around and see the bully shaking with anger. Even if you're not being physically threatened or threatening anyone else, when you tremble, you feel helpless. This lack of firmness and stability, of course, takes your confidence away and makes the problem worse.

Breathe From Your Belly

When you breathe with the diaphragm and not with the chest, you can warm up the *tan tien,* the Chinese word for "field of elixir." This spot is thought to be the center of the physical and emotional body, and by directing your attention to this point, you can strengthen the whole. Put your hands and fingers around your rib cage to keep it still and then muscularly move your stomach in and out. You will find that exerting pressure on this area tends to focus you, and slowly your limbs will stop shaking.

Open Your Voice

When you are scared and nervous, you tend to speak in a breathy, frightened tone, hardly big enough to make a difference. To counteract that weak feeling, you are going to chant at the top of your lungs. Pick one note in the middle of your natural range and let the sound pour out. It makes no difference if your teeth are chattering—once you open your mouth and throat, the violent movement of your jaw will stop. (The idea is not to make a pretty sound, just to make a *lot* of sound.) Keep the note going as long as you can and imagine that the volume itself is forming into a rope that you can grab onto. Steady the rope by expanding your belly, pushing your stomach muscles out as far as they can go. When you run out of steam, take another breath and start a new sound. Get louder and fuller. You will find that you cannot tremble when you roar like a lion.

Inhale a Strong Scent

Trembling responds well to ammonia ampules (available in most pharmacies). Crack one under your nose when you are shaking—the strong odor will go straight up your nasal passages to the pituitary gland in your brain and stimulate it intensely. Stress hormone production will be reduced and you will soon stop trembling.

Get a Hug

The sense of touch is extremely powerful, and you can use a strong hug similar to the way a doctor might use a straitjacket on a patient who is out of control. If you're wrapped in someone's arms, you are sheltered and feel nourished, as though no harm can come to you. Your body is steadied and held together by someone else's protecting arms. Make sure you ask for a hug the next time you can't stop shaking and quaking.

Homeopathic Help

The homeopathic remedies for fear and trembling are: Aconite, Belladonna, Causticum, Ignatia, Silica, Lycopodium, Phosphorus, and Pulsatilla.

Use Chinese Wisdom

Traditional Chinese medicine would diagnose trembling from fear as a malfunction of the Kidney organ network. The nature of fear is cold, so you would be advised to keep a hot-water bottle on your lower back and keep the bottoms of your feet warm. Press the following acupuncture points:

> For chills: T.B. 5 (in the hollow on the outer aspect of the forearm, between the radius and ulna, about an inch and a half up from the crease of the wrist)
>
> For weakness and fatigue: Ki. 7 (on the inner aspect of the leg, in the hollow between the muscle and the Achilles tendon, about four inches up from the heel)
>
> St. 36 (on the outside of the leg with the knee slightly bent, on the edge of the shinbone three inches down from the kneecap)

*V*ICTIM *M*ENTALITY

see also Aging, page 17; Anxiety; page 43; Stress, page 407

A person with particularly low self-esteem may develop a belief system that circles around being maligned, attacked, and persecuted. Many individuals who really are victims as children because they've been abused physically or emotionally never get free of the feeling that "nobody likes me, and everybody hates me." But you don't have to have suffered abuse to feel as though you deserve it. The unfortunate part of having a victim mentality is that it sticks out all over you, and you may have a greater propensity for becoming a victim. The fear that others are out to get you becomes a self-fulfilling prophecy. All self-defense courses teach a person not to act like a victim—not to walk hesitantly or to shrink away when others approach—so as not to become the prey of bullies who are on the lookout for weak, helpless individuals.

Having a victim mentality is a disability not only in situations where physical violence is threatened. Being a victim on the job makes others lose respect for you and keeps you from raises and promotions; being a victim at home means that you may open yourself up for abuse or allow the rest of the family to pile on the chores and criticize your performance.

▓ *What Happens When You Have a Victim Mentality*

You feel like a pushover, as if anyone could come along and just blow on you and you'd fall down. You're convinced that you are the target; you feel that everyone is out to get you, and they will probably succeed. You constantly look over your shoulder for danger, and whether it's real or imaginary, you feel powerless to combat it.

It is not easy to lose this way of thinking, and it can take years to muster the bravery to stand up for yourself. But when you do, you'll be treated as a formidable and worthy opponent. Learning to defend yourself—physically, mentally, and emotionally—is the key to improving your mental and emotional outlook.

Say a Daily Affirmation

Tell yourself that you are worthy, and you will hear it from a very important source. Tape record the following messages and play them back to yourself before you go to sleep at night and when you awaken in the morning.

I am a worthwhile individual.

I have a lot of standing in my community, at my job, and in my home.

I am worthy of other people's interest and admiration.

By becoming aware of my thoughts and actions I can raise myself to a position of respect.

I am not the target.

Don't Consider Every Meeting a Confrontation

Most people who think of themselves as victims look at every situation as a potentially threatening one. It's time to reevaluate your dealings with others and see them as a meeting of equals. When your spouse accuses you of going over budget in the household accounts, don't feel picked on. Instead, suggest that you both look at your spending patterns and readjust them, maybe checking with each other weekly to see how you're doing. If your boss demands to know where you are with a certain project, don't immediately take it as criticism. Rather, give a full report on what you've been doing and how long you expect it will take—then ask if that fits with his or her schedule.

Whenever You Feel Afraid . . . Whistle

Acting totally in charge when you feel threatened is one of the best ways to distract yourself from the tension you feel.

The old Rogers and Hammerstein lyric, "Make believe you're brave and the trick will take you far; you may be as brave as you make believe you are," makes a lot of sense. When you think someone's out to get you, whistle a happy tune no matter how ridiculous it makes you feel. It will point out to you that life has ups and downs, and nothing is as serious as you tend to think it is.

Learn Self-defense

There are many excellent courses offered at Ys, private martial arts schools, and at police academies that will teach you not just physical but emotional self-defense. By learning to use your voice loudly and to attack sensitive areas on your partner, you come to understand your own power. Most courses include a full-fledged attack of a person in a completely padded suit as a graduation ceremony. You are allowed to punch, kick, hit, and do anything else you need to defend yourself. This type of exercise can be extremely beneficial in real life—even if you never use the physical fighting skills you've learned.

Be Sexually Forthright

If you are being victimized sexually, it's time to take a stand. Make a concerted effort to put forward your own feelings if you're being taken advantage of, because you, and nobody else, are the boss of your body.

If your partner demands sexual favors and humiliates you into giving when you don't feel like it, you can do anything—bar the door to the bedroom, stop shopping and cooking meals, take the kids and go to your mother's house—to alter the behavior. If you are really in danger, you should immediately get out of the house and into a shelter. You must not think about hurting your partner's feelings—all you have to do is save yourself.

And even if you're not being threatened, but feel as though you are, you have every right to reclaim your sexuality. If the two of you get together only when your partner initiates the action, turn the tables and create your own intimate moments. By saying, in effect, "this is what I want and how I want it," you stop being a victim and start being an equal partner.

Flower Power

There are several Bach flower remedies that will change a victim mentality. Take 5 or 6 drops under the tongue or mixed with half a glass of water as needed. (If several remedies apply, you may take 2 drops from no more than three remedies at a time in combination.)

> Try Larch for despondency and an expectation of failure due to lack of self-confidence
>
> Try Mimulus for fear of known things, shyness, and timidity
>
> Try Walnut for protection from powerful influences and difficulty with transitions
>
> Try Willow for resentment and bitterness or if you have a "poor me" attitude

The Aroma of Life

Try a massage with an uplifting essential oil such as Tangerine, Orange, Cedar, Lemon, Fir, Spruce, Pine, or Rosewood. Use two or three drops mixed with a carrier oil (Almond or Jojobe), or place a couple of drops in your bathwater.

Stop Abusing Substances

Very often, it's easier to close your eyes to feelings of self-loathing when you fog out your mind and emotions. It's common to overeat, stop eating, drink too much alcohol, and abuse recreational, over-the-counter, or prescription drugs.

If you want to stop the cycle, you have to take care of yourself. That means treating yourself as though you counted, not as though you wanted to escape reality. The next time you feel as if you're backed up against a wall and the firing squad is about to appear in front of you, walk as far from the medicine or liquor cabinet as can you, take a breath, and drink a tall glass of water. You are instantly changing your status from victim to victor.

VIOLENCE/AGGRESSIVE BEHAVIOR

see also Depression, page 112; Impulse Control, page 246

When anger and rage can no longer be contained, they explode in violent or aggressive behavior. The individual with a very short fuse is a threat to himself or herself and to others. Underneath violence, however, usually lurks depression and a very poor self-image. The batterer is the flip side of the victim (see Victim Mentality, page 433) and also tends to think life is unfair and that others are "out to get" him or her.

Violent people are usually taught about violence at a very early age—they have been told from childhood that they are "chicken-shit," "dumb," "stupid," or "bad," and their behavior tries to reverse the power struggle they've had with an abusive parent. They lack a feeling of empathy and can't relate to another's pain, because they themselves are numb, anesthetized by the blows they've taken throughout life.

What Happens When You Are Violent

You feel anger bubbling up in you, taking over your mind and body until it spews out all over the place. You may throw objects with everything you've got, breaking them apart to show how strong you are. You may stop traffic, getting out of your car to pound on the hood of a driver who has cut you off or given you the finger. You may physically beat and batter another individual to release the incredible feeling of tension inside. As soon as you can intimidate your victim, you start to feel a little easier, because now you have control and your victim doesn't.

Violence is mindless—the perpetrator often has no idea that he or she has injured others or destroyed property. It's only sometimes in the aftermath of a wave of aggressive behavior that the individual can look back and reflect on this explosion and try to pinpoint the cause. Violent feelings can bring terrifying thoughts—murder and mutilation fantasies are not uncommon. It's important to tell yourself that even when you're out of control, you will not allow yourself to go over the limits of reason. In treating your aggressive behavior, you need as much awareness of what you're doing as why you're doing it.

Get Help

Behavioral therapy will create an environment in which you must change what you're doing. Chart your progress with a daily diary and write down setbacks as well as triumphs.

The first step, of course, is an awareness of the way you react when you're angry (or even when you're not angry but act aggressive with no trigger at all). When you feel overwhelmed, you will need an intervention to stop your habitual behavior. You can try snapping a rubber band on your wrist to remind yourself not to get violent, but if this isn't enough, you may need a buzzer you can sound at the same time. These will be your cues to start counting to ten, doing some yoga or Taoist breathing (see below), or distracting yourself with another activity.

Your goal is not to react aggressively, no matter what happens. At first, of course, you won't be able to completely block the feelings that make all your circuits light up. So for the first week, start with the goal of recognizing the feeling, using the intervention, and performing an activity that will give you time to think about your actions. If you must yell and scream after this, do so, but you may not resort to any physical behavior.

During the second week, your goal will be to think of a calming activity to perform as soon as you get angry. This might be turning on some music, going for a quick jog, or discussing your problem with the person you're mad at.

As you work on changing your behavior, you will sense that your feelings are changing subtly as well. By the third or fourth week of this program, you will still get angry, but you should find it easier not to react with violence.

Breathe!

Yogic alternate nostril breathing is an excellent way to calm down. Cover your left nostril with your right pinky and fourth finger. Inhale into your right nostril, exhale right, then place your right thumb on your right nostril as you release your pinky and fourth finger. Inhale through your left nostril, exhale, then cover it with your pinky and fourth finger as you release your thumb. Continue for ten minutes. This type of breathing aligns the two hemispheres of the brain and allows clearer thinking.

You may also try Taoist (Chinese) prenatal breathing. Inhale and draw your stomach muscles in, trying to pull your bellybutton back to your spine. Exhale, releasing the belly and pushing it out—make a big Buddha belly. Continue for ten minutes.

If you feel at all lightheaded, sit down, relax, and return to normal breathing.

An Eastern Approach

Ayurveda sees violence as a *pitta* imbalance. Pittas tend to be very intense, and their anger (at themselves and at others) can be overwhelming when unchecked. It can also bring on a host of problems such as heartburn, ulcers, heart disease, and other stress-related conditions.

In order to balance pitta, you need to achieve moderation in all aspects of your life. If you're a workaholic, it's time to reassess your priorities. Don't take work home with you and make time to wind down from the frantic pace of your office as you come home. Meditation is almost essential to restore balance to pitta dosha. It's also vital to stay cool—don't overdress, keep your bedroom window open a crack at night, and drink plenty of fluids (cool, but not iced).

Your diet should also show moderation—eat reasonable amounts three times a day. A vegetarian diet is preferable to a meat-centered diet, and you should avoid fried foods, processed foods, and junk food assiduously. Eat bitter greens (such as chard or arugula) and stay away from spices and too much salt. Avoid fermented products such as alcohol, vinegar, pickles, and also try to cut down on or cut out coffee, which is too acidic for this dosha.

Traditional Ayurveda recommends occasional laxatives to reduce excess pitta. You may try 1 tablespoon of castor oil before bed once every four to six weeks *(but no more)*. Drink a glass of warm water after you move your bowels, and the following day, eat very lightly—just fruit juice, a sweet potato, or some brown rice and vegetables.

Avoid any type of entertainment that is too violent or stimulating: Avoid movies and TV programs that feature blood and gore, and turn off the evening news if it upsets you.

Bioenergetic Exercise Makes a Difference in Your Anger

Bioenergetic therapy explores the body language that we show when we're angry or depressed. Stand in front of a mirror and thrust your jaw forward as far as you can—you'll see that just by doing this, anger will spark in your face and eyes. Now clench your fists and shout at the mirror, "I hate you!" "I could kill you!" Feel how these words affect the tension in your body.

Now thrust the jaw forward and move it right and left. Open your mouth wide and try to put your three middle fingers in between your teeth. (If you're terribly tense, you won't be able to open that far.) Take your fingers out and try saying, "No! I won't!" as loudly as you can.

This time, try yawning as you thrust your jaw forward. Relax it and drain all the tension from it. Make a long "aah" sound and let the anger run out of you.

Finally, go to your bed. Stand in front of it and raise your arms, interlacing your fingers. Pound down on the bed and yell, "No!" Raise the arms again and pound again, establishing an even rhythm. Pound the bed between 20 and 50 times.

At the end of this, you should be panting and very loose, having released a lot of your anger. Sit quietly for a moment and take in the peacefulness of your body and mind.

Scream When You Want to Let Go

Instead of taking your rage out on someone else, give it to the cosmos. A wonderfully cathartic activity is to go to a train track or underground in the subway and, as the train is whizzing past, let go and try to drown out the sound with your own voice. When you really commit yourself to this type of release, you dampen the need to express yourself in a violent or aggressive way.

Homeopathic Help

The homeopathic remedies for violence are

Stramonium, Tarantula hispanica, Silica, and Aurum metallicum

Herbal Tension-Relievers

Various nervine relaxants will help in the treatment of violence and aggressive tendencies. Skullcap, pasque flower, and valerian will all calm nervous tension. Take 2 to 4 ml. of tincture three times daily, or 2 to 4 teaspoons of dried herb infused in a cup of water three times daily or 1–2 teaspoons root (valerian) infused in a cup of water three times daily.

Get off Drugs

Several prescription medications used to treat depression and anxiety can trigger aggressive behavior if overused. The family of drugs known as *benzodiazepines* (Xanax, Ativan, and Serax are short-acting versions of the drug; Valium and Librium are long-acting benzodiazepines) have been shown to create unusual excitement and even violent behavior. There have also been rare reported cases of Prozac, a serotonin reuptake inhibitor, causing aggressive and violent behavior.

Dream Relaxers

Your dreams will give you a lot of information about your violent tendencies. Keep a pad and pen next to your bed and decide before you go to sleep that you will jot down any images that come to you. If you wake in the middle of the night, tap into the feeling you have—are you angry, scared, overwhelmed? Who was in your dream? Were you there? What did you do?

If there was a violent component to the dream, write down exactly what happened without judging it. You want to explore the themes of the dream when you're fully conscious and then, the next night, try to take this dream in another direction. If there was torture, humiliation, or evil in the dream, ask the characters what you can do to change their attitude and their actions. Go back into the dream with an open mind, remembering that you are the dream and the dreamer, and you have ultimate control over what happens in the scenario. If you choose to, you can tone down the violence or remove it entirely.

VISUALIZATION

Visualization is a proven relaxation technique that involves imagining a scene and putting yourself in it. The better you can create the details of where you are and how you are feeling, the more relaxed and calm you can feel. Visualization has been shown to alter what used to be thought of as involuntary physiological response. Studies have shown that cancer patients who used guided imagery in addition to their chemotherapy were able to reduce the size of their tumors over a six-month period faster than those who used chemotherapy alone with no imagery. The picture most of them used was the tumor as a black granite mountain and the macrophages (white blood cells that act as disease fighters) as white knights on horseback attacking the mountain with powerful spears. By concentrating on this scene every day, they actually made the mountain shrink.

In a recent study in a Harvard neuroscience lab, a particular type of brain scan was used on patients who had been asked to visualize emotionally neutral subjects and very negative subjects. It was found that a part of the brain known as the insula was most active—the insula has strong neural connections to the limbic system, which is the seat of the emotions right in the center of the brain. It also has connections with the stomach and intestines, via the vagus nerve pathways. (The vagus nerve also connects with the thymus gland, a chief seat of immune-boosting white blood-cell production.)

Animal studies indicate that you can stimulate the insula directly in order to raise or lower heart rate and blood pressure. This means that both physical and mental stimulation can trigger activity throughout the body. If you constantly imagine your boss walking into your office to fire you, you can actually think yourself into an ulcer. But if you see yourself getting a raise and promotion, you can conceivably lower your blood pressure and heart rate, reduce muscle tension throughout your body, and possibly prevent the development of any stress-related disorders.

CASE HISTORY

Sylvia learned about her cancer after a mammogram showed a small lump on the left breast. A needle biopsy confirmed that it was malignant.

"The doctors and nurses kept rushing me—I had so much to do, and all they could say was, 'We have to operate immediately.' I was terribly scared; nothing seemed real. I just kept thinking that I didn't want to die, and I couldn't wait five years to find out if I was going to make it. So I chose a mastectomy.

"The night before my surgery, I was skimming through Bernie Siegel's book *Love, Medicine, and Miracles,* and I came upon this passage where he suggests you imagine yourself on a beach with the seagulls flying overhead. The idea is to feel as if you're a part of nature.

"I was sitting in my living room and I sat there with the book in my lap and closed my eyes. I had this vision of myself with my arms outstretched, reaching up to the sky, and I could see my shadow on the sand. My arms were infinite, they just went on forever. And I suddenly knew that *I* would go on forever. I was comforted and perfectly calm about the surgery. I knew I was going to make it."

Visualization allows you to focus and problem-solve without the added distraction of the many thoughts that too often get in the way when we're trying to concentrate on one thing. It lets you reach goals you may not believe you can really achieve, giving you control where you thought you had none.

You can become much more positive-thinking using this therapy, creatively and confidently dispelling fears that might have stopped you from getting ahead. When you visualize, you go inside and reflect on who you are and how you came to be the person living in your body. It also is wonderful for pain relief—the agony of a headache can vanish within moments when you are an accomplished visualizer.

The technique requires you to imagine your illness or problem in terms of a concrete object and change it in your mind. For example, if you have an eating disorder such as bulemia, where you gorge and purge, you might think of your problem as a bulldozer, scooping up massive quantities of dirt (food) and depositing them in a landfill. But since you are the operator of the bulldozer, you are in charge of just how much you take out in the bucket and how much you place in the hole. As you work on the visualization, you can take out less and less.

If you have a fear of public speaking that makes you hyperventilate when you stand up in front of a roomful of people, you can imagine your voice and thoughts as a lake and the people as the shore. The lake naturally washes up on the shore without even trying.

To get rid of that headache, see it as a package inside your brain. You can take paper and string and wrap it up completely, then draw it out by the ends of the string through the top of your head and throw it away.

Like most natural therapies in which you learn a skill that will help you to heal, you get better at this one the more often you practice. You can use your breathing (see page 76) to synchronize your body with your mind while you visualize.

Use the sample visualization that follows or create your own. There are just a few things to keep in mind.

- Give yourself at least 20 minutes for each visualization.
- Practice in a quiet, calm place with good ventilation and dim lighting.
- Breathe calmly and slowly throughout the exercise.
- Each visualization needs a beginning, middle, and end. At the end of the visualization, allow yourself to come back slowly to real time before you become aware of your surroundings and open your eyes.

Sample Visualization: Calming the Spirit

Sit quietly and concentrate on your breath. You will notice various thoughts passing through your mind—allow them to come in and leave freely. It's as though you were sitting on a train, watching the scenery come and then go.

Inhale easily, imagining the air as a healing tonic running through your system. Exhale, and let out any toxins you may have stored inside. Don't let out all the air in a rush— some should stay behind as a core of energy you can tap into when you need it.

Now bring the breath up to your mind and let it form into a spiral that will delve deeper into the limbic system, the brain's storehouse for emotions. See this "house" as a cozy and comfortable space; for some, it may be a cabin in the woods, for others a sprawling seaside mansion.

The door to this house is open, and you can walk inside. Make a full tour—see the details in the hallway, the fire in the living room fireplace, smell the aroma of dinner wafting in from the kitchen. See yourself setting things right if they are out of place, but don't be too much of a perfectionist about it. This is *your* house, and you can keep it as neat or messy as you please.

Spend some time looking out the window, enjoying the view, perhaps a wooded lot or a picturesque city skyline, depending on your preference. Understand that you have the right to this home and to the space beyond it when you move out into the world. This is your kingdom, your land of plenty.

Sense your breath growing deeper and fuller as you enjoy the experience of owning your own space. You can keep this with you even as you return to real time and become aware of your surroundings. Slowly allow your eyes to relax open.

VULNERABILITY

see also Anxiety, page 43; Broken Heart, page 78; Depression, page 112; Shyness, page 400

If you are vulnerable, your flank is unprotected and the enemy can come right in and spear you. The origin of the word actually means capable of being wounded, and therefore, being vulnerable can put you in the position of being victimized. Vulnerability differs from having a victim mentality, however—vulnerable individuals don't feel like victims. Rather, they are open to experience and often neglect to shield themselves from attack.

■ *What Happens When You Are Vulnerable*

You tend to trust to fate, thinking that things will work out. You don't see the venal side of people, who often take advantage of you. You wear your heart on a sleeve, and it's ripe prey for anyone who thinks it might be fun to see you suffer a little. And you don't learn by your mistakes—even if your heart is broken, you might just as easily fall into another inappropriate relationship a week or a month from now. It's easy for people to hurt your feelings: You are particularly sensitive to criticism and may chew over casual comments as though they were gospel.

Being vulnerable is not necessarily a terrible thing. In this jaded world, where most people walk around wearing emotional armor to protect them from any feeling, we need the humility and trust of a vulnerable individual who still believes that people are really good at heart.

Toughen up a Little

You must start to approach life with a little more awareness. This is not to suggest that you should doubt people's intentions, but rather, that you should examine your own belief system and your own propensity to "go with the flow." If you are in the middle of a meeting in which your boss is tearing your ideas apart, ask yourself if every criticism is justified, or if, in fact, your boss is just having a bad day. Try a response such as, "I'm listening, and I think you have a few good points," that doesn't make you seem as if you're caving in.

If you are knocked off your feet by a devastating individual who woos you with flowers, candy, and flashing eyes, stop and ask yourself how much you know about this person and what you want out of the relationship. As you start to initiate activities or withdraw a little from such immediate intimacy, you'll find that you gain more respect from the person—and more time to establish a good groundwork for a relationship together.

Make a Battle Plan

Since the word "vulnerable" actually means the physical openness that can put us in danger, construct a war game for yourself. You can use dollhouse figures or stuffed animals, but be certain that the figurine representing you is always protected. You can devise a shield and sword out of tin foil, and as you act out the aggressions of the other characters, always give yourself a chance to fight back. You don't necessarily need to win this battle, but you should come out of the game feeling competent and secure in your own maneuvers.

Another possibility for "war games," if you are in good physical shape, is that you attempt a difficult physical feat, such as climbing a mountain or swimming a lake and ask a friend to put obstacles in your path that you must overcome in order to proceed. (Certain corporations offer structured weekends for their employees in which they pose similar challenges—Outward Bound runs many of these programs.)

Work on Your Self-Esteem

Tell yourself that you're in charge. The next time someone is "dissing" you or insisting that you're worthless and no good, talk back. You don't have to counter with insults, but instead, you should counter with all your good points. You can say that you're good-natured, easy to get along with, a hard worker, that you're able to accept criticism, and that you never shy away from responsibility. The more you stand up for yourself, the more you can stay vulnerable when it's safe for you to do so and put up your defenses when you need them.

Do Some Tai Chi Push Hands

Pushing hands is a two-person tai chi exercise in which you learn to keep your balance even as your partner tries to upset it. Ask a friend to help you and start by standing with your right feet parallel to each other, and your left about two feet back, angled 45 degrees to the left. Join your right hands at the wrist. The arms should be loose and relaxed—you don't need more than four ounces of pressure on each other.

Partner A will begin by pushing toward B's chest. When A is just about to touch, B will sink her left hip and circle around, yielding away from A's energy and beginning to bring in the push as she completes the circle. As long as both partners push with the same energy and keep the circle completely round, they are in harmony.

To test your ability, you can start pushing a little harder or angling the push up or down as you come toward your partner's chest. If you are very sensitive to the amount of weight your partner is putting on you, and she's pushing hard, you can simply take her pushing arm and pull her off balance. Or, as she is coming in, you can quickly sink your hip and reverse the circle, pushing her over.

The object is to stay rooted and grounded, always protecting your flank by yielding away from aggression and turning the body to your own advantage. As you practice pushing hands, you will find the subtleties of pressure and body mechanics match completely your psychological attitude toward pushing or getting pushed.

WEIGHT **L**OSS/**G**AIN

see also Anorexia, page 34; Anxiety, page 43; Depression, page 112; Eating Disorders, page 139; Overeating, page 331

One of the chief signs of depression is a change in eating habits. Since food can often be a substitute for love, we can overindulge in it or withhold it, depending on whom we're trying to hurt.

Women more than men tend to over- or undereat when they're upset, because our society puts such a high valuation on a woman's physical body. If she can't handle the relationship problems, the pressure to study harder and get better grades, or the job search, this is one way to say to the world that you can't cut it, and they shouldn't expect you to.

▪ *What Happens When You Gain Weight*

You feel upset and can't think logically about what you're doing. You aren't really hungry, but you go to the refrigerator time and again, looking for answers. You put anything and everything into your mouth, trying to assuage the gnawing feeling inside, and when it goes away slightly, you throw up your hands and decide that it's too late to stop the behavior, you might as well get some pleasure out of life. You keep eating because it hurts too much to stop. A fat suit can't be permeated by sadness, fear, or anger. Gaining a lot of weight is often bound up with a feeling of self-loathing—if you despise the person you are, you can't love the body you're in.

Weight gain happens normally at three stages in a woman's life and should *not* be a cause for concern. At puberty, as the body begins to change hormonally, women increase their fat stores; during pregnancy, the body naturally gains weight to support the new life inside; and at menopause, when the body's proportion changes to become more fat and less fiber, many women also gain.

Although men do not have the same life events that might put weight on them, they tend to follow patterns in later life that they've established in their early years. A beefy football player will probably get fatter as he ages if he doesn't keep up his exercise.

What Happens When You Lose Weight

At first it feels great—everyone tells you look marvelous, and your clothes fit you as though they'd been drawn on you. But if you become compulsive, you continue to lose and you notice the hollows in your cheeks; the way your hipbones and ribs stick out. You have to force yourself not to eat at first, but then it gets easier. Why should you conform to what other people expect of you? It's impossible to be as perfect as most parents, spouses, or bosses want you to be. Undereating is a way to spite the world around you—almost as if you were trying to vanish so that you wouldn't have to deal with your problems. Undereating can be an extremely hostile act if you carry it to the extreme of anorexia (see page 34), since refusing to take food is refusing to survive. When your family and friends are trying to save your life and you're trying to take it, you are in effect in control of everyone else's emotions and fears.

Undereating that results from serious illness, such as cancer or AIDS, is a difficult problem to tackle, because the less you eat, the less energy you have, the harder it is to get better, and the more depressed you become. IT IS ESSENTIAL THAT YOU CONSULT A PHYSICIAN IF YOU FEEL YOU CANNOT OR WILL NOT EAT.

Make an Eating Plan

Whether you're gaining or losing, it's vital that you chart exactly what goes into your mouth so that you can determine whether it's the calories you're ingesting, your mood, or a serious clinical problem. Be sure your diet is well balanced, filled with fresh fruits and vegetables, whole grains and cereals, sufficient protein (one meat, chicken, or fish meal daily), and no junk food. Cut out or cut down on refined sugar and high-fat foods. Stick to about 1,800 to 2,500 calories daily.

At the end of a month, you should notice that your weight has stabilized. If it hasn't, consult a physician.

Eat with a Friend

It's hard to gain or lose a lot of weight when you always have company at meals. If you can see that you and your friend or family member are consuming about the same amount, you shouldn't see a lot of fluctuation on the scale. Remember, seconds count and thirds are not allowed if you've been gaining, and cleaning your plate is a good idea if you've been losing.

Get Out and Exercise

Whether you're too heavy or too light, exercise will make a definite improvement in your eating habits. If you're concerned that the amount of food you eat seems too small to warrant a big gain, you'll start to see the pounds come off when you burn more calories by jogging, dancing, biking, swimming, or doing martial arts.

If you can't understand why the pounds roll off you when you hardly lift a finger, see whether moderate exercise (*not* a killer aerobic schedule, but a brisk walk or bike ride daily) will increase your appetite and encourage you to eat more carbohydrates and proteins that will stick with you.

Get on the Scale Daily

Although it's common practice for dieters *never* to weigh themselves, it's essential that you get on the scale every day if you've been subject to big swings in weight. By monitoring yourself at the same time, wearing the same clothing daily, you'll see if anything radical is happening and can stop the pattern in its tracks.

Supplement Your Meals

Vitamin and mineral supplementation are extremely important when you're concerned about rapid shifts in weight.

If you're gaining weight, try a multivitamin plus a B-complex supplement (100 mg. daily) plus magnesium (750 mg. daily), plus chromium (200 mg. daily).

If you're losing weight, try zinc (50 mg. daily), niacin (40 mg. three times daily), Vitamins B_2 and B_6 (200 mg. daily), and evening primrose oil (500 mg. three times daily).

Offer a Prayer

When you can't seem to control your body, it can be useful to allow a higher power to take over and do the work for you. You may wish to ask for guidance in your eating habits, or to alter your metabolism slightly to make it easier for you to remain at one steady weight.

Prayer doesn't have to be directed at a specific goal in order to work. Just a few moments of quiet appreciation of the joys of nature or the wonder of being alive—no matter what body you're in—can be fulfilling and helpful in your attempt to calm down and adjust your nutrition accordingly.

WORRYING

see also Anxiety, page 43; Nervousness, page 304

Worry is closely related to fear, especially about the future. Worriers never take a coming event at face value. Instead, they imbue it with all kinds of awful expectations—most of which are detrimental and unnecessary—deciding beforehand everything that might go wrong. If you're a worrier, you immediately categorize events, deeming them difficult, anxiety-producing, or problematic. But when you constantly paint your thoughts with a negative feeling, you color them unfairly.

What Happens When You're Always Worried

You start sweating days before a test, sure that you'll flunk it no matter how much you study. You mull over and over the comment you made to your spouse the night before, sure that it will sour your marriage and probably lead to its ultimate demise. You can't bear to see your child go off to school in the morning because you imagine what might happen—car accident, kidnapping, bully taking his lunch money, mud on his new shoes.

When you're worried, you're in a highly aroused anxious state that is fairly constant. This reaction is often connected with depression and is very common in people who can't seem to relax, no matter what they do. Worrying is also universal—it can be done on your own behalf (hypochondria, agoraphobia, and other phobias are common personal worries) and on behalf of those you love, as well as for the general community (maybe a hurricane will strike; maybe a bomber will demolish Washington, D.C.).

Worriers and nonworriers have little difference in their cognitive processes when neutral activities are going on; however, when there is any ambiguity in the situation and it's necessary to come to a decision, nonworriers perform much faster and better. They don't doubt their choices, and even when they do, they never fret that the world will fall apart if they're wrong. Worriers have so much at stake they are often paralyzed by their negative thoughts so they cannot function efficiently. They fear that they'll make the wrong choice, but at the same time, they fear that they may fail to respond at all. In several studies on worry-related cognition, it was found that when worriers were taught how to relax and let their minds wander, their performance improved.

Gang up on Your Worries

If you have to worry, do it all at once. Train yourself to make a mental note of things you have to worry about later on, and then at the end of the day, spend a full 20 minutes devoted to these concerns. You will have to discipline yourself at other times to acknowledge that you are worried but you just aren't going to think about the problem right then because you've allotted time later on. This will clear your mind the rest of the day for efficient thinking.

Over several weeks, reduce your daily worry time to 15, 10, and then 5 minutes. As you cut down on your allotment, you'll see that you have to worry about the most important elements and let the rest go. In so doing, you may be able to break yourself of the habit of taking every petty little incident to heart.

Learn a Relaxation Skill

Any one of the techniques discussed in this book will be helpful: meditation (see page 292), visualization (see page 442), progressive relaxation (see page 361), or autogenics (see page 481) can enhance alertness as it teaches you to let go of tension. So that the treatments stay fresh and useful to you, alternate your practice daily. You'll probably find one that works best in terms of reducing your worries—when you do, stick with it.

Have a Trash Day

Write down your worries on separate pieces of paper. Be sure to detail all the possible problems, glitches, hassles, and annoyances you can think of. Spread the pieces of paper out in front of you in order—most to least important. Now crumple them up, one at a time, and deliberately throw them into the garbage pail. You'll find an enormous sense of relief—perhaps mixed with some anger—as you let go physically. Realizing that your worries are trash to be disposed of, nothing more, may help you to fret less and enjoy life more.

Practice Mindfulness

Select one activity that is difficult for you to accomplish without worrying, such as bathing your infant (you might turn around and she could slip under the water and drown), cleaning the turtle tank (you might drop it and smash glass all over the floor), or preparing a meal for your boss (you might ruin everything and lose your job).

Let's do a mindfulness exercise on bathing an infant. First, undress your baby, delighting in the smooth, warm skin that begins to emerge as you undo each snap or fastener. First peel off the tiny overalls, then pull off the sweet-smelling T-shirt, and finally, rip open the tabs on the diaper. Feel the heaviness and wetness pull away from your baby as you discard it.

Now luxuriate in the beauty of your baby's naked body. See how carelessly but deliberately she waves arms and legs in the air. Reach down and scoop your hands under her armpits, then support her head as you snuggle her against your neck and chest. Breathe in her essence and find the part of her that is you and the part that is completely her own.

Bring her into the bathroom and place her in the infant seat as you turn each tap, feeling its cold, metal resistance to your hand. The rush of water makes a comforting sound, almost as flowing as your baby's delighted gurgling. Keep your hand under the water and your eyes on her while you adjust the temperature. Compare the warmth of the water to the warmth of your child's body. Put in just enough water and then listen to the silence as you close the faucets.

Lift your child and place her either in her bathing seat or in the tub itself. Feel how you can cradle her in one arm as you use a washcloth or the soap on her skin with your other hand. You are completely balanced together, your weight equally distributed. Watch her face as she is surprised and pleased by the water streaming down her head to her stomach and then to her legs.

Soap her lavishly, seeing the rainbows form in the bubbles just before they pop on her creamy skin. Wash the creases and planes of her body, paying attention to the ears, like little apricots, and the adorable toes, like delicate radishes.

At last you can rinse her off. Holding her securely, you can reach back and grab for a towel, then lift her into it and lay her on the bathmat to dry her. Cuddle her to your body and feel how different she is now, washed and polished, from the way she was when you first came into the bathroom. She is safe and sound, and so are you.

Let a Flower Bring Peace to Your Mind

White chestnut is the Bach flower remedy for someone who is a prisoner of his or her thoughts and who can't turn off the worrying, which preoccupies him or her constantly. Take 5 or 6 drops under the tongue or mixed with water as needed.

Use the Power of Touch

Have a massage with an essential oil, either Geranium, Neroli, Clary Sage, or Ylang-clang mixed with a carrier oil such as Almond or Jojobe. You should ask a friend or massage therapist to allot a long time (perhaps an hour) to work slowly on each body part, gently manipulating muscles, tendons, and ligaments to alleviate stress. An essential part of this treatment for worrying should be a facial massage—light pressure should be placed on the forehead, temples, bridge of the nose and along the sides of the nose, around the mouth and jaw (where a lot of tension is held), and ears. Think about letting go as these practiced hands work on you.

Ayurvedic Assistance

The *vata* personality tends to worry a great deal. The healthy nature of vata (which is characterized by changeability and movement) is to be enthusiastic and buoyant, very clear thinking and alert. But when vata is out of balance in the area of *prana*, the element of thought and spirit in the brain, nervous disorders may result. A disruption of prana vata may also lead to symptoms such as insomnia, tension headaches, hiccups, asthma, and other respiratory problems.

You must balance vata by becoming regular and evenly paced in everything from your diet and exercise regimen to the herbs you take. You need lots of rest; at least 7 hours' sleep a night, and a 20-minute period of meditation daily.

You should keep warm and dry and avoid drafts and humidity. Drink lots of herb teas (gotu kola tea is particularly warming for vata) and make sure you consume lots of hot, nourishing food and drink, starting with hot cereal with warm milk for breakfast and moving onto soups or stews for lunch and dinner. Use lots of stimulating spices and herbs. Tahini (sesame paste), used in the Middle Eastern dish hummus, is one of the best foods for balancing vata. Lassi, a traditional Indian drink made of half a cup plain yogurt mixed with half a cup of water, spiced with ginger or cumin, sweetened with mango pulp, is excellent for vata worriers. Because various substances prevent you from calming your mind, it's important to cut out caffeine, alcohol, and tobacco.

Gentle yoga postures (avoid the stimulating ones such as the Plough, Locust, and Headstand) are the perfect exercise for vata, as are walking and dancing. In the winter, it's best to exercise indoors to avoid getting chilled. Warm baths and showers will soothe and support your system.

YOGA

The practice of yoga, which means "yoke" or "union" in Sanskrit, dates back to the third century B.C., according to most sources. This meditative system of postures (called *asanas*) developed in India as a means of unifying mind and body, using mental power to bring about healing—both internal and external. These postures stretch and condition the muscles, bring a fresh flow of blood to the various organs, improve circulation throughout the body, and calm the mind and spirit. The element of prana, (like the Chinese qi), the life energy that supports us, is strengthened during yoga practice.

The relaxation and energy flow that come as we assume the various postures one after another can actually alleviate stress-related diseases such as headache, gastrointestinal disorders, and allergies, and can help to prevent or reverse heart disease and certain cancers when used in an all-around program of diet, exercise, and other stress-management techniques found in this book. The power of yoga to change the mind and emotions is now well documented—it is among the most popular and effective bodywork techniques practiced throughout the world.

When practicing and holding the postures, you begin to feel a certain stillness, an ability to breathe through whatever problems or fears you have. If you can stay calm and alert through the petty annoyances and large problems you encounter, you know you have a new tool that will alleviate stress and relax you whenever you need it most. The balance yoga affords is complete relaxation alternating with the tension necessary to achieve and maintain the postures.

When you start practicing yoga, you will feel the tug and pull of muscles you haven't used in a very long time. Your initial impulse will be to get out of the posture before it has done its good work. But as you practice longer and understand how to use your breath in conjunction with the movements, you will see that the longer you stay in the posture, the more benefits you receive. When you stop thinking of the process as holding a posture and begin *releasing* into it, you will have grasped the concept of how yoga heals. At first the poses may seem stiff and awkward, as you breathe into them, you will find that you can let go a bit more, and then a bit more.

As you become more skilled at assuming and moving through the postures, you will sense that your body is one whole rather than an unrelated group of limbs and organs. You will unify all the structures of your body and be able to rally the strengths of healthy areas to compensate for the weaknesses you may have elsewhere.

Yoga benefits the mind as it causes a release of neurotransmitters and endorphins that act as natural opiates. You will find a calm awareness when you practice that feels quite different from your mental state after conventional exercise. The practice of yoga keeps the prana, or body's energy, in balance, which in turn keeps the entire cycle of mind and body in balance.

Yoga uses several different types of directed breathing. The easiest one to master is the three-level breathing. First, take a breath and expand your stomach. Let it out. Next, take a breath, expand the stomach, and allow the breath to continue up to expand the lungs. Let it out. Finally, take a breath and expand stomach, lungs, and throat. Feel how much more open you are as you expand every cavity with oxygen and prana. Let the breath out.

A particularly good breathing technique to promote relaxation is alternate nostril breathing. Place the thumb of your right hand on your right nostril and inhale, then exhale through your left. Close off your left nostril with your fourth and fifth fingers and lift your thumb. Inhale and exhale on the opposite side. This technique centers the mind and actively integrates right- and left-brain function—this appears to give better electrical conductivity throughout the brain, which is a balancing and calming effect.

Yoga classes are available at most local YMCAs and health clubs and are offered privately by many excellent teachers around the country. Many corporations currently offer it as a lunchtime option for stress management. You can also find information about classes on the bulletin boards of health-food stores or alternative bookstores.

Yoga is performed barefoot; all you need to get started is a thin mat or blanket to work on. IF YOU HAVE ANY BACK OR NECK PROBLEMS, CHECK WITH YOUR PHYSICIAN BEFORE DOING ANY YOGA POSTURES THAT MIGHT STRAIN THEM.

The following sequence of yoga exercises will give you a series of easy postures you can perform every day without strain. Always work slowly, breathing into each asana. As you breathe, try to take the posture a little deeper and release into it a little longer. Sense the air circulating throughout your body with each pose and inhale and exhale several times before returning to center.

Follow the sequence of these postures, or purchase a basic yoga videotape and use it to guide your practice. End your yoga session with a quieting time of about ten minutes in which you assume "Corpse Pose." As you might imagine, this posture is flat on your back, hands at your sides, legs relaxed outward, looking like a corpse but being very alive indeed, with a feeling that you are sinking into the floor. You may wish to cover yourself with a light blanket as you center your mind and allow your respiration and heart rate to come into harmony.

COBRA

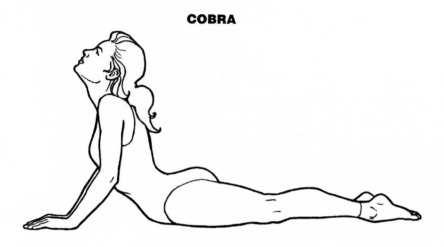

FISH

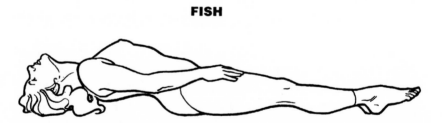

YOGA MUDRA

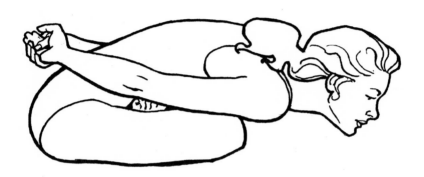

BOW

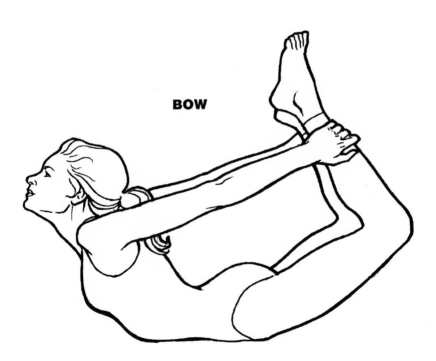

G*ETTING OFF* M*EDICATION*

■ *What Medication Does to the Mind and Body:*

Drugs that affect the brain and central nervous system are designed to alleviate symptoms that are upsetting and difficult to deal with. If you can't get out of bed in the morning, if you are so anxious that you compulsively tear your hair, if you find yourself enraged to the point of violence when your boss criticizes your work, you need some intervention. Although the body and mind do heal themselves, most people in our culture feel they cannot wait for nature to take its course. If they are really miserable, they visit a medical doctor, who generally prescribes medication.

But why do these medications change us and our feelings? And what do drugs accomplish in the great chemical scheme of things? In order to understand, we must look at the structure of brain cells.

The brain contains billions of neurons that are joined to one another across a web of connections called synapses. The incoming chemical messenger seems to change the composition of a secondary messenger who delivers the information to the next cell at the synapse. Then that messenger takes off for the next cell, where the same process occurs again. Messages that we need to function ("Move your right arm to scratch your nose." "Feel pain because you have just stubbed your toe." "Start to smile when you see your child running toward you.") jump across synapses through the advent of neurotransmitter secretion. These are brain hormones that assist the passage of information from one neuron to another.

About 5 percent of neurotransmission occurs via substances known as *biogenic amines,* which are complex chemicals similar to ammonia in structure. These substances are many-faceted in function: They affect mood, but they also affect heart rate and gut motility as well as alertness and drowsiness. Many antidepressants work by holding the amine right at the synapse for a longer period of time before it moves onto the transmitting cell. Since the amines tend to make most people feel better, having them stick around longer can alleviate depression. It doesn't always work this way, however, since there are many other chemical reactions going on at the same time; if you alter the function of one chemical, you very often alter a bunch of chemicals simultaneously. Regulating neurotransmitter movement is a very imprecise art, as has been learned by those who take drugs to alter their moods. Sometimes it works brilliantly, sometimes it doesn't work at all, and sometimes it gives the opposite reaction to the desired one.

The neurotransmitters most involved in relaying emotional information are norepinephrine and serotonin. When scientists decided to invent medications that would change the way we feel, they vacillated between trying to change one or the other of these. Some drugs are "dirty," that is, they affect many neurotransmitters simultaneously. Naturally, medical science strives for the "clean" drug, which goes right to the target and knocks it out, while leaving all the other neurological functions and responses untouched.

One of the biggest hitches in medicating your problems away is that changing the chemistry of the brain has far-reaching implications. If you feel down and draggy in the morning but anxious and overstimulated by the time you're ready for bed, do you have to take one drug to stimulate and one to sedate? Or, since medications usually have long half-lives (that is, they stay in the body even after their initial effectiveness wears off), are you really just compensating for one drug by dosing with another? This would seem to constitute overmedicating.

Remember, too, that every body is different and the number of chemicals at play is never the same twice. If you think about the random ways that the same amount of alcohol affects people, making some cuddly and adorable and others aggressive and nasty, you will have a pretty good idea of what psychiatric medicines may or may not do.

One individual may be exceptionally sensitive to a synthetic preparation, whereas others would need triple dosage in order to get any effect at all. Some people find that an antidepressant drug makes them feel better within a few days of taking it, and others never respond to it at all. Some individuals report good emotional results; however, they are so plagued with side effects (dry mouth, racing heart, grogginess, lack of sex drive, gastrointestinal upset) that they can't enjoy the good feelings the drug supplies.

One enormously important factor in drug treatment is the interactions that occur among different drugs. Two drugs that work on the central nervous system cannot happily coexist in the body, which means that taking an antihistamine for allergies when you're already taking a tricyclic antidepressant could prove disastrous. Some drugs enhance the effects of an antidepressant; others diminish or cancel out the effects. Drinking alcohol, taking diuretics, pain relievers, and certain blood-pressure medications can be strictly contraindicated, depending on which antidepressant you're taking. Those individuals who try to deceive their physicians or merely forget (which is often the case with elderly patients) can get into real trouble by mixing and matching drugs.

Below are the major medications that your physician may have discussed or prescribed for you, depending on your symptoms. Remember that you can always change your mind about drugs—even if you've been a Prozac pro for years, there is no harm in telling your physician that you would like to be weaned off it as you begin to use natural therapies. Once you have found holistic treatments that work in conjunction with your personality and lifestyle, you may be able to create the same positive feelings and experiences you have learned to rely on from the medication.

The Mood-Altering Drugs:

Anti-Anxiety Drugs (long-acting such as Valium or Librium; short-acting such as Xanax or Ativan; pro drugs such as Paxipam):

In the 1960s, medical science developed a range of drugs to calm those who were overwrought and continually stressed out. Originally known as "tranquilizers" (Miltown and Equanil were two of the most popular of the now obsolete drugs), they had a sedative effect that was difficult for most people to manage during their daily routine.

The newer anti-anxiety drugs, made from a chemical known as *benzodiazepine,* tend to decrease activity of a certain neurotransmitter known as *gaba-ergic,* thereby reducing anxiety and relaxing muscle tension.

These drugs are good for short-term use—they might be taken before a plane ride if you're phobic, during short-term therapy for a panic disorder, or after a traumatic experience such as the sudden death of a spouse. Long-term use can increase the likelihood of dependence.

SIDE EFFECTS: Any of these drugs can cause dizziness, drowsiness, restlessness, and hangover. If you take these for more than a week to 10 days, they may cause the very problems—anxiety and insomnia—that you have taken them to cure. Over-use of short-term anti-anxiety drugs can cause addiction, depression, and behavioral abnormalities, and the withdrawal process is exceptionally difficult.

Hypnotic Sedatives (barbiturates such as Nembutal and Seconal; nonbarbiturates such as Placidyl and Doriden; and benzodiazepines such as Dalmane and Halcion):

There are three classes of hypnotics on the market. Barbiturates were first developed in the 1920s and are used for insomnia as well as anxiety. These drugs tend to lower the pulse and breathing rate and leave you with a hangover.

The nonbarbiturate drugs shorten the amount of time it takes you to fall asleep and tend to keep you asleep through the night. The benzodiazepines are short-acting sedatives as well as anti-anxiety drugs, and have the fewest side effects; however, they tend to encourage dependency because their reaction is predictably so good. These should not be used over a period greater than two weeks. There is a short latency period to these drugs; that is, they don't work right away because it takes a while for them to get into your system and become effective.

One of the chief problems of hypnotics is tolerance. This means that the more you take the drug, the more your body becomes accustomed to it and the less well it works. You need increasingly more of the drug to do the same thing that initially was done at a lower dose.

Barbiturates also cut down on the ability of your gut to absorb Vitamins D and C, which means it's important to supplement these if you're on medication. You should not mix barbiturates and alcohol, pain relievers, tranquilizers, and antihistamines. Another drawback of this type of medication is that it alters your sleep cycles and suppresses REM sleep, the beneficial stage in which you dream. After discontinuing this medication, you may experience nightmares or increased dreaming as your system gets back to normal.

SIDE EFFECTS: Drowsiness, dizziness, confusion, overstimulation, anxiety, insomnia, and hallucinations.

First Generation Tricyclic Antidepressants (Elavil, Tofranil):

These drugs, developed in the 1960s, are so named because their chemical structure involves three rings joined together. They were a welcome change from the old anti-anxiety drugs because they lifted depression and elevated mood, improved sleep, appetite, and exercise potential, and increased mental acuity and a sense of hopefulness about daily life. The generic drug, *imipramine,* was a nonstimulating antidepressant and replaced the use of antihistamines and opium in the treatment of depression. Some people are overstimulated by these drugs to the point of delirium or mania—they must be very carefully prescribed and monitored by a physician.

SIDE EFFECTS: Dry mouth, palpitations, sweating, constipation and urinary retention, dizziness, and drowsiness.

MAOIs (Monoamine Oxidase Inhibitors) (Marplan, Nardil, Parnate):

These drugs were developed to respond to certain amines that affect mood, and they often work for patients who don't respond to tricyclics. Unfortunately, however, because of their chemical composition, the dangers of interactions are substantial. This drug inhibits the release of a chemical called tyramine that causes nerve cells to release complex amines, and certain foods such as aged cheese, red wine, fava beans, and figs contain massive amounts of tyramine. MAOIs are contraindicated for anyone with high blood pressure. Signs of overdose are difficult to recognize, since the drug may cause you to feel high, even manic one moment, fatigued and weak the next.

SIDE EFFECTS: Drowsiness, dizziness (particularly getting up too fast from sitting or lying down), weakness, dry mouth, insomnia, trembling, restlessness, increased appetite or weight gain, headache, and sexual dysfunction.

ADVERSE REACTIONS: Severe reactions from combination with any food that contains tyramine might include pounding heartbeat, skin rash, edema, hypertension with nosebleed, chest pains, enlarged pupils, severe headache, nausea and vomiting.

Second-Generation Tricyclics (Wellbutrin, Pamelor, Sinequan, Norpramin):

These drugs improved the original tricyclics and generally cause fewer side effects. Although they were designed to get to work in your system faster, they actually have the same latency period as the first-generation drugs. The purpose of these drugs is to increase the amounts of norepinephrine or serotonin or both in your central nervous system.

SIDE EFFECTS: Dizziness, drowsiness, dry mouth, excessive sweating, weight gain, and fatigue.

Serotonin Reuptake Inhibitors (Prozac, Paxil, Zoloft, Luvox, Effexor, Serzone):

The advent of these mood-changing, antidepressant drugs caused a surge of excitement on the psychopharmaceutical front—here were "clean" drugs that affected only the targets they aimed at. These medications have few side effects (no more dry mouth, sweating, dizziness, and urine retention), and for many individuals they appear to be very effective in relieving depression and other mental and emotional problems.

Unlike any of the other anti-anxiety drugs on the market, Prozac has the added advantage of one daily dose, easing compliance for the patient. (That one capsule, by the way, costs $2 a day, or $730 a year, in most parts of the country.)

Serotonin reuptake inhibitors work by prolonging the amount of time serotonin spends in the synapse between nerve cells. Depression is relieved since the neurotransmitter hangs around at the target site long enough to achieve a good balance of brain chemistry and electrical activity.

Prozac has been extolled, cursed, and otherwise made into a media spectacle. Many people who have "failed" at other drug therapies say that they didn't know how they managed before Prozac—the classic statement of those who love the drug is that it "makes them more themselves." For individuals who were severely handicapped by obsessions, compulsions, black moods, and incomprehensible behavior, Prozac appears to alleviate or obliterate unpleasant symptoms, and in addition, it adds vitality and color to their lives. As described by its first champion Peter D. Kramer in *Listening to Prozac,* the medication is an agent of "personal transformation." "Prozac," he says, "can induce the sort of widespread change ordinarily brought about by [years of] psychotherapy."

The old beliefs that personality was responsible for "characterologic depression" changed under the sway of Prozac and its progenitors. Some experts now believe that mental illness and personality disorder may be one and the same—both conditions arising from a chemical imbalance in the brain. So if you could take care of the occasional bouts of depression that left many people feeling fatalistic about their ability to ever feel good again, you could change personality. A chronically sad person may then be not so different from a chronically happy person—it's just that the latter has a built-in mechanism that allows neurons to make allowances for changes in mood. What if Prozac were like a starter in an automobile? If you could install a new mechanism in a terribly depressed person, you might be able to alter his or her personality. But human beings are maddeningly, wonderfully elastic in their reactions, which means that every model won't start all the time, even with a brand new piece of machinery in place.

One enormous and generally acknowledged flaw in Prozac is its ability to rob men and women of their natural, God-given sex drives, and this is a very serious problem when you're talking about personality change. In order for us to feel aroused and sense desire, we need fluctuating serotonin levels that move through our nervous system on an as-needed basis. When the neurotransmitter is altered chemically, we don't experience those highs and lows, that buildup and release of tension. Zoloft, Effexor, and Serzone appear to return some erotic feeling, and Luvox gets the best reviews for the sexually deprived, except that it puts most people to sleep before they get to enjoy themselves. So the problem persists. Many mostly satisfied customers bounce on and off these drugs simply because they miss that exuberant thrill of the chase and capture that fills most people's lives with joy. (Not to mention the fact that they are depriving their loved ones of the same joy.)

Then too, there are those individuals for whom Prozac does nothing at all. They may be biochemically resistant or have such low serotonin levels naturally that the medication can't touch them. Some individuals do experience side effects: There are reports of nausea, nervousness, loss of appetite, drowsiness, excessive sweating, allergic rashes, dizziness, and headaches, as well as arrhythmias and thyroid and liver dysfunctions. There are others for whom Prozac has brought on disastrous results—some people abandon Prozac (usually switching to another, newer serotonin reuptake blocker) because it made them manic or very aggressive, often toward themselves. The case histories that link Prozac and suicide or violent behavior toward others are few; however, they are one indication of the fact that no drug, however perfect seeming, can be taken without consequences.

What's probably the most disturbing fact is that serotonin uptake inhibitors are not addictive—there is no withdrawal period from the drug. So there's a built-in incentive to stay on it forever if it makes you feel good. (These drugs have been on the market too short a time to be able to predict whether there may be long-term dangers.) But knowing that a drug can't hook you biochemically doesn't mean that you won't feel a definite longing for it if you've experienced its beneficial effects. And do you really want to be that dependent on any synthetic palliative for your lifelong well-being?

Taking medication is only one way to raise serotonin levels and keep the balance of dozens of other brain chemicals on an even keel. But taking medication does not guarantee happiness or good health. The continuing search for a "magic bullet" that will alleviate all symptoms and provide the best of all possible mental states will go on until human beings blow themselves off the planet or evolve into some kinder, wiser creatures.

We have always longed for ecstasy. Since the dawn of civilization, we have sought spiritual relief from emotional problems, by staring into a fire, by whirling madly into a trance state, by chewing mushrooms, and by ingesting herbs that appear to alter animal behavior. The excitement of being human involves the search for something better.

But probably, it's not in a pill.

▨ *How to Get off Medication Safely and Onto Natural Therapies:*

Drugs that affect the mind and emotions are strong medicine, indeed. It can be very dangerous to muck around with synthetic mood alteration. If you're currently taking any antidepressant, you undoubtedly know that abrupt withdrawal can give you a rebound effect, that is, your symptoms may return with a vengeance as you bounce off the drug and onto real life. You should also know that most antidepressants have a half-life (some longer than others), so that you may be fooled into thinking that you can quit cold turkey after a couple of days of laying off them. In fact, you're still on them. Four days or two weeks later, however, you may have a very bad reaction.

The general rule of thumb is that whatever drug you're on, you should wean yourself off it very slowly under a doctor's support and supervision. And at the same time, you should be substituting one or several of the natural therapies that are targeted to your condition.

Let's say that you have been depressed and your doctor has you on the standard daily dose of 20 mg. of Prozac. (If you are taking the drug to treat an obsessive-compulsive disorder, you may be prescribed 40 to 80 mg. daily.) You've been on it for six months, and you do feel brighter, more mentally alert and more vivacious, but your sex life is at a standstill and you are concerned about not truly experiencing the deeper aspects of your life and the significant issues you had the way you did before you were taking Prozac.

Your doctor will probably advise you to cut the medication by one eighth every two to four weeks until you can finally stop. (If you're on a high dosage, you would be weaned by stepping down the daily dosage by one eighth every two to four weeks). If you're currently on a low dose of Prozac, start by cutting out one pill a week. After two or three weeks, cut out a second pill, and after two more weeks, a third pill. At this rate, it will take from 10 to 16 weeks to get off the medication.

Many medications require a washout period, that is, a week or two in which you eliminate not only the drug you're taking, but all other drugs that might cause similar reactions or with which you might have an adverse reaction were you still taking your former medication. Your body is not free of the chemical input of Prozac, for example, for one week after you've stopped taking it. If you are making a change from MAOIs to Prozac, a washout period of two weeks is possible. You may experience urine retention, constipation, or dry mouth as you are coming off the medication, so you want to be sure to drink plenty of pure water and fruit juices while you are cleaning out your system.

Herbal remedies can help you get through withdrawal symptoms, but you should never take herbs and drugs in the same time period (always space them at least five hours apart). Many experts recommend taking scullcap and valerian to ease anxiety and tension as well as oat tea to get your nervous system in shape, passionflower if you're having palpitations or feel very agitated, motherwort for your circulation, and pasque flower for nervous exhaustion. In addition, exercise, vitamin and mineral supplementation, qi gong breathing, meditation, massage, homeopathy, and acupuncture should help you have a nearly painless drug withdrawal.

It is important to keep in mind that natural therapies do not function as one-to-one substitutes for a drug. In a sense, that type of thinking is what led you to rely on medication in the first place. And because there are no FDA regulations

on herbs, amino acids, vitamins and minerals, and homeopathics, you must use good judgment and, probably, the
advice of a professional when you select the treatments you're
going to try. Too much of a "natural" herb can make you nauseated and dizzy; an overdose of amino acids can damage your
kidneys. Recent shocking evidence about the product called
Herbal Ecstasy (ephedra or ma huang) link it to heart attacks,
seizures, strokes, and psychotic breaks. Several deaths have
been attributed to overuse of this product.

The point of holistic treatment is that you want to
encourage the body and mind to heal themselves, and usually the smallest amounts of these various natural substances
are sufficient to accomplish that.

So you want to wean yourself off drugs as you learn
more about the way you function without drugs. It may feel
strange—you will probably say that you don't feel "like yourself." After a couple of weeks on your new regimen, you may
find that you are having more bad days than good ones, and
the lure of going back on the medication will be very strong.
Remember, however, that you can have (and *did* have) bad
and good days when you were on Prozac, but the overall feeling you had was optimistic and clear thinking. You had an
expectation of being able to cope and of doing better tomorrow.

In order to get over your nostalgia for the drug, you are
going to have to prove to yourself that there are other things
in life that can give your spirits that lift. This is the time to
intensify your efforts, with nutrition and exercise, with meditation and yoga, with support groups and the healing power
of sex. There is no reason why natural therapies can't make
you into the person you believed you became when you took
the drug.

You were there all the time, waiting to emerge, like a but-
terfly from its cocoon. When you can see the sun shining
through the rain, it's because you chose to notice. Make that
choice once, and it will be easier the next time. The brain is
a magnificent system—it will remember the hard work you
put in and reward you amply with a new perspective and,
possibly, a new life.

*W*HERE TO *G*O FOR *H*ELP

Understand that you are not alone. There are hundreds of individuals, groups, and other resources to make your healing journey easier. You just have to know whom to call when you're depressed or anxious and feel stranded. With the right names, addresses, and phone numbers at your fingertips, you will never be at a loss for a therapy, an organization, or a book that might help you get back on track. Following is a listing of resources—books, support groups, and items to make life easier—that will assist you on your road to good mental and emotional health.

▣ *Insurance for Complementary Therapies*

Wellness Plan
100 Foster City Blvd.
Foster City, CA 94040
(800) 925-5323

The American Western Life Insurance's Wellness Plan is available to residents of California, Utah, Colorado, New Mexico, and Arizona. You must choose a primary-care physician from their network; however, you also have a choice of alternative and allopathic doctors on this plan. You must have an annual "wellness" exam and appropriate testing, and you are then covered for 12 visits per year to a variety of specialists, including acupuncturists, Ayurvedic doctors, hypnotherapists, and others. The plan pays for herbal and homeopathic remedies and vitamins that are prescribed for particular conditions.

Alternative Health Plan
PO Box 6279
Thousand Oaks, CA 91359-6279
(800) 966-8467

Alternative Health Services' Alternative Health Plan is available to subscribers all over the country, and there is greater freedom of choice with practitioners than there is in the Wellness Plan. The specialists you may see include acupuncturists, Ayurvedic doctors, homeopaths, naturopaths, chiropractors, and doctors of traditional Chinese medicine. The plan does not cover vitamins, but will pay up to $500 per year for homeopathic and herbal remedies prescribed by one of their physicians. They also cover 12 sessions of bodywork when prescribed by a physician. Major medical, hospitalization, and surgery are all included.

Oxford Health Plans
(800) Connecticut Avenue
Norwalk, CT 06854
(800) 444-6222

Oxford Health Plans, the fastest growing HMO in the Northeast, covers members in Connecticut, New York, New Jersey, and Pennsylvania. Oxford is currently developing a program, set to go into effect in 1997, that will offer its members the option of selecting a naturopath or homeopath as well as a primary-care physician.

National Organizations

Nutrition

American Dietetic Association
216 W. Jackson Blvd., Suite 800
Chicago, IL 60606
(312) 899-0040

Center for Science in the Public Interest
1501 16th Street, NW
Washington, DC 20036
(202) 332-9110

Aromatherapy

National Association for Holistic Aromatherapy
3072 Edison Ct.
Boulder, CO 80301
(303) 444-0533

Herbalism

American Herbalists Guild
PO Box 1683
Soquel, CA 95073
(408) 469-4372

Northeast Herbal Association
PO Box 146
Marshfield, VT 05658-0146

Bach Flower Remedies

Ellon (Bach USA)
463 Rockaway Ave.
Valley Stream, NY 11580
(516) 593-2206

Homeopathy

International Foundation for Homeopathy
2366 East Lake E., No. 301
Seattle, WA 98192
(206) 324-8230

National Center for Homeopathy
801 Fairfax St., Suite 306
Alexandria, VA 22314
(703) 548-7790

Homeopathic Educational Services
(800) 359-9051 (orders)
(510) 649-0294 (information)

They will send you books, remedies, tapes, software, and home-study courses on homeopathy.

Feldenkrais Therapy

The Feldenkrais Guild
P.O. Box 489
Albany, OR 97321
(800) 775-2118

Alexander Technique

The Alexander Society
129 W. 67th St.
New York, NY 10023
(212) 799-0468

Magnetic Healing

Neuro Magnetic Systems
c/o Leane E. Roffey
8011 N. New Braunfels #208
San Antonio, TX 78209
(210) 824-5352

The Magnetic Wellness and Fitness Center
9711 Montgomery Rd.
Montgomery, OH
(513) 793-5332

Nikkey, Inc.
10866 Wilshire Blvd. #250
Los Angeles, CA 90024

Craniosacral Therapy

The Upledger Institute, Inc.
11211 Prosperity Farms Rd.
Palm Beach Gardens, FL 33410-3487
(407) 622-4706

Mental Health

National Alliance for the Mentally Ill
2101 Wilson Blvd. Suite 302
Arlington, VA 22201
(800) 950-NAMI

National Institutes of Mental Health
5600 Fishers Lane, Room 7C-02
Rockville, MD 20857
(301) 443-4513

National Mental Health Association
1021 Prince St.
Alexandria, VA 22314-2971
(800) 969-NMHA

National Anxiety Foundation
3135 Custer Dr.
Lexington, KY 40517-4001
(800) 755-1576

Anxiety Disorders of America
6000 Executive Blvd., Suite 200
Rockville, MD 20852-3801
(301) 231-9350

Panic Disorder Education Program
National Institutes of Mental Health
5600 Fishers Lane, Rm. 7C-02
Rockville, MD 20857
(800) 64-PANIC

Depression

Depression/Awareness, Recognition and
Treatment Education Program (DART)
National Institute of Mental Health
(800) 421-4211

National Alliance for Research on Schizophrenia and Depression
60 Cutter Mill Rd., Suite 200
Great Neck, NY 11021
(516) 829-0091

National Depressive and Manic Depressive Association
730 N. Franklin St., Suite 501
Chicago, IL 60610
(800) 826-3632

National Foundation for Depressive Illnesses
PO Box 2257
New York, NY 10116
(800) 248-4344

Society for Light Treatment and Biological Rhythms
10200 W. 44th Ave., Suite 304
Wheat Ridge, CO 80033
(303) 422-8527

Seasonal Affective Disorder (SAD) and Light Therapy

National Organization for SAD
PO Box 40133
Washington, DC 20016

Depression and Related Affective Disorders Association (DRADA)
John Hopkins University School of Medicine
Meyer 3-181
600 N. Wolfe St.
Baltimore, MD 21287-7381
(410) 955-4647

Center for Environmental Therapeutics
Box 532
Georgetown, CO 80444
(303) 569-0910

Aging and Mental Health

American Association of Geriatric Psychiatry
PO Box 376A
Greenbelt, MD 20768
(301) 220-0952

National Association of Area Agencies on Aging
600 Maryland Avenue SW, Suite 208
Washington, DC 20024
(202) 484-7520

American Association of Retired Persons (AARP)
1909 K St., NW
Washington, DC 20049
(202) 872-4700

Eating Disorders

American Anorexia/Bulemia Association, Inc.
293 Central Park West, Suite 1R
New York, NY 10024
(212) 501-8351

Anorexia Nervosa and Related Eating Disorders, Inc.
PO Box 5102
Eugene, OR 97405
(503) 344-1144

National Association of Anorexia Nervosa and Associated
Disorders (ANAD)
PO Box 7
Highland Park, IL 60035
(708) 831-3438
HOTLINE: (847) 831-3438

Obsessive Compulsive Disorder

Obsessive Compulsive Information Center
Dean Foundation
8000 Excelsior Drive, Suite 302
Madison, WI 53717-1914
(608) 836-8070

Trichotillomania (Hair-Pulling) Learning Center
1215 Mission Street, Suite 2
Santa Cruz, CA 95060
(408) 457-1004

Obsessive Compulsive Foundation
PO Box 60
Vernon, CT 06066
(203) 772-0565

ADD and ADHD

The Feingold Association
56 Winston Drive
Smithtown, NY 11787
(516) 543-4658
Send a SASE for their brochure

Children and Adults with Attention Deficit Disorders
499 NW 70th Avenue, Suite 109
Plantation, FL 33317
(305) 587-3700

Posttraumatic Stress Disorder

National Center for Posttraumatic Stress Disorder
VA Medical and Regional Office Center, 116D
White River Junction, VT 05001
(802) 296-5132

Sleep Disorders

Narcolepsy Network
PO Box 42460
Cincinnati, OH 45242
(513) 891-3522
(914) 834-2855 (for lay counseling)

National Sleep Disorder Foundation
122 S. Robertson Blvd., 3rd Fl.
Los Angeles, CA 90048
(310) 288-0466

National Sleep Foundation
1367 Connecticut Ave., NW
Dept. NT1
Washington, DC 20036
(202) 785-2300

The RLS (Restless Leg Syndrome) Foundation
304 Glenwood Ave.
Raleigh, NC 27603
(919) 834-0821

Send $25 for membership and the annual medical bulletin, as well as four newsletters a year. The Foundation will also refer you to practitioners who treat restless leg and other sleep disorders.

Headache

National Headache Foundation
5252 N. Western Ave.
Chicago, IL 60625
(800) 843-2256

Holistic Health Care
Center for Natural Medicine, Inc.
1330 SE 39th Ave.
Portland, OR 97214
(503) 232-1100

A consultation, research, and diagnostic center run by naturopathic physicians offers a range of therapies from naturopathy to chiropractic, acupuncture, homeopathic, and botanical medicine.

Rise Institute
PO Box 2733
Petaluma, CA 94973
(707) 765-2758

This educational organization offers courses, workshops, and seminars to help people cope with chronic disease. The physical, emotional, and spiritual approach of the healing is based on the work of Sri Eknath Easwaren, a meditation teacher who created a program of holistic healing.

American Holistic Health Assoc.
PO Box 17400
Anaheim, CA 92817
(714) 779-6152

This organization publishes information on holistic approaches to health care.

American Holistic Medical Assoc.
4101 Lake Boone Trail, Suite 201
Raleigh, NC 27607
(919) 787-5146

This group of physicians dedicated to holistic medical practices may offer referrals to doctors in your area who are members.

Center for Mind-Body Studies
5225 Connecticut Avenue, NW, Suite 414
Washington, DC 20015
(202) 966-7338

The Center provides education and information for anyone wishing to explore his or her capacity for self-care and self-healing. They also sponsor self-help groups for people with chronic illness.

Stress

Center for Stress and Anxiety Disorders
Dr. David Barlow and Dr. Edward Blanchard
(affiliated with SUNY/Albany)
1535 Western Ave.
Albany, NY 12203
(518) 456-4127

Stress Reduction Clinic/Department of Medicine
University of Massachusetts Medical Center
55 Lake Avenue North
Worcester, MA 01655-0267
(508) 856-1616

This outpatient clinic offers an eight-week course for those with a chronic or acute medical condition. Mindfulness meditation and hatha yoga are taught as the tools to allow the patient to control his or her stress.

TM TRAINING/STRESS-MANAGEMENT COURSES: Your local community college probably offers several different stress-reduction and/or meditation programs. Most offer a ten-week beginner course so you can see how you like it and what benefits it offers.

Acupuncture and Chinese Medicine

Council of Colleges of Acupuncture and Oriental Medicine
8403 Colesville Rd., Suite 370
Silver Spring, MD 20910
(301) 608-9175

This council will refer you to a Chinese medical practitioner or school of Oriental medicine near you.

National Commission on the Certification of Acupuncture
1424 16th St., NW, Suite 501
Washington, DC 20036
(202) 232-1404

This organization offers information on professional standards and licensing requirements for acupuncturists.

American Association of Acupuncture and Oriental Medicine
(address same as above)
(202) 265-2287

This group, which shares the same offices, will give you referrals to practitioners.

Ayurveda

If you wish to find an Ayurvedic practitioner, you may call one of the Maharishi Ayurveda Health Centers around the country. The number to call for a referral is (515) 472-5866.

Biofeedback

Biofeedback practitioners, hospitals, and pain management centers can be found through

> American Association of Biofeedback Clinicians
> 2424 South Demptster Ave.
> Des Plaines, IL 60016
> (312) 827-0440

▓ *Ingredients for Good Mental Health*

Mail-Order Essence Companies (Aromatherapy)

> Aroma Vera
> 5901 Rodeo Rd.
> Los Angeles, CA 90016
> (800) 669-9514

> Simplers Botanical
> PO Box 39
> Forestville, CA 95436
> (707) 887-2012

Mail-Order Vitamin Companies

> Bronson
> PO Box 46903
> St. Louis, MO 63146-6903
> (800) 235-3200

> Eclectic Institute
> 14385 Lusted Road
> Sandy, OR 97055
> (800) 332-HERB

> NF Formulas
> 9775 SW Commerce Circle
> Wilsonville, OR 97070
> (800) 547-4891

Thorne Research
PO Box 3200
Sandpoint, ID 83864
(800) 228-1966

Tyler Encapulations
2204-8 NW Birdsdale
Gresham, OR 97030
(503) 661-5401

L&H Vitamins
37–10 Crescent St.
Long Island City, NY 11101
(800) 221-1152

Nutrition Warehouse
106 East Jericho Turnpike
PO Box 311
Mineola, NY 11501-0311
(800) 645-2929

Mail-Order Homeopathic Remedies

Boiron-Borneman
1204 Amosland Rd.
Norwood, PA 19074
(800) BLU-TUBE

Dolisos
3014 Rigel Ave.
Las Vegas, NV 89102
(800) DOLISOS

Standard Homeopathics
(800) 624-9659
Retail brand name is Hyland, Los Angeles, CA.

Mail-Order Herb Companies

Nature's Way Products, Inc.
10 Mt. Springs Pkway.
Springville, UT 84663
(801) 489-1520
(dried herbs, tinctures, capsulated herbs)

Wild Weeds (dried herbs and herbal products)
PO Box 88
Ferndale, CA 95560
(707) 786-4906

International Traditional Medicines (Chinese herbs)
Portland, OR
(800) 544-7504

Eclectic Institute
14385 Lusted Rd.
Sandy, OR 97055
(800) 332-HERB

Herbs of Grace
Division of School of Natural Medicine
PO Box 7369
Boulder, CO 80306-7369
(303) 443-4882

NF Formulas
9775 SW Commerce Circle
Wilsonville, OR 97070
(800) 547-4891

Herb Pharm
PO Box 116-N
Williams, OR 97544
(800) 348-4372

Herbalist & Alchemist, Inc.
PO Box 553
Broadway, NJ 08808
(908) 689-9020

Earth's Harvest
2557 NW Division
Gresham, OR 97030
(800) 428-3308

Chinese Herbs

East Earth Trade Winds
PO Box 493151
Redding, CA 96049-3151
(800) 258-6878

Nuherbs Company
3820 Penniman Ave.
Oakland, CA 94619
(800) 233-4307

These companies have a full catalog of Chinese herbs, books, and supplements.

Ayurvedic Products

The various oils, herbs, raw-silk gloves for massage, and other Ayurvedic products are available from

Maharishi Ayurveda Products International, Inc.
PO Box 541
Lancaster, MA 01523
(800) 255-8332
(508) 368-8101
(Massachusetts, Alaska, and Hawaii)

■ Available Libraries And Databases

If you're online with any computer network such as Medline, Grateful Med, or Paperchase on Compuserve, you can look up articles from medical libraries all over the country, including scientific journals that cover alternative health care.

You may also wish to contact the following groups:

Center for Medical Consumers/Health Care Library
237 Thompson Street
New York, NY 10012
(212) 674-7105

This is an excellent resource for books and the latest articles on traditional and alternative medicine. They also publish a monthly newsletter called *Healthfacts.*

World Research Foundation
15300 Ventura Blvd., Suite 405
Sherman Oaks, CA 91403
(818) 907-5483

This organization provides information packs on health subjects. For a fee of $45 plus shipping, they will research either standard or alternative medical approaches to any disease or condition, calling on information from 5,000 medical journal articles and a variety of books on complementary treatments.

Planetree Health Resource Center
2040 Webster St.
San Francisco, CA 94115
(415) 923-3681

Planetree offers an In-Depth Information Packet for $100 that offers a selection of up-to-date medical references, or you can order a $20 bibliography of source materials. They can also supply you with their directory of physicians and other healthcare practitioners, organizations, and support groups.

The Health Resource
Janice R. Guthrie
209 Katerine Drive
Conway, AZ 72032
(501) 329-5272

They will provide reports on traditional and alternative treatments of specific medical problems for a fee of $195 plus shipping.

Recommended Reading

Newsletters

The Panic Relief News
981 Shepard Ave.
North Brunswick, NJ 08902-2252
(908) 937-4832

Magazines

Natural Health
PO Box 1200
Brookline Village, MA 02147

For a subscription ($24 a year) write to:

PO Box 7440
Red Oak, OA 51591-0440

Books:

Altman, Nathaniel, *Everybody's Guide to Chiropractic Care,* Los Angeles: Jeremy P. Tarcher, Inc., 1990.

Austin, Phyllis, and Agatha M. Trash, *Natural Remedies: A Manual,* Santa Cruz, CA: NewLife Books, 1983.
—— *More Natural Remedies,* NewLife Books, 1984.

Balch, James F., M.D., and Phyllis A. Balch, CNC, *Prescription for Nutritional Healing,* Garden City Park, NY: Avery Publishing Group, Inc., 1990.

Baumel, Syd, *Dealing with Depression Naturally,* New Canaan, CT: Keats Publishing Company, 1995.

Benson, Herbert, *The Relaxation Response,* New York: Morrow, 1975.

Bock, Steven J., M.D., and Michael Boyette, *Stay Young the Melatonin Way,* New York: Dutton/Penguin, 1995.

Borland, Douglas, M.D., *Homeopathy in Practice,* New Canaan, CT: Keats Publishing, Inc., 1982.

Boyd, Hamish W., M.D., *Introduction to Homeopathic Medicine,* New Canaan, CT: Keats Publishing, Inc., 1981.

Breggin, Peter, *Toxic Psychiatry,* New York: St. Martin's Press, 1991.
—— *Talking Back to Prozac,* New York: St.Martin's Press, 1994.

Buchman, Dian Dincin, *Herbal Medicine: The Natural Way to Get Well and Stay Well,* New York: Gramercy Publishing Co., 1980.

Burton Goldberg Group, *Alternative Medicine: The Definitive Guide,* Payallup, WA: Future Medicine Publishing, 1993.

Chang, Dr. Stephen Thomas, *The Complete Book of Acupuncture,* Berkeley, CA: Celestial Arts, 1976.

Chappell, Peter, BSc, *Emotional Healing with Homeopathy,* Rockport, MA: Element, Inc., 1994.

Chopra, Deepak, M.D., *Perfect Health,* New York: Bantam Books, 1990.

Connery, Donald S., *The Inner Source: Exploring Hypnosis with Dr. Herbert Spiegel,* New York: Holt, Rinehart & Winston, 1982.

Dossey, Larry, *Healing Words,* New York: Bantam Books, 1994.

Feldenkrais, Moshe, *Awareness Through Movement,* New York: Harper & Row, 1972.

Gash, Michael Reed, *Acupressure's Potent Points,* New York: Bantam Books, 1990.

Girdano, Daniel A., et al., *Controlling Stress and Tension,* 4th ed., Englewood Cliffs, NJ: Prentice Hall, 1993.

Goodwin, Donald W., M.D., *Anxiety,* New York: Ballantine Books, 1986.

Greist, John H., M.D., et al., *Anxiety and Its Treatments,* New York: The Warner Home Medical Library, 1986.

Grossman, Richard, *The Other Medicines,* New York: Doubleday & Co., 1985.

Harding, D. E., *Head Off Stress,* London: Arkana/Penguin Group, 1990.

Hoffmann, David, *The Holistic Herbal,* Rochester, VT: Healing Arts Press, 1990.
—— *An Herbal Guide to Stress Relief,* Healing Arts Press, *1991.*

Horan, Paula, *Empowerment Through Reiki,* Wilmot, WI: Lotus Light/Shangri-La, 1992.

Kabat-Zinn, Jon, *Full Catastrophe Living,* New York: Delta Books, 1990.
—— *Wherever You Go, There You Are,* New York: Hyperion Books, 1994.

Kaptchuk, Ted, O.M.D., *The Web That Has No Weaver: Understanding Chinese Medicine,* New York: Congdon & Weed, 1983.

Kramer, Peter D., *Listening to Prozac,* New York: Viking/Penguin, 1993.

Krochmal, Arnold, and Connie Krochmal, *A Field Guide to Medicinal Plants,* New York: Times Books, 1973, 1984.

LeCron, Leslie M., *Self-Hypnotism: The Techniques and Its Use in Daily Living,* Englewood Cliffs, NJ: Prentice Hall, 1964.

Lowen, Alexander, M.D., *Love, Sex and Your Heart: The Health-Happiness Connection,* New York: Penguin USA, 1988.
—— *The Spirituality of the Body,* New York: Macmillan, 1990.

Mabey, Richard, *The New Age Herbalist,* New York: Collier Books, Macmillan Publishing Co., 1988.

Mindell, Earl, *Earl Mindell's Herb Bible,* New York: Fireside/Simon & Schuster, 1992.

Mowrey, Daniel B., Ph.D., *The Scientific Validation of Herbal Medicine,* New Canaan, CT: Keats Publishing, Inc., 1986.

Murray, Michael T., N.D., and Joseph E. Pizzorno, N.D., *An Encyclopedia of Natural Medicine,* Rocklin, CA: Prima Publishing, 1991.

Murray, Michael T., N.D., *Stress, Anxiety, and Insomnia,* Prima, 1995.

Natural Medicine Collective with Diana L. Ajjan, *Stress, Anxiety, and Depression,* New York: Dell Natural Medicine Library, 1995.

Olshelvsky, Moshe, et al., *Manual of Natural Therapy,* New York: Facts on File, 1989.

Panos, Maesimund B., and Jane Heimlich, *Homeopathic Medicine at Home,* Los Angeles, CA: J.P. Tarcher, Inc., 1980.

Papolos, Demitri F., M.D., and Janice Papolos, *Overcoming Depression,* Mt. Vernon, NY: Consumers Union, 1987.

Parker, Alice Anne, *Understand Your Dreams,* Tiburon, CA: HJ Kramer, Inc., 1995.

Quillan, Patrick, Ph.D., R.D., *Healing Nutrients,* Chicago, New York: Contemporary Books, 1987.

Salzman, Bernard, M.D., DABPN, *The Handbook of Psychiatric Drugs,* New York: Henry Holt & Co., 1991.

Spiegel, Herbert, and Spiegel, David, *Trance and Treatment: Clinical Uses of Hypnosis,* New York: R. R. Bowker, 1987.

Stern, Robert M., and William J. Ray, *Biofeedback,* Homewood, IL: Dow-Jones Irwin, 1977.

Tisserand, Robert, *Aromatherapy,* Rochester, VT: Healing Arts Press, 1985, 1988.

Ullman, Dana, *Discovering Homeopathy,* Berkeley, CA: North Atlantic Books, 1988, 1991.

Weed, Suan S., *Healing Wise,* Woodstock, NY: Ash Tree Publishing, 1989.

Weil, Andrew, M.D., *Natural Health, Natural Medicine,* Boston, MA: Houghton, Mifflin Co., 1990.

Werbach, Melvyn R., M.D., *Nutritional Influences on Illness,* Tarzana, CA: Third Line Press, Inc., 1987, 1988.

Zhou, Dahong, M.D., *The Chinese Exercise Book,* Roberts, WA: Hartley & Marks, Pt., 1984.

INDEX

Printed in the United States
136987LV00003B/52/P